From Genes to Phenotypes
The Basis of Future Allergy Management

From Genes to Phenotypes

The Basis of Future Allergy Management

Proceedings of the 25th Symposium of the
Collegium Internationale Allergologicum

Edited by Henning Løwenstein, John Bienenstock,
and Johannes Ring

Allergy & Clinical Immunology International –
Journal of the World Allergy Organization, Supplement 2, 2005

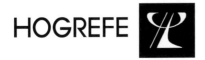

HOGREFE

Library of Congress Cataloguing-in-Publication Data

is available via the Library of Congress Marc Database
under the LC Control Number 2005932713

Library and Archives Canada Cataloguing-in-Publication Data

Collegium Internationale Allergologicum. Symposium (25th : 2004 : Bornholm, Denmark)
From genes to phenotypes : the basis of future allergy management : proceedings of the 25th
Symposium of the Collegium Internationale Allergologicum / Henning Løwenstein, John Bienenstock,
Johannes Ring (editors).

Symposium held Aug. 24–30, 2004.
Includes bibliographical references.
ISBN 0-88937-298-5

1. Allergy—Congresses. I. Løwenstein, Henning   II. Bienenstock, John   II. Ring, Johannes, 1945–
II.   IV. Title.

RC583.2.C64 2004   616.97   C2005-906342-4

Copyright © 2006 by Hogrefe & Huber Publishers

PUBLISHING OFFICES
USA: Hogrefe & Huber Publishers, 875 Massachusetts Avenue, 7th Floor,
              Cambridge, MA 02139
              Tel. (866) 823-4726, Fax (617) 354-6875, E-mail info@hhpub.com
Europe: Hogrefe & Huber Publishers, Rohnsweg 25, 37085 Göttingen, Germany
              Tel. +49 551 49609-0, Fax +49 551 49609-88, E-mail hhpub@hogrefe.de

SALES AND DISTRIBUTION
USA: Hogrefe & Huber Publishers, Customer Service Department, 30 Amberwood
              Parkway, Ashland, OH 44805, Tel. (800) 228-3749, Fax (419) 281-6883
              E-mail custserv@hhpub.com
Europe: Hogrefe & Huber Publishers, Rohnsweg 25, 37085 Göttingen, Germany
              Tel. +49 551 49609-0, Fax +49 551 49609-88, E-mail hhpub@hogrefe.de

OTHER OFFICES
Canada: Hogrefe & Huber Publishers, 1543 Bayview Avenue, Toronto, Ontario, M4G 3B5
Switzerland: Hogrefe & Huber Publishers, Länggass-Strasse 76, CH-3000 Bern 9

Hogrefe & Huber Publishers
Incorporated and registered in the State of Washington, USA, and in Göttingen, Lower Saxony,
Germany

Printed and bound in Germany
ISBN 0-88937-298-5

Table of Contents

Allergens

Infection and Allergy

Skin, Nerves, and Allergy

Asthma

Preface

Allergy and allergic diseases have dramatically increased in prevalence in recent decades and represent a major health problem in most countries of the world. It is no longer true that only privileged "Western" societies are affected – alarming prevalence rates of eczema and asthma are now being reported from Africa and Latin America. At the same time, while the genetic basis and the mechanisms of allergic reactions are becoming ever clearer, there is still a tremendous gap as regards actual practice in many allergists' offices.

One of the aims of this book and of the Collegium Internationale Allergologicum (CIA) is to help bridge this gap.

The Collegium comprises a group of leading experts from all over the world who meet for an outstanding scientific symposium every other year in order to exchange ideas and discuss the recent developments in research and practice in the field of allergy and clinical immunology. This volume stands in a long tradition of monographs featuring the highlights of allergy research over the decades. It reflects the most important discussions and summarizes the state of the art across the wide spectrum of experimental and applied, clinical research, as presented at the latest CIA symposium. In doing so it covers a wide range of topics, with special emphasis being given to basic mechanisms, dentritic cells, mast cells, neuro-immune interactions, as well as to clinical aspects of asthma, food allergy, eczema, and anaphylaxis, and the most recent developments in diagnosis of allergic diseases.

Finally, many thanks to Henning Løwenstein and his team for so splendidly organizing the CIA symposium on the beautiful Baltic island of Bornholm, and also to Christina Sarembe and Robert Dimbleby of Hogrefe & Huber Publishers for their help in preparing this book.

Munich, Fall 2005

Johannes Ring
President
Collegium Internationale Allergologicum

Allergy Is in the Blood at Birth

J.A. Denburg

Department of Medicine, Division of Clinical Immunology & Allergy,
McMaster University, Hamilton, ON, Canada

Summary: Alterations in numbers and phenotype of peripheral blood, bone marrow and airways tissue eosinophil-basophil (Eo-B) progenitors parallel clinical and physiological changes related to allergic *disease expression*, indicating the contribution of systemic processes to allergic tissue inflammation, which include both hemopoietic and chemokinetic events. We have examined whether or not alterations in numbers, differentiation pattern, and cytokine receptor expression on CD34⁺ cord blood (CB) progenitors at birth might relate to the *development* of the allergic diathesis. In a preliminary study, we had previously shown that a *reduction* in CD34/45⁺ cell expression of GM-CSFRa was associated with increased risk for atopy, as defined by parental questionnaire. In more recent studies, we have investigated whether phenotypic switching of CB hemopoietic progenitor differentiation towards the Eo-B pathway is a predictor of allergy in early infancy and childhood. These and other findings are discussed in support of the overall concept that *dysmature hemopoietic processes at birth may play a key role in the subsequent development of atopy*. Targeting these processes may be helpful in the prevention and treatment of allergic disease.

Keywords: atopy, cord blood progenitors, cytokine receptors

A growing body of research currently addresses the role of both genetic and environmental factors in the development of allergic disease in childhood, focusing especially on the expression of clinical symptoms related to *acquired* immune (T-cell) responses to *in utero* and *ex utero* stimuli. However, there has been no examination of the potentially important, *innate* immune mechanism of hemopoiesis, which is critically involved in the elicitation and maintenance of allergic diseases, and their "systemic" nature; we have termed this the "bone marrow hypothesis of atopy and asthma."

The Bone Marrow Hypothesis of Atopy and Asthma

An atopic donor can transfer skin test responses as well as asthma to a nonatopic recipient [1]. While the transfer of IL-4-producing Th2 cells to the recipient could lead to upregulation of IgE responses [2–4], transfer of upregulated, CD34⁺/IL-5Rα⁺ or CD34⁺/CCR3⁺ eosinophil-basophil (Eo-B) myeloid progenitors could also promote allergic tissue inflammation [5, 6], leading to ongoing asthma and rhinitis. Thus, hemopoietic progenitors in the neonatal period could predict atopic disease independent of, or in addition to, T-cells and adaptive immune responses. Our recent studies performed on the cord blood of infants at high risk for developing atopy suggest a dysregulation of hemopoietic progenitors, in particular *down*regulated expression of GM-CSFRα and IL-5Rα [7].

Development of Allergic Disease and Asthma

It is thought that the development of allergic disease or asthma results from the interaction of environmental stimuli in individuals with genetic susceptibility. Genetic linkage analysis has identified a number of loci, which are likely to contain causal polymorphisms contributing to the expression of allergy and of asthma phenotypes, including loci for important hemopoietic cytokines or transcription factors for eosinophil lineage commitment: e.g., the GATA family, FOG, PU.1, and c/EBPs [8, 9]. Likewise, abnormalities in Toll-like Receptors (TLR) might determine immune responses, through TLR-mediated events on nonimmunocompetent, inflammatory effector cells such as mast cells [10], basophils, eosinophils, or their progenitors.

Clinical Investigative Studies of Cord Blood Eo/B Progenitors: Hemopoietic Immaturity as a Basis for Atopy

Prescott et al. originally demonstrated that children who developed atopic symptoms produced significantly *lower* levels of allergen-specific cytokines, implying delayed or altered postnatal maturation of T-cell function [11]. Our pilot studies suggest that altered cord blood eosinophil progenitor phenotype (i.e., expression of cytokine receptors) may also predict the subsequent development of atopic disease. For example, cord blood CD34$^+$/CD45$^+$ cell Eo-B differentiation-specific cytokine receptor expression–GM-CSFRα, IL-5Rα, but *not* IL-3Rα–is *downregulated* when compared to low risk infants [7]. These studies suggest that *hematologic immaturity* may represent a counterpart to the T-cell "immaturity" seen in at-risk atopic infants.

We, and the Australia group, have recently investigated the effects of maternal dietary supplementation with n-3 PUFA during pregnancy on developing immunity in the neonate. We have confirmed the inverse correlation between measures of atopic risk in the infant (i.e., the number of maternal skin test responses) and GM-CSFRα and/or IL-5Rα (but not IL-3Rα) expression on CD34$^+$ cord blood

cells. Maternal dietary supplementation, which lowered risk of atopic symptoms at 1 year [12, 13], was accompanied by increased numbers of CD34$^+$ cells in neonatal cord blood and increased progenitor responsiveness to IL-5 in the functional culture assay, consistent with the hypothesis that infants at risk of atopy have delayed innate immune maturation which can be "unmasked" *in vitro/ex vivo*. The studies provide novel, preliminary findings concerning the responsiveness of progenitors to changes in the maternal *in utero* milieu.

The cellular and molecular mechanisms underlying any hemopoietic progenitor phenotypic and/or functional changes associated with atopic risk and the development of atopy and asthma require elucidation.

References

1. Agosti JM, Sprenger JD, Lum LG, Witherspoon RP, Fisher LD, Storb R, Henderson WR: Transfer of allergen-specific IgE-mediated hypersensitivity with allogeneic bone marrow transplantation. N Engl J Med 1988; 319:1623–1628.
2. Hogan SP, Koskinen A, Matthaei KI, Young IG, Foster PS: Interleukin-5-producing CD4$^+$ T-cells play a pivotal role in aeroallergen-induced eosinophilia, bronchial hyperreactivity, and lung damage in mice. Am J Respir Crit Care Med 1998; 157:210–218.
3. Mehlhop PD, van de Rijn M, Goldberg AB, Brewer JP, Kurup VP, Martin TR, Oettgen HC: Allergen-induced bronchial hyperreactivity and eosinophilic inflammation occur in the absence of IgE in a mouse model of asthma. Proc Natl Acad Sci USA 1997; 94:1344–1349.
4. Eum S-Y, Hailé S, Lefort J, Huerre M, Vargaftig BB: Eosinophil recruitment into the respiratory epithelium following antigenic challenge in hyper-IgE mice is accompanied by interleukin 5-dependent bronchial hyperresponsiveness. Proc Natl Acad Sci USA 1995; 92:12290–12294.
5. Sehmi R, Wood LJ, Watson R, Foley R, Hamid Q, O'Byrne PM, Denburg JA: Allergen-induced increases in IL-5 receptor α-subunit expression on bone marrow-derived CD34$^+$ cells from asthmatic subjects. A novel marker of progenitor cell commitment toward eosinophilic differentiation. J Clin Invest 1997; 100:2466–2475.
6. Sehmi R, Dorman S, Baatjes A, Watson R, Foley R, Ying S, Robinson DS, Kay AB, O'Byrne PM,

Denburg JA: Allergen-induced fluctuation in CC chemokine receptor 3 expression on bone marrow CD34⁺ cells from asthmatic subjects: Significance for mobilization of hemopoietic progenitor cells in allergic inflammation. Immunology 2003; 109:536–546.

7. Upham JW, Hayes LM, Lundahl J, Sehmi R, Denburg JA: Reduced expression of hemopoietic cytokine receptors on cord blood progenitor cells in neonates at risk for atopy. J Allergy Clin Immunol 1999; 104:370–375.

8. Cookson WOCM, Sharp PA, Faux JA, Hopkin JM: Linkage between immunoglobulin E responses underlying asthma and rhinitis and chromosome 11q. Lancet 1989; I:1292–1295.

9. Laitinen T, Polvi A, Rydman P, Vendelin J, Pulkkinen V, Salmikangas P, Mäkelä S, Rehn M, Pirskanen A, Rautanen A, Zucchelli M, Gullstén H, Leino M, Alenius H, Petäys T, Haahtela T, Laitinen A, Laprise C, Hudson TJ, Laitinen LA, Kere J: Characterization of a common susceptibility locus for asthma-related traits. Science 2004; 304:300–304.

10. McCurdy JD, Olynych TJ, Maher LH, Marshall JS: Cutting edge: distinct toll-like receptor 2 activators selectively induce different classes of mediator production from human mast cells. J Immunol 2003; 170:1625–1629.

11. Holt PG, Macaubas C, Prescott SL, Sly PD: Primary sensitization to inhalant allergens. Am J Respir Crit Care Med 2000; 162:S91–S94.

12. Denburg JA, Hatfield HM, Cyr MM, Hayes L, Holt PG, Sehmi R, Dunstan JA, Prescott SL: Fish oil supplementation in pregnancy modifies neonatal progenitors at birth in infants at risk of atopy. Pediatr Res, in press.

13. Dunstan JA, Mori TA, Barden A, Beilin LJ, Taylor AL, Holt PG, Prescott SL: Maternal fish oil supplementation in pregnancy reduces interleukin-13 levels in cord blood of infants at high risk of atopy. Clin Exp Allergy 2003; 33:442–448.

Judah A. Denburg

Department of Medicine, HSC-3V46, McMaster University, 1200 Main Street West, Hamilton, ON L8N 3Z5, Canada, Tel. +1 905 521-2100 × 76714, Fax +1 905 521-4971, E-mail denburg@mcmaster.ca

Interleukin-4/13-Induced Activation of STAT 6 Is Regulated by SOCS

D. Hebenstreit, P. Luft, A. Schmiedlechner, J. Horejs-Hoeck, and A. Duschl

Department of Molecular Biology, University of Salzburg, Austria

Summary: *Background:* IL-4/IL-13 stimulate activation of signal transducer and enhancer of transcription 6 (STAT6) in, essentially, all cells, but the resulting changes in gene transcription are highly selective depending on the cell type. We have investigated inhibition of STAT6 by suppressors of cytokine signaling (SOCS) factors, which may provide one of the mechanisms involved in cell-specific reactions. *Methods:* The promoters of the STAT6 regulated genes eotaxin-3/CCL26 and SOCS-1 were cloned into an expression construct to regulate expression of the reporter gene Luciferase. The STAT6 dependence of this transcriptional regulation was verified and expression constructs for the negative regulator proteins SOCS-1, SOCS-2, or SOCS-3 were cotransfected. *Results:* The promoter of eotaxin-3/CCL26 contains a single STAT6 binding site, which is required for transcriptional activation. Cotransfection with SOCS-1 or SOCS-3 expression constructs obliterated gene regulation. The SOCS-1 promoter is regulated by STAT6 through three binding sites and in this case too, overexpression of SOCS-1 inhibits expression. *Conclusions:* We have shown previously that IL-4 and IL-13 signaling via STAT6 induces expression of SOCS-1, and we show here that SOCS-1 suppresses STAT6-mediated gene expression of an allergy-associated target gene and in SOCS-1 itself. The resulting negative feedback loops may contribute to modulations of STAT6 activity. Negative regulation by specific SOCS factors could provide one of the mechanisms for modifying STAT6 induced gene regulation depending on cell type or differentiation stage.

Keywords: IL-4, IL-13, STAT6, SOCS-1, SOCS-3, eotaxin-3/CCL26, transcriptional regulation

Essentially all cells respond to IL-4 and IL-13 with STAT6 regulated changes in gene expression. There are very few exceptions, such as cells from transgenic mice, the cell line HEK293, and erythrocytes. The Jak/STAT system provides a straightforward mechanism for receptor-induced signal transduction; nevertheless, gene regulation by STAT6 depends on cell type and differentiation stage, as shown, for example, by microarray studies of IL-4 induced gene expression in B-cells [1] and T-cells [2]. One possible mechanism to introduce additional layers of regulation on a simple Jak/STAT signaling system is selective inhibition. It has been reported that members of the SOCS family of negative regulatory proteins are differentially expressed by Th1 and Th2 cells [3]. We have shown previously that IL-4 and IL-13 upregulate SOCS-1 expression via binding of STAT6 to three independent binding sites in the SOCS-1 promoter [4]. Recently we have investigated the effects of SOCS proteins on a representative target gene of IL-4/IL-13 in allergy and asthma, the chemokine CCL26/eotaxin-3 [Hebenstreit et al., submitted], and on the promoter of SOCS-1.

Materials and Methods

CCL26/eotaxin-3 gene expression was studied in the human embryonic kidney cell line HEK293, which endogenously expresses an inactive version of STAT6, but can activate

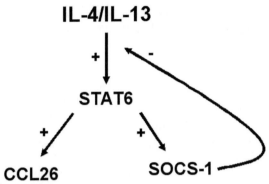

Figure 1. Negative regulation of IL-4/IL-13-induced gene regulation by SOCS-1.

exogenous STAT6 derived from an expression construct [5]. SOCS-1 expression was studied in the human lung epithelial cell line A549 [4]. HEK293 or A549 cells were cotransfected with (1) a reporter gene expressing Luciferase under the control of a CCL26/eotaxin-3 promoter or a SOCS-1 promoter, (2) an expression vector for STAT6, and (3) expression vectors for SOCS-1, SOCS-2 or SOCS-3. Protein secretion was detected by ELISA using cell culture supernatants.

Results

The CCL26/eotaxin-3 promoter contains a single functional STAT6 binding site. Active STAT6 is required for CCL26/eotaxin-3 expression, since normal HEK293 cells were unable to express Luciferase under control of the CCL26/eotaxin-3 promoter, while HEK293 cells transfected with a STAT6 expression construct expressed high levels of Luciferase.

Cotransfection of expression constructs for SOCS-1 and SOCS-3, but not for SOCS-2 inhibited the expression of Luciferase. The same was observed when CCL26/eotaxin-3 secretion from HEK293 cells was measured by ELISA: Only cells transfected with a STAT6 expression vector secreted CCL26/eotaxin-3, and overexpression of SOCS-1 or SOCS-3, but not of SOCS-2, inhibited IL-4/IL-13 induced CCL26/eotaxin-3 secretion. The effects of SOCS-1 and SOCS-3 on CCL26/eotaxin-3 did not reflect a general repression of chemokine expression and secretion, since TNF-α induced expression of the chemokine CCL-

7/MCP-3 was not affected by overexpression of SOCS-1, SOCS-2, or SOCS-3.

Cotransfection with SOCS-1 or SOCS-3 expression vectors prevented binding of STAT6 to DNA oligonucleotides representing the single STAT6 binding site in the CCL26/eotaxin-3 promoter. Again, SOCS-2 had no effect.

The SOCS-1 promoter was used for reporter gene studies in A549 cells and was found to be inducible by IL-4 and IL-13, in a mechanism that depended on an intact STAT6 binding site. Cotransfection of a SOCS-1 expression construct inhibited expression of endogenous SOCS-1.

Discussion

SOCS and STAT proteins perform specific interactions, which may result in selective regulation of gene expression. The present study presents examples: SOCS-1 and SOCS-3 are negative regulators of STAT6, but SOCS-2 is inactive. Also, none of the three SOCS proteins studied affected CCL-7/MCP-3 expression. Since SOCS-1 is upregulated by IL-4 and IL-13 via STAT6 [4], STAT6 and SOCS-1 are participants in a negative feedback loop, which may limit effects of proallergic cytokines. However, since SOCS-1 blocks STAT6-dependent SOCS-1 expression, the effects of SOCS-1 will be dampened by product inhibition.

SOCS-1 is considered to be associated with IFN-γ signaling, and SOCS-1 knockout mice die from a number of symptoms associated with inflammation caused by overactive IFN-γ

[6,7]. Nevertheless, SOCS-1 inhibits not only IFN-γ signal transduction, but IL-4 signaling as well [8]. Knockout of SOCS-3 in mice is embryonically lethal, but mice overexpressing SOCS-3 show increased Th2 response. Overall, the effects of the various SOCS proteins are complex but certainly relevant for the Th1/Th2 balance.

The various incarnations of the Jak/STAT pathway provide targets for diseases including allergy, asthma, cancer, and transplant rejection [9]. In this context, targeting SOCS proteins is also considered, both for general immunosuppression or for a more selective modulation of immunity. At present, the complex interactions of SOCS proteins with their target pathways and their indiscriminate use by many cytokines and noncytokines do not encourage hope for therapeutic applications. Much more will need to be learned about the mechanisms and effects of SOCS proteins in the regulation of specific genes.

Acknowledgments
This work was supported by the University of Salzburg through the research program "Biomedicine and Health." DH is supported by the Doctoral Scholarship Program of the Austrian Academy of Sciences.

References

1. Schroder AJ, Pavlidis P, Arimura A, Capece D, Rothman PB: STAT 6 serves as a positive and negative regulator of gene expression in IL-4-stimulated B lymphocytes. J Immunol 2002; 168:996–1000.
2. Chen Z, Lund R, Aittokallio T, Kosonen M, Nevalainen O, Lahesmaa R: Identification of novel IL-4/Stat6-regulated genes in T lymphocytes. J Immunol 2003; 171:3627–3635.
3. Egwuagu CE, Yu CR, Zhang M, Mahdi RM, Kim SJ, Gery I: Suppressors of cytokine signaling proteins are differentially expressed in Th1 and Th2 cells: Implications for Th cell lineage commitment and maintenance. J Immunol 2002; 168: 3181–3187.
4. Hebenstreit D, Luft P, Schmiedlechner A, Regl G, Frischauf AM, Aberger F, Duschl A, Horejs-Hoeck J: IL-4 and IL-13 induce SOCS-1 gene expression in A549 cells by three functional STAT6-binding motifs located upstream of the transcription initiation site. J Immunol 2003; 171:5901–5907.
5. Hoeck J, Woisetschläger M: Stat6 mediated eotaxin-1 expression in IL-4 or TNF-α-induced fibroblasts. J Immunol 2001; 166:4507–4515.
6. Alexander WS: Suppressors of cytokine signalling (SOCS) in the immune system. Nat Rev Immunol 2002; 2:410–416.
7. Kubo M, Hanada T, Yoshimura A: Suppressors of cytokine signaling and immunity. Nat Immunol 2003; 4:1169–1176.
8. Losman JA, Chen XP, Hilton D, Rothman P: Cutting edge: SOCS-1 is a potent inhibitor of IL-4 signal transduction. J Immunol 1999; 162:3770–3774.
9. O'Shea JJ, Pesu M, Borie DC, Changelian PS: A new modality for immunosuppression: targeting the JAK/STAT pathway. Nat Rev Drug Discov 2004; 3:555–564.

Albert Duschl

Department of Molecular Biology, University of Salzburg, Hellbrunner Str. 34, A-5020 Salzburg, Austria, Tel. +43 662 8044-5731, Fax +43 662 8044-5751, E-mail albert.duschl@sbg.ac.at

Th1-Mediated Inflammation as a Potential Pathogenic Factor in Allergic Disease

P.G. Holt

Telethon Institute for Child Health Research and Centre for Child Health Research, Faculty of Medicine and Dentistry, University of Western Australia, Perth, Western Australia

Summary: *Background:* Our earlier description of sluggish Th1 maturation in CD4$^+$ T-cells as a determinant of atopic risk has been independently confirmed. The "window" period of attenuated Th1 function in high-risk children is restricted to infancy, during which time diminished IFN-γ feedback may contribute to preferential development of Th2-polarized memory against allergens. Th1 maturation frequently accelerates in atopics beyond infancy, resulting in high-level expression of Th1 immunity. Recent studies suggest a contribution from Th1 immunity allergic inflammation, but the limited data available precludes firm conclusions regarding the role of individual Th1 cytokines. *Methods:* We are investigating this issue via two prospective cohort studies spanning the period birth-high school, employing populations of $n \approx 170$. The first study comprises children in whom atopic outcomes at 2 years have been related to cytokine response patterns in peripheral blood mononuclear cells (PBMC) collected between birth and outcome age. The second focuses on a cohort sampled at 11 years, involving detailed analysis of immune responses in relation to current asthma/allergy phenotypes. *Results:* In the infants, regression modeling identified IFN-γ production by CD8$^+$ T-cells as the strongest independent predictor of atopy. In the older cohort, IL-5 and/or eosinophilia most strongly associated with skin prick test (SPT) wheal size and with bronchial hyperresponsiveness (BHR), in each case in independent association with IFN-γ reactivity. *Conclusion:* Beyond the period of allergen-specific Th-memory priming during which Th1 cytokines are atopy-antagonistic, Th1 cytokine production (including from CD8$^+$ T-cells) may synergize with Th2 cytokines to drive atopy pathogenesis.

Keywords: atopic inflammation, Th1 immunity, IFN-γ

The original observation from our group linking attenuated postnatal maturation of the IFN-γ response capacity of CD4$^+$ Th-cells with increased risk for atopic disease [1] has been subsequently confirmed in a range of independent laboratories (reviewed in [2]). The precise mechanism underlying this association remains to be confirmed, but the available information from animal model systems indicates that cross-regulation between Th1 and Th2 cytokines during the early stages of Th-memory generation plays an important role in shaping long term Th-memory phenotype [3]. This suggests that reduced IFN-γ responsiveness in infants at high risk of atopy may increase the likelihood that the differentiation of CD4$^+$ T-cells, which are primed with allergen during this period, will default down the Th2 pathway, resulting eventually in consolidation of Th2-polarized allergen-specific memory.

However, the association between IFN-γ response capacity in atopics and the ultimate expression of atopic disease, post the sensitization phase, is less clear. In particular, once immunological maturity is reached, the expression of Th1 immunity in a large proportion of atopics appears at least equivalent to nonatopics [4, 5]. We are readdressing this complex issue in a series of prospective and cross-sectional cohort studies, relating immune response phenotypes to clinical phenotypes. Underlying the strategy of these investigations is acceptance of the reality that the high levels of genetic diversity within our study populations necessitates the use of sample sizes as large as possible, in order to obtain sufficient statistical power to detect subtle clinical/immunological associations.

Material and Methods

The priming methodology for the studies discussed here is detailed in our recent publications [6, 7], and is summarized below.

Infant Cohort

Cord blood mononuclear cells (CBMC) were cryobanked from 175 newborns at high risk (HR) of atopic disease. The latter classification was based on a standardized questionnaire [8], plus positive doctor diagnosis of asthma, hay fever, or AD for one or both parents. Atopic outcomes in the cohort were obtained by SPT to a panel of inhalant and food allergens; atopy at outcome age 2 years was defined as any SPT wheal diameter $\geq 2\,mm$. CBMC were cultured with PHA[**please define**] or staphylococcal enterotoxin B (SEB) for 48 h, and levels of IL-5, IL-10, IL-13, and IFN-γ protein in culture supernatants were determined by standardized ELISA. CD4$^+$ and CD8$^+$ cell purifications were performed on CBMC samples employing DYNA beads.

11-Year-Old Cohort

These children are part of an ongoing birth cohort study and were not selected via any criteria related to atopy status. The children were assessed for SPT reactivity to a panel of allergens, and asthma status determined by doctor diagnosis. BHR to inhaled histamine was determined by standard methodology [7].

Results and Discussion

The salient findings from the infant cohort study [6] indicate that positive atopic outcomes at age 2 years are associated with elevated IFN-γ responses to either PHA or SEB in CBMC (atopic > nonatopic at outcome age; PHA: $p < 0.002$, SEB: $p < 0.005$). This finding appears counterintuitive, given the earlier literature associating diminished IFN-γ responsiveness at birth with increased susceptibility to atopic sensitization. However, the key study defining this latter relationship focused on CD4$^+$ Th-cell clones. In a more recent study from our laboratory, we demonstrated that in the neonatal period expression of the IFN-γ gene in CD4$^+$ T-cells was regulated in a unique fashion relative to other IFN-γ-producing cell types such as NK and CD8$^+$ T-cells. Notably, IFN-γ production in CD4$^+$ T-cells in CBMC was tightly (negatively) regulated via an epigenetic mechanism involving hypermethylation of CpG sites in the proximal promoter of the gene [9]. This process results in chromatin remodeling, which restricts access of necessary transcription factors to binding sites in the promoter, thus, inhibiting gene activation. In contrast, levels of CpG methylation in CD8$^+$ T-cells in neonates are relatively low, permitting IFN-γ gene transcription in these cells at levels approximately one log-fold greater than in CD4$^+$ T-cells [9]. Accordingly, when the overall T-cell population present in CBMC is separated into its CD4$^+$ and CD8$^+$ components, and the latter assessed independently for capacity to produce IFN-γ in response to mitogenic stimulation, on the order of 90% of production is attributable to the CD8$^+$ population [6, 9].

This finding suggests that the association between atopic outcome status in the infants and their IFN-γ response capacity in early postnatal life relates to CD8$^+$ T-cell function, as opposed to an activity of the CD4 Th-cell subset, which are involved in conventional Th-memory generation. It should also be emphasized that the association pertains to a prese-lected population of children at high genetic risk of atopy, and at this stage there is no evidence available to indicate whether children at low risk of atopy who become sensitized display comparably elevated CD8+ T-cell IFN-γ responses during infancy.

The precise mechanism underlying this association also remains to be defined. High IFN-γ responder phenotype within the CD8+ T-cell compartment expressed early in life may, for example, equate to a constitutively proinflammatory milieu at the mucosal surfaces at which allergen exposure occurs, thus, enhancing the likelihood of local Th-cell priming. This and related possibilities require more detailed follow-up studies.

The results of immunoprofiling studies on 11-year-olds are reported in detail in [7]. The key findings pertaining to this discussion are as follows. Firstly, positive IFN-γ responses to allergens such as HDM are observed in PBMC samples from nonatopic and atopic children at essentially equivalent intensities and frequencies. However, once the population is stratified on the basis of HDM responsiveness, and the SPT+ subgroup is analyzed in isolation, multiple logistic regression (controlling for multiple potential confounders including titres of HDM-specific IgG and IgG4) identifies the IFN-γ component of the *in vitro* PBMC response to HDM as independently associated (along with the IL-5 component) with wheal size ($p = 0.003$ by multiple linear regression). This finding is consistent with that detailed above in neonates, and again indicates that in the group most likely to express severe allergic disease, the IFN-γ component of the host T-cell response is positively associated with atopy intensity.

The second association detected in this study pertains to BHR to inhaled histamine. A hallmark of the immunoprofile of 11-year-olds with BHR is elevated polyclonal T-cell responses [7], which include IL-5 (BHR+ > BHR-; $p < 0.002$), IL-13 ($p < 0.016$), TNF-α ($p < 0.004$), and IFN-γ ($p < 0.015$). Further analysis of these associations by logistic regression, including a broad range of potential confounders in the model, identified the com-bination of Eosinophilia (OR 29.09 [7.01–120.69]; $p = 0.000$) and the polyclonal IFN-γ response (OR 1.55 [1.06–2.27]; $p = 0.023$) as independently associated with BHR.

There are a variety of precedents for this finding in the literature. Firstly, experimental animal data clearly demonstrates the potential of IFN-γ producing Th1 cells to synergize with Th2 cells in BHR induction [10]. Additionally, elevated levels of IFN-γ have been detected in BAL fluid [11] and blood [12] of adults during asthma exacerbations. Moreover, increased numbers of IFN-γ secreting CD8+ T-cells have been documented in airway biopsies in fatal asthma [13] and in the blood of children with BHR [14].

It is also noteworthy that elevated polyclonal TNFα responses were also a feature of the immune response profiles of 11-year-olds with BHR [7], and this cytokine is also present in BAL in adults during asthma attacks [11]. Collectively, these data are consistent with an important ancillary role for Th1 effector mechanisms in the pathogenesis of one or more of the clinical phenotypes in atopic asthma. Development of more precise methods to detect and enumerate these patients within the overall atopic asthmatic population may provide novel opportunities for more targeted interventions in the future.

Acknowledgment

The majority of the studies reviewed involved collaborations with PD Sly, J Rowe, M Kusel, T Heaton, GP White, P Lesouef, and S Turner.

References

1. Holt PG, Clough JB, Holt BJ, Baron-Hay MJ, Rose AH, Robinson BWS, Thomas WR: Genetic "risk" for atopy is associated with delayed post-natal maturation of T-cell competence. Clin Exp Allergy 1992; 22:1093–1099.

2. Holt PG, Macaubas C: Development of long term tolerance versus sensitisation to environmental allergens during the perinatal period. Curr Opin Immunol 1997; 9:782–787.

3. O'Garra A, Arai N: The molecular basis of TTh and Th2 cell differentiation. Trends in Cell Biol 2000; 10:542–550.

4. Holt PG, Rudin A, Macaubas C, Holt BJ, Rowe J, Loh R, Sly PD: Development of immunologic memory against tetanus toxoid and pertactin antigens from the diphtheria-tetanus-pertussis vaccine in atopic versus nonatopic children. J Allergy Clin Immunol 2000; 105:1117–1122.

5. Smart JM, Kemp AS: Increased Th1 and Th2 allergen-induced cytokine responses in children with atopic disease. Clin Exp Allergy 2002; 32: 796–802.

6. Rowe J, Heaton T, Kusel M, Suriyaarachchi D, Serralha M, Holt BJ, de Klerk N, Sly PD, Holt PG: High IFN-γ production by CD8⁺ T-cells and early sensitization among infants at high risk of atopy. J Allergy Clin Immunol 2004; 113:710–716.

7. Heaton T, Rowe J, Turner S, Aalberse RC, de Klerk N, Suriyaarachchi D, Serralha M, Holt BJ, Hollams E, Yerkovich S, Holt K, Sly PD, Goldblatt J, Le Souef PN, Holt PG: An immunoepidemiological approach to asthma: identification of in vitro T-cell response patterns associated with different wheezing phenotypes amongst 11-year-olds. Lancet, 2005; 365:142–149.

8. Prescott SL, Macaubas C, Smallacombe T, Holt BJ, Sly PD, Holt PG: Development of allergen-specific T-cell memory in atopic and normal children. Lancet 1999; 353:196–200.

9. White GP, Watt PM, Holt BJ, Holt PG: Differential patterns of methylation of the IFN-γ promoter at CpG and non-CpG sites underlie differences in IFN-γ gene expression between human neonatal and adult CD45RO⁻ T-cells. J Immunol 2002; 168:2820–2827.

10. Hansen G, Berry G, DeKruyff RH, Umetsu DT: Allergen-specific Th1 cells fail to counterbalance Th2 cell-induced airway hyperreactivity but cause severe airway inflammation. J Clin Invest 1999; 103:175–183.

11. Calhoun WJ, Murphy K, Stevens CA, Jarjour NN, Busse WW: Increased interferon-γ and tumor necrosis factor-α in bronchoalveolar lavage (BAL) fluid after antigen challenge in allergic subjects. Am Rev Respir Dis 1992; 145:A638.

12. Corrigan CJ, Kay AB: CD4 T-lymphocyte activation in acute severe asthma: relationship to disease severity and atopic status. Am Rev Respir Dis 1990; 141:970–977.

13. O'Sullivan S, Cormican L, Faul JL, Ichinohe S, Johnston SL, Burke CM, Poulter LW: Activated, cytotoxic CD8⁺ T lymphocytes contribute to the pathology of asthma death. Am J Respir Crit Care Med 2001; 164:560–564.

14. Magnan AO, Mely LG, Camilla CA, Badier MM, Montero-Julian FA, Guillot CM, Casano BB, Prato SJ, Fert V, Bongrand P, Vervloet D: Assessment of the Th1/Th2 paradigm in whole blood in atopy and asthma. Increased IFN-γ-producing CD8⁺ T-cells in asthma. Am J Respir Crit Care Med 2000; 161:1790–1796.

P.G. Holt

Division of Cell Biology, Telethon Institute for Child Health Research, PO Box 855, West Perth WA 6872, Australia, Tel. +61 8 9489 7838, Fax +61 8 9489 7707, E-mail patrick@ichr.uwa.edu.au

Healthy or Allergic Immune Response Characterized by Fine Balance Between Specific T-Regulatory 1 and T-Helper 2 Cells

M. Akdis, K. Blaser, and C.A. Akdis

Swiss Institute of Allergy and Asthma Research (SIAF), CH-7270 Davos, Switzerland

Summary: *Background:* Immune response to nonpathogenic environmental antigens and molecular mechanisms, which lead to either allergy or normal immunity appears a crucial question. *Methods:* We investigated the immunoregulatory mechanism to the major house dust mite (HDM), pear, hazelnut, and birch pollen allergens – Der p 1, Pyr c 5, Cor a 1, and Bet v 1, in healthy and allergic individuals, respectively, by direct purification of allergen-specific T-cells. *Results:* Single allergen-specific T-cells constitute less than 0.1% of the whole CD4+ T-cell repertoire and can be isolated from peripheral blood of humans according to their cytokine profile. Freshly purified IFN-γ-, IL-4-, and IL-10-producing allergen-specific CD4+ T-cells display characteristics of Th1-, Th2-, and T-regulatory 1 (Tr1)-like cells, respectively. Tr1 cells suppress Th2 cells by using multiple suppressive mechanisms, including IL-10 and TGF-β as secreted cytokines and CTLA-4 and PD-1 as surface molecules. Neutralization of cytokine activity showed that T-cell suppression was mainly mediated by IL-10 and TGF-β during allergen-specific immunotherapy SIT and in normal immunity to mucosal allergens. *Conclusions:* Together these results demonstrate a deviation to a regulatory/suppressor T-cell response during SIT and the decisive role of the fine balance between allergen-specific Tr1 cells and Th2 cells in the generation of a healthy or an allergic immune response. Although in different proportions, healthy and allergic individuals exhibit all three allergen-specific subsets, suggesting that a change in the dominant subset may lead to allergy development or recovery.

Keywords: T-regulatory cells, immunotherapy, tolerance, anergy, IgE, T-cells

Introduction

Anergy, tolerance, and active suppression may not be independent events, but rather involve similar mechanisms and cell types in immune regulation. T-cell tolerance is characterized by induced unresponsiveness of surviving T-cells when subject to antigen encounter [1]. Anergy entails a process by which presentation of an antigen to T-cell clones in the absence of professional antigen-presenting cells (APC) re-sults in the induction of a hyporesponsive state affecting IL-2 production and proliferation upon restimulation [1–3]. Anergic T-cells can be characterized by their reversible functional limitations, including cell division, cell differentiation, and cytokine production [1–3]. It is important to note that in earlier studies, which provide a basis for the definition of anergy/tolerance, functional unresponsiveness was analyzed by nonsophisticated assays such as antigen-induced [³H] thymidine incorporation,

IL-2, and total IgG production. Furthermore, until recently, the antigens used in mouse models contained high amounts of impurities, such as LPS and other innate immune-response stimulating substances, which may have influenced experimental outcomes.

Type1 T-Regulatory Cells (Tr1)

The idea of T-regulatory (T_{Reg}) cells suppressing immune responses via cell-cell interactions and/or the production of suppressor cytokines is well established. However, many mechanisms behind these aspects remain to be unraveled [3–5]. Tr1 cells, which are also-called inducible T_{Reg} cells, are defined by their ability to produce high levels of IL-10 and TGF-β [6, 7]. Tr1 cells specific for a variety of antigens arise in vivo, but may also differentiate from naive CD4+ T-cells in vitro. It has been reported that stimulating naive CD4 T-cells in the presence of IL-10, IFN-α, or a combination of IL-4 and IL-10, dexamethasone, and vitamin D3 leads to the in vitro generation of a Tr1 cell subset [4, 8, 9]. It is now clear that IL-10- and/or TGF-β-producing Tr1 cells in humans are generated in vivo during the early course of allergen-SIT, implying that high and increasing doses of allergens induce Tr1 cells [5, 6, 10]. These Tr1 cells downregulate allergen-specific Th1 and Th2 responses [7].

Tr1 Cell-Mediated Peripheral T-cell Tolerance in Allergen-Specific Immunotherapy (SIT) and the Healthy Immune Response to Allergens

Allergen-SIT has been most successfully applied in the treatment of insect venom allergy and allergic rhinitis in clinical practice during the last century. Successful allergen-SIT is associated with an increase in allergen-blocking IgG antibodies (mainly IgG4) [11], the generation of IgE-modulating CD8+ T-cells [12], and a decline in the number of mast cells and eosinophils as well as the release of mediators [13]. The induction of peripheral T-cell tolerance plays a crucial role in allergen-SIT [3, 5, 6, 14]. T-cell tolerance is initiated by the autocrine action of IL-10 and TGF-β, which are increasingly produced by antigen-specific T-cells [3, 5, 6]. Reactivation of tolerized T-cells can result in the distinct production of either Th1 or Th2 cytokine profiles depending on cytokines present in the tissue microenvironment, and can, therefore, direct allergen-SIT toward either successful or unsuccessful treatment [14].

Analysis of responses to various food and inhalant antigens has shown the healthy immune response to mucosal antigens to have a similar mechanism of immunological unresponsiveness [7]. By using interferon (IFN)-γ, IL-4-, and IL-10- secreting allergen-specific CD4+ T-cells that resemble Th1, Th2, and Tr1-like cells, respectively, it was demonstrated that healthy and allergic individuals exhibit all three subsets, but in different proportions. In healthy individuals Tr1 cells represent the dominant subset for common environmental allergens, whereas a high frequency of allergen-specific IL-4 secreting T-cells (Th2-like) is found in allergic individuals. Hence, a change in the dominant subset may lead to either the development of allergy or recovery [7].

Allergen-Specific Peripheral T-cell Tolerance is Associated with Antibody Isotype Regulation and Effector Cell Suppression

Although peripheral tolerance was demonstrated in specific T-cells, the ability of B-cells to produce specific IgE antibodies was not eliminated during SIT [14]. In fact, during the early phase of treatment, specific serum levels of both IgE and IgG4 antibodies increased. However, the increase in antigen-specific IgG4 was more striking and the ratio of specific IgE to IgG4 decreased. IL-10 potently suppresses both total and allergen-specific IgE, whereas it simultaneously increases IgG4 production [5]. Therefore, IL-10 not only generates T-cell tolerance, it also regulates specific isotype formation and skews the specific

IgE response toward an IgG4-dominated phenotype. The induction of specific IgA and IgG4 in serum coincides with increased TGF-β and IL-10, respectively. This may account for the role of IgA and TGF-β as well as IgG4 and IL-10 in mucosal immune responses to allergens in healthy individuals [5, 15].

An obvious decrease in IgE antibody levels and IgE-mediated skin sensitivity normally requires several years of SIT, however, most patients are already protected against bee stings at an early stage of BV-SIT. The reason for this could be: (1) the effector cells (mast cells, basophils, and eosinophils) are desensitized during the induction phase; (2) they require T_cell cytokines for priming, survival, and activity, which cannot be sufficiently provided by suppressed Th2 and T_{Reg} cells; (3) T_{reg} cell cytokines can directly or indirectly suppress mast cells, basophils, and eosinophils; (4) T_{reg} cells can also downregulate local tissue cells and other inflammatory cells [16]. Therefore, T_{reg} cells can tune the thresholds for type 1 hypersensitivity reactions as well as type 4 hypersensitivity reactions in allergic diseases [16].

Conclusion

The key mechanism in healthy immune responses to noninfectious, non-self-antigens is the induction and maintenance of specific peripheral T-cell tolerance. This hypothesis is clinically well-documented in allergy, transplantation, tumor, and infection. Development of prophylactic vaccines to induce allergen-specific T_{Reg} cells should be considered in addition to the treatment of established allergy. However, caution should be taken concerning the over-activation of T_{Reg} cells, since several studies show that they may be responsible for the chronicity of infections and tumor tolerance; not always a healthy response.

Acknowledgments

The authors' laboratories are supported by the Swiss National Science Foundation Grants No. 32–100266, 32–105865, and 32–65436/2.

References

1. Schwartz RH: T-cell anergy. Annu Rev Immunol 2003; 21:305–334.

2. Faith A, Akdis CA, Akdis M, Simon H-U, Blaser K: Defective TCR stimulation in anergized type 2 T-helper cells correlates with abrogated p56 l^{ck} and ZAP-70 tyrosine kinase activities. J Immunol 1997; 159:53–60.

3. Akdis CA, Blaser K: IL-10-induced anergy in peripheral T-cell and reactivation by microenvironmental cytokines: two key steps in specific immunotherapy. FASEB J 1999; 13:603–609.

4. Groux H, O'Garra A, Bigler M, Rouleau M, Antonenko S, de Vries JE, Roncarolo MG: A CD4$^+$ T-cell subset inhibits antigen-specific T-cell responses and prevents colitis. Nature 1997; 389:737–742.

5. Akdis CA, Blesken T, Akdis M, Wüthrich B, Blaser K: Role of IL-10 in specific immunotherapy. J Clin Invest 1998; 102:98–106.

6. Jutel M, Akdis M, Budak F, Aebischer-Casaulta C, Wrzyszcz M, Blaser K, Akdis AC: IL-10 and TGF-β cooperate in regulatory T-cell response to mucosal allergens in normal immunity and specific immunotherapy. Eur J Immunol 2003; 33:1205–1214.

7. Akdis M, Verhagen J, Taylor A, Karamloo F, Karagiannidis C, Crameri R, Thunberg S, Deniz G, Valenta R, Fiebig H, Kegel C, Disch R, Schmidt-Weber CB, Blaser K, Akdis CA: Immune responses in healthy and allergic individuals are characterized by a fine balance between allergen-specific T-regulatory 1 and T-helper 2 cells. J Exp Med 2004; 199:1567–1575.

8. Levings MK, Sangregorio R, Galbiati F, Squadrone S, de Waal Malefyt R, Roncarolo MG: IFN-α and IL-10 induce the differentiation of human type 1 T-regulatory cells. J Immunol 2001; 166:5530–5539.

9. Barrat FJ, Cua DJ, Boonstra A, Richards DF, Crain C, Savelkoul HF, de Waal-Malefyt R, Coffman RL, Hawrylowicz CM, O'Garra A: *In vitro* generation of interleukin 10-producing regulatory CD4$^+$ T-cells is induced by immunosuppressive drugs and inhibited by T-helper type 1 (Th1)- and Th2-inducing cytokines. J Exp Med 2002; 195:603–616.

10. Nasser SM, Ying S, Meng O, Kay AB, Ewan PW: Interleukin-10 levels increase in cutaneous biopsies of patients undergoing wasp venom immunotherapy. Eur J Immunol 2001; 31:3704–3713.

11. van Neerven RJ, Wikborg T, Lund G, Jacobsen

B, Brinch-Nielsen A, Arnved J, Ipsen H: Blocking antibodies induced by specific allergy vaccination prevent the activation of CD4$^+$ T-cells by inhibiting serum-IgE-facilitated allergen presentation. J Immunol 1999; 163:2944–2952.

12. Rocklin RE, Sheffer A, Greineder DK, Melmon KL: Generation of antigen-specific suppressor cells during allergy desensitization. N Engl J Med 1980; 302:1213–1219.

13. Creticos PS, Adkinson NF, Jr., Kagey-Sobotka A, Proud D, Meier HL, Naclerio RM, Lichtenstein LM, Norman PS: Nasal challenge with ragweed pollen in hay fever patients. Effect of immunotherapy. J Clin Invest 1985; 76:2247–2253.

14. Akdis CA, Akdis M, Blesken T, Wymann D, Alkan SS, Muller U, Blaser K: Epitope-specific T-cell tolerance to phospholipase A2 in bee-venom immunotherapy and recovery by IL-2 and IL-15 I. J Clin Invest 1996; 98:1676–1683.

15. Sonoda E, Matsumoto R, Hitoshi Y, Ishii T, Sugimoto M, Araki S, Tominaga A, Yamaguchi N, Takatsu K: Transforming growth factor β induces IgA production and acts additively with interleukin 5 for IgA production. J Exp Med 1989; 170:1415–1420.

16. Akdis CA, Blaser K, Akdis M: Genes of tolerance. Allergy 2004; 59:897–913.

Mübeccel Akdis

Swiss Institute of Allergy and Asthma Research (SIAF), Obere Strasse 22, CH-7270 Davos, Switzerland, Tel. +41 81 4100848, Fax +41 81 4100840, E-mail akdism@siaf.unizh.ch

Indications for the Existence of an IgE Isotype-Specific Signal Transduction

I. Oberndorfer[1], D. Schmid[1], R. Geisberger[1], R. Crameri[2], and G. Achatz[1]

[1]*Department of Molecular Biology, University of Salzburg, Austria,* [2]*SIAF, Davos, Switzerland*

Summary: *Background:* Immunoglobulins can be expressed in a secreted and in a membrane-bound form (mIg). The mIg molecule associates with the signal transducing molecules Igα and Igβ and forms the B-cell receptor (BCR), which triggers signals that control activation, affinity maturation, memory induction, differentiation, and various other processes. We previously found that truncation of the 28 amino-acid long cytoplasmic tail of mIgE in mice led to reduced levels of serum IgE (sIgE), smaller numbers of IgE-secreting cells, and the absence of a clear secondary response. These findings indicate an active role of the cytoplasmic tail in processes controlled by BCR engagement. In the present publication we report that HAX-1 (hematopoietic lineage cell-specific protein (HS1)-associated protein X-1) interacts with the cytoplasmic tail of mIgE. *Methods:* A phage display experiment used a murine B-cell cDNA library displayed on the surface of phage as prey and the recombinantly expressed cytoplasmic tail of mIgE as bait. *Results:* Phage expressing HAX-1 were selected in phage display biopanning. The interaction of HAX-1 with the cytoplasmic tail could also be shown in surface plasmon resonance measurements. *Conclusions:* We hypothesize that HAX-1 could be involved in transmitting IgE-specific signals from the surface receptor to the B-cell nucleus. Our findings suggest that in mIgE-positive B-cells HAX-1 either directly interferes with BCR-signalling via Igα/Igβ, or signals from the IgE-tail are independently conveyed via HAX-1.

Keywords: mIgE, B-cell receptor, HAX-1

From the numerous surface markers of a B lymphocyte, the BCR complex is probably the most powerful marker influencing the developmental process of the cell. The BCR consists of the membrane-bound immunoglobulin (mIg) but, depending on the state of differentiation, may be associated with other transmembrane proteins, most notably Igα (CD79a) and Igβ (CD79b) [1]. So far, the sheath proteins Igα and Igβ are known as the signal-transducing component of the BCR complex that connects the antigen receptor to the tyrosine phosphorylation pathways in the cell. All isotypes of mIg can form a complex with Igα and Igβ [2], indicating an involvement of all Ig-isotypes in the signal transduction pathway.

Previous work from our lab showed that the truncation of the 28 amino acids long cytoplas-

mic tail of mIgE to three amino acids lead to a 90% reduction of serum IgE, smaller numbers of IgE-secreting cells and the absence of a clear secondary response [3]. These results indicated that the cytoplasmic tail of mIgE is involved in the processes of plasma cell differentiation and memory induction and, therefore, interferes with BCR signalling pathways. We concluded that the tail may interact specifically with proteins that change the outcome of BCR signalling in an isotype specific manner. In the present work we present HAX-1 as a protein interacting with the cytoplasmic tail of mIgE. We used phage display technology to search for proteins interacting with the mIgE-tail. In our phage display experiments we used the recombinantly expressed cytoplasmic tail of mIgE as bait and a murine B-cell cDNA library displayed on the

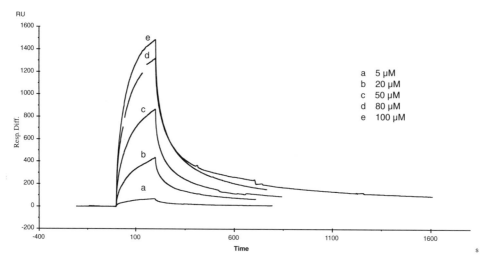

Figure 1. The affinity of recombinant HAX 1 toward the recombinant IgE-tail peptide was measured by surface plasmon resonance analysis with a BIACORE X device. The synthesized IgE-tail peptide (1 mg/mL in PBS; sequence HHHHHHKVKWVFSTPMQDTPQTFQDYANILQTRA) was injected at different concentrations (5 µM – 100 µM). Data were analyzed with the help of BIAevaluation software. Response difference (Resp. Diff.) between signals from the empty flow cell 1 and the flow cell 2 coupled with approximately 4000 RUs of recombinant HAX-1 in RU (response units).

surface of phage as prey. The cytoplasmic tail was expressed as His-tagged fusion protein with globular carrier proteins (IgE constant exon 4 or DHFR) in *E. coli*. For the construction of the murine B-cell cDNA library lymphocytes from spleen and lymph nodes were pretreated for the IgE bias. After stimulation 4×10^7 CD19+ B-cells (93% purity) were sorted by MACS and used for the construction of a murine B-cell cDNA library in a modified pJuFo phagemid vector [4]. After four panning rounds, phage specifically expressing HAX-1 were preferentially found. In the B-cell cDNA library 0.014% of all phagemid vectors encoded the C-terminus of HAX-1 but after the fourth panning round HAX-1 was enriched up to 64%.

His-tagged murine full-length HAX-1 was recombinantly expressed in *E. coli* and the affinity toward the recombinant cytoplasmic tail was measured by surface plasmon resonance analysis. An association constant of 1.4×10^4 1/M and a dissociation constant of 7.55×10^{-5} M were measured (Figure 1). The measured association constant of 1.4×10^4 1/M is an indication of a weak but biologically relevant interaction between recombinant HAX-1 and the recombinant mIgE-tail.

We point to the fact that all experiments were performed with the recombinantly expressed and, therefore, unphosphorylated tail. This indicates that the *in vitro* interaction of HAX-1 with the tail is independent of tyrosine-phosphorylation or other protein modifications.

HAX-1, first identified as HS1 interacting protein, is a 35-kD protein that is expressed ubiquitously among tissues and is localized in the cytoplasm [5] and along the endoplasmic reticulum and the nuclear envelope [6] of cells. HAX-1 shows no clear similarity to known proteins and contains no significant motifs that point to a biochemical function but several publications indicate that HAX-1 is an antiapoptotic protein [5, 7, 8].

Focusing on the antiapoptotic function, HAX-1 is a candidate protein that could confer higher apoptotic resistance to mIgE-positive cells. HAX-1 could be prebound to the unphosphorylated IgE-tail and, thus, influence the outcome of signalling processes that are initiated upon BCR-activation. It has already been hypothesized that HAX-1 may neutralize the proapoptotic function of HS1 [5]. Additionally it was reported that HAX-1 inhibits Bax-induced apoptosis [7] and it was also shown that HAX-1 physically interacts with

B cell lymphoma 2 protein (Bcl-2) [8]. This could give an explanation for the phenotype of the mutant mouse strains carrying a truncated cytoplasmic tail of mIgE. These mice show reduced levels of serum IgE and smaller numbers of IgE-secreting B-cells. B-cells with the mutated mIgE molecule lack the binding site for HAX-1 and could, therefore, be predisposed to undergo apoptosis.

In conclusion, we present evidence that the cytoplasmic tail of IgE has the ability to interact with HAX-1 *in-vitro*.

Acknowledgments

This work was supported by the Austria Science Foundation (S8809-MED) and the Austrian National Bank (OENB grant 9546).

References

1. Reth M: Antigen receptors on B lymphocytes. Annu Rev Immunol 1992; 10:97–121.
2. Venkitaraman AR, Williams GT, Dariavach P, Neuberger MS: The B-cell antigen receptor of the five immunoglobulin classes. Nature 1991; 352:777–781.
3. Achatz G, Nitschke L, Lamers MC: Effect of transmembrane and cytoplasmic domains of IgE on the IgE response. Science 1997; 276:409–411.
4. Crameri R, Achatz G, Weichel M, Rhyner C: Direct selection of cDNAs by phage display. Methods Mol Biol 2002; 185:461–469.
5. Suzuki Y, Demoliere C, Kitamura D, Takeshita H, Deuschle U, Watanabe T: HAX-1, a novel intracellular protein, localized on mitochondria, directly associates with HS1, a substrate of Src family tyrosine kinases. J Immunol 1997; 158:2736–2744.
6. Gallagher AR, Cedzich A, Gretz N, Somlo S, Witzgall R: The polycystic kidney disease protein PKD2 interacts with Hax-1, a protein associated with the actin cytoskeleton. Proc Natl Acad Sci USA 2000; 97:4017–4022.
7. Sharp TV, Wang HW, Koumi A, Hollyman D, Endo Y, Ye H, Du MQ, Boshoff C: K15 protein of Kaposi's sarcoma-associated herpesvirus is latently expressed and binds to HAX-1, a protein with antiapoptotic function. J Virol 2002; 76: 802–816.
8. Matsuda G, Nakajima K, Kawaguchi Y, Yamanashi Y, Hirai K: Epstein-Barr virus (EBV) nuclear antigen leader protein (EBNA-LP) forms complexes with a cellular antiapoptosis protein Bcl-2 or its EBV counterpart BHRF1 through HS1-associated protein X-1. Microbiol Immunol 2003; 47:91–99.

Gernot Achatz

Fachbereich für Molekulare Biologie, Abteilung Allergologie und Immunologie, Hellbrunnerstraße 34, A-5020 Salzburg, Austria, Tel. +43 662 8044-5764, Fax +43 662 8044-144, E-mail gernot.achatz@sbg.ac.at

Studies on the Regulation of IgE Expression by the Use of "Knock-in" Mice

G. Achatz-Straussberger[1], A. Karnowsky[2], M. Lamers[2], and G. Achatz[1]

[1]Department of Molecular Biology, Division Allergology and Immunology, Salzburg, Austria,
[2]MPI for Immunobiology, Freiburg, Germany

Summary: *Background:* IgE is the key effector molecule of allergic reactions. The expression of IgE is tightly regulated on different levels. Preliminary data from our laboratories suggest a regulation based on the expression of the membrane-bound IgE. In further studies we could show that the mRNA for the ε heavy chain gene is expressed at very low levels caused by poor processing and polyadenylation of the transcript. *Methods:* A step forward in the analysis of this tight regulation was done with the construction of "knock-in" mice with composite and/or chimeric poly(A) sites influencing the posttranscriptional regulation. *Results:* Expression of mRNA for the secreted form of IgE is favored over that for the membrane form in resting B-cells. The ratio between the amount of secreted vs. the amount of membrane-bound Ig that is produced by a single cell is determined by the efficiency with which the internal or external polyadenylation sites are used and by the stability of the ensuing mRNAs. *Conclusion:* Factors that influence the alternative polyadenylation are largely unknown. However, because expression of mIgE is essential for recruitment of IgE-producing cells in the immune response, clarification of this issue is of great importance. So far, IgE regulation is evident on the level of DNA recombination (switch), transcription and RNA processing. It is not inconceivably that also posttranslational and post-transcriptional processes may influence the expression of membrane-bound IgE.

Keywords: mIgE, alternative polyadenylation, B-cell receptor

Under normal conditions, our organism tries everything to keep the level of IgE as low as possible. Compared to other Ig isotypes, total IgE serum levels are very low not only under steady-state conditions, but also after immunizations. However, if the decision: "force IgE expression" occurred, the organism sets value on highest quality of the IgE molecules produced [1]. The biological mechanism of this dangerous migration is unknown, but obviously several independent mechanisms are responsible for this fact. First, serum IgE has a very short half-life [2], which contrasts with the other immunoglobulin classes that form a substantial component of serum proteins. Second, IgE expression seems to be regulated by a negative feedback mechanism

committed by CD23, the low affinity IgE receptor [3]. Third, our previously published [1, 4] experiments show very clearly that the IgE antigen receptor (mIgE) itself plays a significant role in the maturation process and the expansion of antigen-specific IgE B-cells. Fourth, *in vitro* data from our laboratories indicate an influence of an inefficient processing of the mRNA transcripts for the membrane form of IgE [5, 6]. By constructing mouse lines, expressing IgE antigen receptors, chimeric for their transmembrane and cytoplasmic tails, we investigated *in vivo* the direct influence of the processing efficiency of the transcript coding for the membrane form of IgE and its effect on the later recruitment of IgE secreting cells.

Materials and Methods

Construction of the Target Vectors

The target vectors consist of genomic DNA, spanning a region from the ε constant exon 3 and 4 to the exchanged γ1 membrane exons M1 and M2. Downstream of the polyadenylation signals of εor γorigin we introduced a neomycin resistance gene for positive selection. A herpes simplex virus thymidine kinase gene for negative selection was introduced 5' of the ε constant region 3. Targeting was performed as previously described [4].

Examination of Correct Splicing

For verification of correct splicing of the γ1 membrane exons to the last constant exon of ε, we constructed a eukaryotic expression vector (pGA139), expressing ε constant exon 3 and 4 followed by the γ1 membrane exons M1 and M2 (see Figure 3). K46 cells were transfected, RNA was isolated, and cDNA was constructed using oligo(dT) priming. RT-PCR was performed with primers: 201: 5'-GAGGCACTTCAGAAACCCAGGAAAC T-3'; 232: 5'-GTGACAGCAGCGCTGTAG-

CAC-3'; PCR products were recloned and sequenced.

Results

Alternative Polyadenylation of IgE

With the exception of IgE, for the *secreted* and the *membrane* polyadenylation signals, the consensus sequence AATAAA is used. However, the ε membrane locus uses three crytic polyadenylation signals (Figure 1). These signals (AGTAAA, AAGAAA, and ATTAAA) are in considerable disagreement with the consensus sequence. The ratio of transcripts for the secreted and the membrane form of immunoglobulin reflects the usage of either polyadenylation signal. The choice depends normally on the developmental stage of the B lymphocyte. Therefore, the production of the two types of RNA are determined by alternative splicing or rather, alternative polyadenylation [7, 8]. The ratio between the amount of secreted vs. the amount of membrane-bound Ig that is produced by a single cell is determined by the efficiency with which the two polyadenylation sites are used and by the sta-

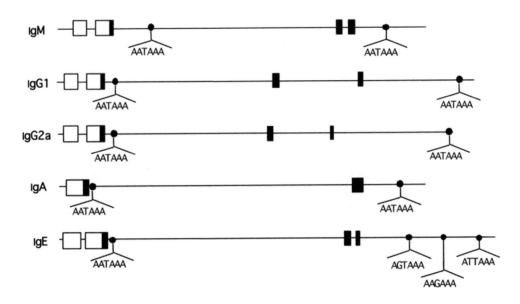

Figure 1: External and internal poly(A) signals in different Ig-isotypes.

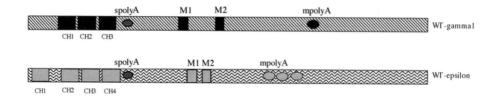

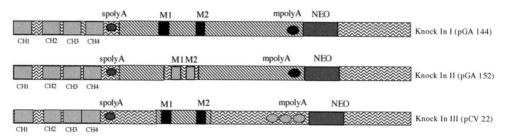

Figure 2: Germline situation of the three "knock-in" strains.

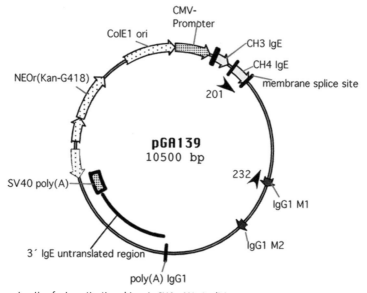

Figure 3: Vector construction for investigating chimeric *CH4-ε-M1-γ1* splicing.

bility of the ensuing mRNA's. In resting B-cells the ratio is about 1, but in activated lymphoblasts more mRNA for secretory Ig can be found.

In vitro Polyadenylation Studies

Spleen cells from CD23-deficient mice [3] were stimulated for 4 days with LPS and IL-4. mIgE+ and mIgG1+ B-cells were isolated from these cultures by fluorescence activated cell sorting. RNA was extracted from the sorted cells and the relative number of transcripts for the secreted and membrane form of ε and γ1 were determined by quantitative real-time PCR [6]. In the mIgE+ B-cells 100 times more transcripts for sε than for mε were found. In contrast, in mIgG1+ B-cells we detected 140 times more transcripts for mγ1 than for sγ1. We conclude that the variant structure of the

3'UTR of the ε HC gene is reflected in an expression pattern of the mRNA for sε and mε that differs significantly from that of the other HC gene isotypes, and that is also reflected in the expression of the mIgE and mIgG1 protein on B-cells.

Construction of Functional Chimeric "Knock-in" Mice

The logical next step in the investigation of the regulation of IgE expression concerning alternative polyadenylation was the extension of the *in vitro* results for *in vivo* situations.

Therefore, we constructed three "knock-in"mice strains, carrying chimeric IgE-IgG1 antigen receptors. Figure 2 shows the principle germline situation of the three mice strains.

Examination of CH4-ε-M1-γ1 Chimeric Splicing

We first investigated if chimeric *CH4-ε-M1-γ1* splice donor and acceptor sites were spliced correctly to form functional chimeric B-cell receptors. We constructed an eukaryotic expression vector harboring the CH3 and CH4 exon of the germline ε locus followed by the complete 3'-γ1-membrane locus (Figure 3). The vector was transiently transfected to K46 B-cell lymphoma lines. After 2 days, RNA was isolated and cDNA was constructed by oligo(dT) priming. Chimeric splicing was checked by subsequent PCR amplification using CH4-ε sense and M1-γ1 antisense primer pairs. Correct splicing was shown by sequencing the PCR products.

Serum IgE levels of Chimeric "Knock-in" Mice

So far, germline transmission could be reached for all three mouse strains. However, because of low offspring rates, preliminary data can only be presented for "knock-in" mouse I. In this mouse strain we could measure a 1000-fold increase of membrane IgE transcript in real time experiments (data shown elsewhere). This increase of membrane IgE transcript is also reflected by a tremendous increase of specific serum IgE if compared to a wild type strains (data shown elsewhere).

Discussion

In vitro data of our group and others [5, 6] unambiguously show that a fundamental difference between IgE and other immunoglobulins lies in the pattern of expression of the mRNA for the secreted and membrane form. The poor expression of the mRNA for the membrane form of IgE is responsible for this difference. Deletion of the "internal" polyadenylation signal results in a shift toward the expression of the mRNA for the membrane form of IgE [6], which indicates that the secreted polyadenylation signal is preferentially used. Exchanging the 3'UTR of the εHC gene for that of the μHC gene also causes a shift toward the expression of the mRNA for the membrane form, indicating that the most likely explanation for the results is the poor processing of the mRNA for the membrane form at the deviant polyadenylation signals in the 3'UTR of the ε-heavy chain gene.

The logical next step in the investigation of the regulation of IgE expression concerning alternative polyadenylation was the extension of the *in vitro* results for *in vivo* situations. Therefore, we decided to start with the construction of three mice strains, carrying chimeric IgE antigen receptors. With these mice, we are able to study the changed transcriptional prerequisites in regard to the new germline situation and the resulting effect on the quantity and quality of the IgE response. Indeed, the "sIgE–mIgE total" mouse strain showed a dramatic increase of membrane IgE transcript if compared to wild type strains. This effect is further reflected by a 5-fold increase of specific serum IgE after immunization experiments. Our preliminary *in vivo* data clearly showed that the unusual polyadenylation of the membrane IgE transcript and the dedicated extremely low membrane IgE expression present an additional regulatory mechanism, which keeps serum IgE in healthy individuals at a very basal level. The consequences of a possible uncontrolled IgE secretion warrant an in-depth study of these processes. Therefore, we think that the knowledge about the basic mechanisms of IgE expression, including transcription, posttranscriptional processing, translation, and posttranslation, opens a completely new field in the study of allergy.

Acknowledgments
Animal experiments were conducted in accordance with guidelines provided by the Austrian law on experimentation with live animals. The work was supported by the Austrian Science Foundation (Hertha Firnberg Program T166-B12; S8809-MED) and the Austrian National Bank (OENB grant: 9546).

References

1. Luger E, Lamers M, Achatz-Straussberger G, Geisberger R, Infuhr D, Breitenbach M, Crameri R, Achatz G: Somatic diversity of the immunoglobulin repertoire is controlled in an isotype-specific manner. Eur J Immunol 2001; 31:2319–2330.
2. Haba S, Ovary Z, Nisonoff A: Clearance of IgE from serum of normal and hybridoma-bearing mice. J Immunol 1985; 134:3291–3297.
3. Yu P, Kosco-Vilbois M, Richards M, Kohler G, Lamers MC: Negative feedback regulation of IgE synthesis by murine CD23. Nature 1994; 369: 753–756.
4. Achatz G, Nitschke L, Lamers MC: Effect of transmembrane and cytoplasmic domains of IgE on the IgE response. Science 1997; 276:409–411.
5. Achatz G, Luger E, Geisberger R, Achatz-Straussberger G, Breitenbach M, Lamers M: The IgE antigen receptor: a key regulator for the production of IgE antibodies. Int Arch Allergy Immunol 2001; 124:31–34.
6. Karnowski A, Achatz-Straussberger G, Achatz G, Lamers MC: Inefficient processing of mRNA transcripts for the membrane form of the IgE heavy chain: impact on serum IgE levels. Submitted 2004.
7. Colgan DF, Manley JL: Mechanism and regulation of mRNA polyadenylation. Genes Dev 1997; 11:2755–2766.
8. Edwalds-Gilbert G, Veraldi KL, Milcarek C: Alternative poly(A) site selection in complex transcription units: means to an end? Nucleic Acids Res 1997; 25:2547–2561.

Gernot Achatz

Fachbereich für Molekulare Biologie, Abteilung Allergologie und Immunologie, Hellbrunnerstraße 34, A-5020 Salzburg, Austria, Tel. +43 662 8044-5764, Fax +43 662 8044-144, E-mail gernot.achatz@sbg.ac.at

Differential Expression of IgA-Positive Plasma Cells in Palatine Tonsils of Bet v 1-Allergic Patients and Healthy Individuals

E.O. Luger[1], G. Achatz[2], C. Meco[3], A. Radbruch[1], and H. Olze[4]

[1]DRFZ, German Rheumatism Research Center Berlin, Germany, [2]University of Salzburg, Department of Allergology and Immunology, Austria, [3]St. Johann Hospital Salzburg, ENT Department, Austria, [4]Charité Campus Virchow Klinikum Berlin, ENT Department, Germany

Summary: *Background:* Clinical manifestations of type 1 hyperreactivity are triggered when allergens cross-link effector cell-bound IgE and aggregate the underlying high affinity FcεRI. While the IgE antibody-mediated release of mediators constitutes the immunopathological basis for immediate symptoms, much less is known concerning the role of allergen-specific responses of isotypes other than IgE. Here we investigated the impact of an allergen-specific immune reaction on the presence of IgA plasma cells in palatine tonsils of healthy individuals and Bet v 1 (*Betula verrucosa 1*, major birch pollen)-allergic patients. The position of the tonsils, which belong to the mucosa-associated lymphoid tissues (MALT), implies a key role as secondary lymphoid organs in initiating immune responses against various antigens entering the body through the mouth and nose. *Methods:* Ectomized human tonsils from healthy and allergic individuals were obtained and 7 μm cryosections were prepared. Using immunohistological methods, IgA-positive cells were stained and developed using neufuchsin. Nuclei were counterstained with hematoxilin. *Results:* Our analysis of IgA-positive plasma cells in palatine tonsils of healthy individuals and Bet v 1-allergic patients showed a differential expression and distribution. The amount of IgA-positive plasma cells is diminished in Bet v 1-allergic individuals. They show an increase of faint IgA-staining in the tonsillar crypts, which might be due to soluble IgA sticking to the mucosal surface. *Conclusions:* Altogether, these data may lead to the assumption that the reduction of IgA-positive plasma cells within the epithelial microenvironment of the cryps and the extrafollicular areas in allergic individuals results in a reduced ability of the organism to mount a defensive immune response against allergens.

Keywords: IgA plasma cells, palatine tonsils, Bet v 1

The mucosal surfaces of the respiratory and digestive tract are major entrance sites for various airborne and food-derived antigens. To defend itself against harmful antigens, the organism is equipped with a protective ring of specifically arranged lymphoid tissues (e.g., tonsils, adenoids) in this strategic pharyngeal region called the Waldeyer's ring (for an overview see [1]). The tonsils are located in the lamina propria of the pharyngeal wall and belong to the MALT. The subepithelial lymphoid compartments consist of numerous secondary and primary lymphoid follicles, which are specialized sites of antibody development

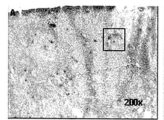
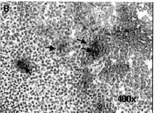

Figure 1. Immunohistochemical staining of palatine tonsils. IgA-positive plasma cell-staining in tonsils from a representative healthy individual (1A, B) and a Bet v 1-allergic patient (1C, D). Figures 1B and D represent marked areas in Figures 1A and C, respectively, at the given magnifications. Single IgA-positive plasma cells are indicated (arrows).

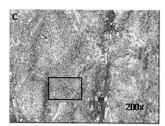
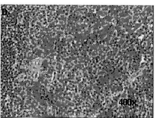

and plasma cell differentiation. The tonsillar epithelium not only provides a protective surface cover, but also invaginates and lines the tonsillar crypts, which are narrow epithelial inlets increasing the available surface for direct antigenic stimulation. In this surrounding, Ig-producing cells are found, including a high percentage of IgA-producing plasma cells, which build up a first line of immune defense at boundaries with the external environment [2]. In this environment we investigated the impact of IgA-positive plasma cells in allergen-specific immune reactions and compared their distribution in tonsils of healthy individuals and Bet v 1-allergic patients.

Material and Methods

Immunohistochemistry

Freshly ectomized human tonsils from healthy individuals ($n = 10$) and allergic patients ($n = 6$) were cut in convenient pieces of approximately 300 mm^3 and embedded in Tissue-Tek® Cryomold® Intermediate. Seven μm cryosections were performed in a microtome (Microm, HM 500 OM) and acetone fixed. Before specific antibody staining and signal amplification by APAAP technology, unspecific binding sites were blocked with PBS/2% BSA. Sections were stained with mouse anti-human IgA antibody (Cymbus). After washing, sections were incubated with the secondary antibody rabbit anti-mouse Ig (DAKO). For signal amplification, APAAP (DAKO) was applied. APAAP consists of soluble complexes of calf intestinal alkaline phosphatase and mouse monoclonal anti-alkaline phosphatase antibodies. Stainings were developed with neufuchsin. Nuclei were counterstained with hematoxylin.

Results and Discussion

Serial tonsillar sections from healthy individuals and Bet v 1-allergic patients were made. As shown in Figures 1A and B, single IgA-positive cells can be stained as indicated by arrows in tonsillar sections of a healthy, non-allergic individual. They are of plasma cell morphology with a characteristic enlarged cytoplasm and a marginal nucleus. Figures 1C and 1D show tonsillar sections of a representative Bet v 1-allergic patient. A faint IgA-staining in the crypts with only a few single IgA-positive plasma cells is detectable. The faint staining may be caused by the sticky mucosal surface and the presence of soluble IgA antibodies. Our analysis of the Bet v 1-specific immune response showed the differential expression and distribution of IgA-positive plasma cells in palatine tonsils of healthy individuals and Bet v 1-allergic patients. The amount of IgA-positive plasma cells is diminished in Bet v 1-allergic individuals. Altogether, these data may lead to the assumption that the reduction of IgA-positive plasma cells within the epithelial microenvironment of the cryps and the extrafollicular areas result in a reduced ability of the organism to mount a defending immune response against allergens.

Acknowledgments
We thank the FWF, the Austrian Science Foundation, which supported this study.

References

1. Perry M, Whyte A: Immunology of the tonsils. Immunol Today 1998; 19:414–421.
2. Lamm ME, Phillips-Quagliata JM: Origin and homing of intestinal IgA antibody-secreting cells. J Exp Med 2002; 195:F5–F8.

Elke O. Luger

DRFZ, Schumannstr 21/22, D-10117 Berlin, Germany, Tel. +49 30 28460-672, Fax +49 30 28460-603, E-mail luger @drfz.de

Survivin – A Key Regulator of Neutrophil and Eosinophil Survival

S. Yousefi, S. Martinelli, F. Altznauer, E. Vassina, and H.-U. Simon

Department of Pharmacology, University of Bern, Switzerland

Summary: Survivin is a member of the inhibitor of apoptosis protein (IAP) family. It stands out for its close association with cancer where its expression correlates with drug resistance and poor prognosis. Survivin expression has been described to be cell-cycle dependent and restricted to the G2-M checkpoint. In agreement with this current view, we found that survivin expression was high in immature granulocytes, which proliferate during differentiation. In contrast, mature blood neutrophils or eosinophils expressed little or no survivin protein. Strikingly, neutrophils derived from patients with cystic fibrosis and eosinophils from patients suffering from the hypereosinophilic syndrome re-expressed survivin. The induction of the survivin gene under inflammatory conditions was mimicked *in vitro* by exposing normal neutrophils to GM-CSF or G-CSF. Similarly, survivin expression was inducible by IL-5 in eosinophils in vitro. The antiapoptotic role of survivin in granulocytes was shown using antisense oligonucleotides in intact cells and an immunodepletion strategy in a cell-free system. Our data provide new molecular insights into the accumulation of granulocytes in bacterial infections and allergic diseases, respectively.

Keywords: apoptosis, cytokines, eosinophils, inflammation, neutrophils, survivin

The proteolytic activity of caspases is tightly controlled by the IAP family of proteins that has evolved to protect cells from unwanted self-execution by fortuitous activation of the death cascade. Survivin is a 17-kDa protein that contains only a single baculovirus IAP repeat (BIR) and no RING domain. It stands out for its close association with cancer where its expression correlates with drug resistance and poor prognosis. In the nucleus, survivin binds to microtubules and assists in chromosomal segregation and cytokinesis during mitosis. In the cytoplasm, survivin inhibits apoptosis by interacting with caspase-9 in the presence of the hepatitis B X-interacting protein HBXIP cofactor, by binding to Smac or associating with XIAP [1].

Here, we report that survivin is highly expressed in immature neutrophils, whereas in mature neutrophils as well as in eosinophils survivin expression is absent or only marginal. Strikingly, however, hematopoietic growth factors reactivated the survivin gene in these terminally differentiated cells, which are unable to resume cell cycle progression at G2-M, and high levels of survivin were expressed in both mature neutrophils and eosinophils under inflammatory conditions *in vivo*.

Survivin expression seems to be a matter of active regulation in granulocytes during differentiation and inflammation. Reduced expression in mature compared to immature neutrophils was associated with caspase-3 activation and spontaneous apoptosis. Moreover, anti-

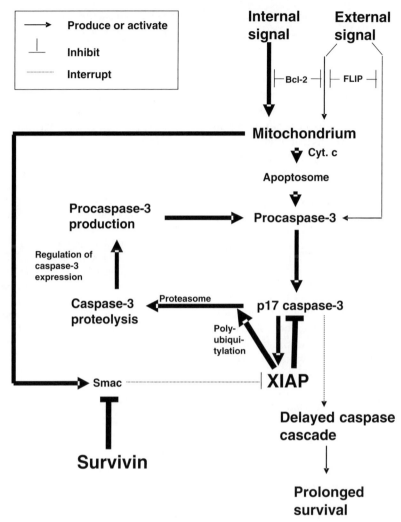

Figure 1. The potential role of survivin in controlling caspase activation in neutrophils and eosinophils under inflammatory conditions. Normal granulocytes are prone to caspase activation. For full caspase-3 activation, however, Smac is required in many experimental systems, including neutrophils [12]. The fully functional active 17-kDa fragment of caspase-3 is blocked by XIAP, and the caspase-3 – XIAP – complex is degraded via the ubiquitin-proteasome system. The balance between caspase-3 activation and its immediate inhibition with subsequent degradation and protein replacement, can be disturbed by strong pro-apoptotic stimulation or by insufficient XIAP levels. In either case, full activation of the caspase cascade occurs and the cell undergoes apoptosis. Under inflammatory conditions, however, survivin, which blocks Smac, is overexpressed in both neutrophils and eosinophils due to exposure to hematopoietic growth factors. Consequently, XIAP is further able to prevent the activation of the caspase cascade.

sense-mediated inhibition of survivin expression prevented the antiapoptotic effect of GM-CSF and G-CSF in human neutrophils [2]. When we performed experiments in a cell-free system [3] using eosinophil lysates from patients with the hypereosinophilic syndrome, we also obtained evidence for an antiapoptotic role of survivin: Immunodepletion of survivin was associated with rapid activation of caspase-3. Moreover, survivin was inducible in normal eosinophils by short-term exposure with IL-5. Therefore, although survival cytokines may also increase the ratio between anti- and proapoptotic Bcl-2 family members [4, 5], their ability to increase survivin levels seems to be crucial for delayed granulocyte apoptosis.

Because of the many virtues of survivin and the increasing number of interactions [1], it remains elusive how this molecule prevents or delays apoptosis. The presence of a BIR domain in survivin suggests a potential role in caspase inhibition. Indeed, survivin does show an ability to bind to effector caspases under cell-free conditions [6]; in more physiological systems, however, it seems to inhibit apoptosis by binding to the second mitochondrial activator of caspases (Smac) [7], but not to caspases directly [8, 9]. This potential scenario is indicated in Figure 1. Another recent study showed that survivin forms complexes with the HBXIP, which is expressed in various cell types independent of hepatitis infection [10]. Interestingly, complexation of survivin with its cofactor was required for binding to procaspase-9 and preventing its recruitment to Apaf-1, thereby suppressing mitochondrial apoptosis downstream of cytochrome c release. In response to cell death stimulation, survivin and XIAP were also shown to associate via their conserved BIR domains to form a survivin-XIAP complex that increases XIAP stability and leads to synergistic inhibition of caspase-9 activation [11].

Taken together, this study demonstrates the importance of survivin in the regulation of neutrophil as well as eosinophil apoptosis and confirms its role as an antiapoptotic protein. Elevated survivin levels represent a physiologic response in mature terminally differentiated granulocytes under inflammatory conditions. Therefore, survivin might represent a novel target for antiinflammatory therapy. Moreover, and in contrast to previous reports, we demonstrate that survivin expression and its function as an IAP does not require cell cycle progression and mitotic spindle formation.

References

1. Zangemeister-Wittke U, Simon HU: An IAP in action: the multiple roles of survivin in differentiation, immunity, and malignancy. Cell Cycle 2004; 3:1121–1123.
2. Altznauer F, Martinelli S, Yousefi S, Thürig C, Schmid I, Conway EM, Schöni MH, Vogt P, Mueller C, Fey MF, Zangemeister-Wittke U, Si-

mon HU: Inflammation-associated cell cycle-independent block of apoptosis by survivin in terminally differentiated neutrophils. J Exp Med 2004; 199:1343–1354.
3. Murphy BM, O'Neill AJ, Adrain C, Watson RWG, Martin SJ: The apoptosome pathway to caspase activation in primary human neutrophils exhibits dramatically reduced requirements for cytochrome c. J Exp Med 2003; 197:625–632.
4. Moulding DA, Akgul C, Derouet M, White MRH, Edwards SW: Bcl-2 family expression in human neutrophils during delayed and accelerated apoptosis. J Leukoc Biol 2001; 70:783–792.
5. Simon HU: Neutrophil apoptosis pathways and their modifications in inflammation. Immunol Rev 2003; 193:101–110.
6. Shin S, Sung BJ, Cho YS, Kim HJ, Ha NC, Hwang JI, Chung CW, Jung YK, Oh BH: An antiapoptotic protein human survivin is a direct inhibitor of caspase-3 and -7. Biochemistry 2001; 40:1117–1123.
7. Song Z, Yao X, Wu M: Direct interaction between survivin and Smac/DIABLO is essential for the antiapoptotic activity of survivin during taxol-induced apoptosis. J Biol Chem 2003; 278:23130–23140.
8. Banks DP, Plescia J, Altieri DC, Chen J, Rosenberg SH, Zhang H, Ng SC: Survivin does not inhibit caspase-3 activity. Blood 2000; 96:4002–4003.
9. Verdecia MA, Huang H, Dutil E, Kaiser DA, Hunter T, Noel JP: Structure of the human antiapoptotic protein survivin reveals a dimeric arrangement. Nat Struct Biol 2000; 7:602–608.
10. Marusawa H, Matsuzawa S, Welsh K, Zou H, Armstrong R, Tamm I, Reed JC: HBXIP functions as a cofactor of survivin in apoptosis suppression. EMBO J 2003; 22:2729–2740.
11. Dohi T, Okada K, Xia F, Wilford CE, Samuel T, Welsh K, Marusawa H, Zou H, Armstrong R, Matsuzawa S, Salvesen GS, Reed JC, Altieri DC: An IAP-IAP complex inhibits apoptosis. J Biol Chem 2004; 279:34087–34090.
12. Altznauer F, Conus S, Cavalli A, Folkers G, Simon HU: Calpain-1 regulates Bax and subsequent Smac-dependent caspase-3 activation in neutrophil apoptosis. J Biol Chem 2004; 279: 5947–5957.

Hans-Uwe Simon

Department of Pharmacology, University of Bern, Friedbühlstrasse 49, CH-3010 Bern, Switzerland, Tel. +41 31 632-3281, Fax +41 31 632-4992, E-mail hus@pki.unibe.ch

Expression of CD8-α on Human Monocytes and Alveolar Macrophages

D. Gibbings and A.D. Befus

Pulmonary Research Group, University of Alberta, Canada

Summary: *Background:* Originally characterized as being restricted to T-cells, CD8-α has since been described on some NK cells and dendritic cells, as well as rat macrophages and mast cells. Ligation of CD8-α on rat alveolar macrophages (AM) induces release of TNF and nitric oxide (NO). Whether CD8-α on myeloid cells is involved in various diseases is unknown. Moreover whether or not human macrophages express CD8-α is poorly known. *Methods:* RT-PCR, flow cytometry, confocal microscopy, western blot, affinity purification, MHC class I tetramers. *Results:* Using RT-PCR we demonstrated expression of CD8-α mRNA by the human monocyte (THP-1) cell line. Flow cytometry of human AM from BAL and peripheral blood monocytes demonstrated expression of a form of CD8-α that bound three of five anti-CD8-α mAb. Western blot analysis showed expression of two forms (32 kDa and 52 kDa) of CD8-α by peripheral blood monocytes. Intriguingly, only the 52 kDa form of CD8-α could be detected among monocyte (THP-1) plasma membrane proteins purified after biotinylation. This suggests the 52 kDa form of CD8-α accounts for binding of anti-CD8 mAb by myeloid cells. Anti-CD8-α mAb could block binding of MHC class I tetramers to monocytes and augment monocyte TNF production. *Conclusion:* CD8-α is expressed on human monocytes and AM and may be involved in allergic and other diseases.

Keywords: human, CD8-α, macrophage, monocyte, expression, TNF, MHC class I tetramer

While allergy is often dependent on mast cell activation through IgE, IgE-independent allergic reactions can occur in occupational asthma or hypersensitivity pneumonitis and involve other inflammatory processes. The involvement of CD8-α⁺ cells in both types of asthma has been noted. An increased number of CD8-α⁺ cells is found in asthma fatalities [1]. In hypersensitivity pneumonitis there is an inverted CD4/CD8 ratio [2]. Interestingly, in a mast cell-dependent rat model of asthma, depletion of CD8-α⁺ cells with systemic administration of mAb enhanced lung inflammation but not airway responsiveness [3]. In a mouse model of allergic asthma, CD8-α⁺ T-cells were important in development of both airways responsiveness and inflammation [4].

CD8-α is expressed by T-cells in all mammals, and is expressed by NK cells in humans and rats, but not in mice [5]. We identified CD8-α on rat AM and demonstrated that ligation of CD8-α activated several macrophage functions [6]. Early literature suggested that human monocytes (Mo) and AM from victims of Sudden Infant Death Syndrome express CD8-α [7]. The expression of CD8-α by Mo and AM suggests that the established relationships of CD8-α to several diseases may involve CD8-α⁺ myeloid cells as well as T-cells.

CD8-α is involved in T-cell responses and in cytotoxic responses to MHC class I-antigen complexes, partially via CD8-α binding intracellularly to the src kinase lck and the adaptor protein Linker for Activation of T-cells (LAT). Interestingly, a signaling complex homologous to TCR, and involving LAT, is used by several myeloid cell receptors, some of which may be evolutionary precursors of TCR (e.g., SIRPβ

[8], FcR [9]). Thus, CD8-α may control activation of myeloid cells by means similar to its regulation of T-cells. Here we describe studies of CD8-α expression by human Mo and AM and activation of these cells through CD8-α.

Materials and Methods

Isolation of PBMC

Blood was collected in heparin-coated tubes and RBC were removed by separation in 6% dextran for 30 min. Mononuclear cells were enriched on a Ficoll density gradient and washed in PBS three times prior to use. When necessary, Mo (CD14 hi) were gated for analysis from PBMC.

Flow Cytometry

Live cells were used at 4²C. Anti-CD8-α mAb (10 µg/mL) were allowed to bind cells. After three washes anti-mouse Ig-FITC or Tri-color was used to detect anti-CD8-α mAb.

Confocal Microscopy

Cells were fixed with 4% paraformaldehyde (10 min), and permeabilized with 0.1% triton X 100 (10 min).

HLA Tetramer Binding

PE labeled HLA-A *0201 tetramers (a gift of Dr. John Elliott, University of Alberta) were allowed to bind cells at 4²C in the presence of NaN₃. Binding of tetramers was inhibited with 20 µg/mL anti-CD8-α mAb or isotype mAb.

Monocyte Activation with Immune-Complexes and Measurement of TNF Production

Immune complexes were formed by cross-linking anti-CD8-α mAb or isotype mAb (10 µg/mL) with anti-mouse Ig (20 µg/mL) for 10 min. Immune complexes were added to cells for 5 h. Monensin was added for the final 3 h. TNF production was measured by intracellular flow cytometry.

Results

The monocytic cell line THP-1 binds low levels of anti-CD8-α mAb by flow cytometry. In accord with our previous studies of rat AM, THP-1 bound two of three anti-CD8-α mAb (32-M4+, D9+, LT8−). A similar pattern of anti-CD8-α mAb binding was observed in BAL AM from three of five patients (sarcoidosis [2], squamous cancer). Mo and AM (two of five patients, pulmonary nodules, bilateral infiltrates) bound all anti-CD8-α mAb tested. Interestingly, confocal microscopy of THP-1 detected CD8-α intracellularly with an anti-CD8-α mAb (Nu-Ts/c) that did not bind the THP-1 surface. In contrast, confocal microscopy of blood Mo detected CD8-α predominantly at the cell periphery. These findings suggest that there may be structural variants of CD8-α in human Mo and AM with different subcellular localizations.

To investigate potential structural variants of CD8-α (a 32 kDa glycoprotein) we performed Western blot on lysates of THP-1, blood monocytes, thymus, and blood T-cells. Two anti-CD8-α mAb (D9, B9.11) detected two proteins (32 and 52 kDa) in all cell types rather than only one (32 kDa) expected for CD8-α. Furthermore a 52 kDa protein immunoprecipitated by anti-CD8-α mAb 32-M4 could be detected by Western blot with anti-CD8-α mAb D9, suggesting more than one anti-CD8-α mAb recognizes the same 52 kDa protein. Preliminary evidence using surface biotinylation of THP-1 in conjunction with avidin-agarose to purify membrane proteins suggests that the 52 kDa form of CD8-α is predominant on the THP-1 surface. Using mAb affinity chromatography with anti-CD8-α mAb OKT8 we have enriched and analyzed by 2-D electrophoresis and western blot the 32 and 52 kDa proteins recognized by anti-CD8-α mAb. MALDI-QTOF sequencing confirmed that the 32 kDa protein is CD8-α. The identity of the 52 kDa protein is under investigation.

To evaluate whether CD8-α on Mo can interact with MHC class I, we attempted to block binding of MHC class I tetramers to Mo with anti-CD8-α mAb. Two of four anti-CD8-α mAb (B9.11, D9) partially inhibited binding of tetramers to Mo, suggesting

CD8-α on Mo binds MHC class I. Because Mo can signal through LAT when activated through FcR, we postulated that CD8-α may co-activate Mo through Fc receptors (FcR). We activated Mo with immune complexes formed with anti-CD8-α mAb or isotype mAb. Immune-complexes induced significant TNF production from Mo, but immune complexes formed with an anti-CD8-α mAb (32-M4) caused Mo to produce far greater amounts of TNF than isotype antibody containing immune complexes. However, other anti-CD8-α mAb did not enhance Mo TNF production, despite binding to Mo.

Discussion

Early literature identified and discussed a 52 kDa protein, in addition to a 32 kDa protein using anti-CD8-α mAb [10], but the characteristics of the larger molecule were never established. Our evidence demonstrates that several anti-CD8-α mAb bind the same 52 kDa protein (immunoprecipitation 32-M4, OKT8, Western blot D9), or a similar protein (Western blot B9.11). The 52 kDa protein may be a novel form of CD8-α generated by posttranslational modification or alternative splicing of mRNA. We cannot yet conclusively establish which protein (32 kDa or 52 kDa) is found on the surface of various cell types, or recognized by each anti-CD8-α mAb in our experiments, but subcellular localization of the two forms of CD8-α in monocytes and T-cells may vary.

Our evidence suggests CD8-α is found on human AM and Mo where it can bind to MHC class I and activate monocyte proinflammatory mediator production, perhaps in coordination with FcR. This may suggest a novel avenue of research into the role of CD8-α+ cells in diseases such as hypersensitivity pneumonitis, sarcoidosis, and asthma.

Sequencing of proteins bound by anti-CD8-α mAB D9 showed the 32 kDa protein is CD8-α, but the 52 kDa protein is not. Several methods have shown CD8-α on Mo accounts for functions described here.

References

1. O'Sullivan S, Cormican L, Faul JL, Ichinohe S, Johnston SL, Burke CM, Poulter LW: Activated, cytotoxic CD8+ T lymphocytes contribute to the pathology of asthma death. Am J Respir Crit Care Med 2001; 164:560–564.
2. Patel AM, Ryu JH, Reed CE: Hypersensitivity pneumonitis: current concepts and future questions. J Allergy Clin Immunol 2001; 108:661–670.
3. Laberge S, Wu L, Olivenstein R, Xu LJ, Renzi PM, Martin JG: Depletion of CD8+ T-cells enhances pulmonary inflammation but not airway responsiveness after antigen challenge in rats. J Allergy Clin Immunol 1996; 98:617–627.
4. Miyahara N, Swanson BJ, Takeda K, Taube C, Miyahara S, Kodama T, Dakhama A, Ott VL, Gelfand EW: Effector CD8+ T-cells mediate inflammation and airway hyperresponsiveness. Nat Med 2004; 10:865–869.
5. Kieffer LJ, Bennett JA, Cunningham AC, Gladue RP, McNeish J, Kavathas PB, Hanke JH: Human CD8-α expression in NK cells but not cytotoxic T-cells of transgenic mice. Int Immunol 1996; 8:1617–1626.
6. Hirji N, Lin TJ, Bissonnette E, Belosevic M, Befus AD: Mechanisms of macrophage stimulation through CD8: macrophage CD8-α and CD8-β induce nitric oxide production and associated killing of the parasite Leishmania major. J Immunol 1998; 160:6004–6011.
7. Forsyth KD, Bradley J, Weeks SC, Smith MD, Skinner J, Zola H: Immunocytologic characterization using monoclonal antibodies of lung lavage cell phenotype in infants who have died from sudden infant death syndrome. Pediatr Res 1988; 23:187–190.
8. van den Berg TK, Yoder JA, Litman GW: On the origins of adaptive immunity: innate immune receptors join the tale. Trends Immunol 2004; 25: 11–16.
9. Tridandapani S, Lyden TW, Smith JL, Carter JE, Coggeshall KM, Anderson CL: The adapter protein LAT enhances fcSymbol"g receptor-mediated signal transduction in myeloid cells. J Biol Chem 2000; 20480–20487.
10. Martin PJ, Ledbetter JA, Clark EA, Beatty PG, Hansen JA: Epitope mapping of the human surface suppressor/cytotoxic T-cell molecule Tp32. J Immunol 1984; 132:759–765.

Derrick Gibbings

550 Heritage Medical Research Center, University of Alberta, Edmonton, Alberta T6G 2S2, Canada, Tel. +1 780 492-1909, Fax +1 780 492-5329, E-mail dean.befus@ualberta.ca

Autoimmunity and Allergy: A Bioinformatic Approach

B.M. Stadler[1], M.B. Stadler[1], L. Müller[1], R. Truffer[1], A. Mari[2], S. Miescher[1], and M. Vogel[1]

[1]*Institute of Immunology Bern, Inselspital, Bern, Switzerland*
[2]*Allergy Data Laboratories p.s.c., Latina, Italy*

Summary: *Background:* Most allergen sequences can be grouped into approximately 60 motifs by structure-based alignment. These allergen motifs may serve to predict allergens as well as their cross-reactions. Some allergens can be regarded as autoantigens too. Therefore, we studied whether an allergen epitope may be characterized by the same motif as an autoantigen epitope. *Methods:* We have constructed an allergen and an autoantigen database by downloading allergenic and autoantigenic sequences from public databases. Both types of sequences were compared and the homologous protein sequences were used to construct consensus sequences. The consensus sequences were synthesized as DNA-fragments, using overlapping oligonucleotides and expressed as recombinant proteins in E.coli. Recombinant proteins encompassing regions containing both autoantigenic and allergenic motifs were used for immunization purposes in animal models to induce autoimmune reactions. *Results:* Sequence profiles cannot only be used to predict allergenic structures but also to define autoantigenic epitopes. Artificial consensus sequences from either allergenic or autoantigenic motifs represent molecular compromises that are recognized by antibodies from allergic as well as autoimmune patients. *Conclusions:* The study of allergen and autoantigen sequences by bioinformatics is a new approach to improve understanding of molecular and clinical crossreactions. This profile-based allergy prediction is more precise than the proposed regulatory procedures and may even be used to detect new, as yet unknown allergens.

Keywords: autoimmunity, allergy, bioinformatics, epitope, motif, allergy prediction, crossreaction

It is widely accepted that the majority of the clinically relevant allergens are well known and molecularly characterized [1]. Today the most complete allergen database is published at *www.allergome.org* and contains approximately 900 sequences, and it is estimated that this number may represent over 90% of all allergens [2]. The question remains whether the relation among allergens should be purely based on clinical observation or whether a structural approach might deliver a better understanding of crossreactions. We have recently described a method to analyze allergen sequences in order to predict structural relations [3]. The majority of allergen sequences could thereby be grouped into 60 motifs, suggesting that crossreaction among allergens is more common than originally believed and that such an approach may also be used to predict allergenicity. This profile-based method of allergy prediction is also greatly superior to the presently used procedures as proposed by WAO and FAO (Codex Alimentarius Commission, 2003; accessible at http://www.who.int/fsf/GMfood/), which relies on the following parameters: source of the gene, sequence homology, serum testing of patients known to be allergenic to the source organism or to sources distantly related, pepsin resistance, the prevalence of the trait, and assessment using animal models.

Results and Discussion

Motifs vs. Epitopes

Our motif-search was limited to structures spanning 50 amino acids. Thus, it can be argued that such a motif represents a large epitope recognizable by several antibodies, or that it may build only a relatively small surface depending on its molecular folding recognized by few antibodies. Because we intended to focus on epitopes that may be relevant for immediate type reactions, we neglected sequences present in the databases coding for smaller peptides as they may be recognized by T-cells only and will not lead to Type I reactions.

Number of Allergens vs. Number of Motifs

In our first allergen sequence analysis as published in 2003 we used 797 public sequences and detected 52 motifs [3]. Recently we repeated the analysis using the allergen sequences from Allergome, kindly provided by Adriano Mari. This search was based on 875 sequences and delivered 61 motifs. Still there were 165 nonmatching sequences that have not yet produced motifs. Thus, it can be predicted that future motif searches will not yield many more new motifs and that the total number of actual

allergenic epitopes may be below 100. Crossreactions may also be clinically more relevant than previously thought and the recommendation to patients of allergen avoidance may be impractical. On the other hand, crossreactions may also be quantified to generate a hierarchy in relation to the motif. Many of the allergens showing weaker crossreactions may eventually be used for immunotherapy or in immunological terms to induce tolerance.

Allergens and Autoantigens

Even though plant food allergens have been classified into families and superfamilies on the basis of their structural and functional properties [4], our bioinformatic analysis has shown that among allergenic proteins there is no common structural feature to be recognized. However, it is clear that a distinct group of allergens may also be regarded as autoantigens [5]. To further study the question whether motifs may also be defined among autoantigens and whether these sequences may overlap with the allergen motifs we have also constructed an autoantigen database consisting of 348 nonredundant human autoantigens. These sequences were compared to the allergen sequences and we detected all of the already described autoantigen/allergen relations as well as some new candidates.

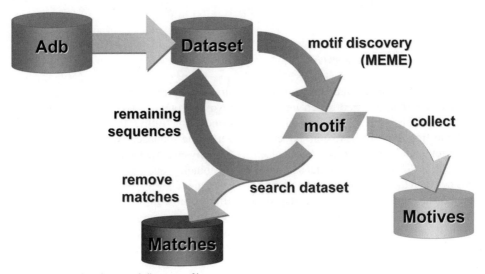

Figure 1. Automatic identification of allergen profiles.

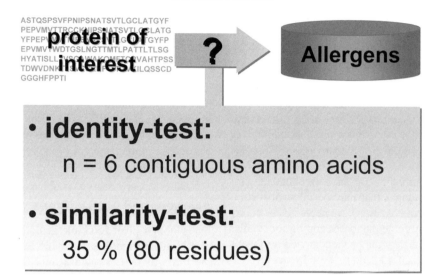

Figure 2. Proposed allergenicity evaluatoin (WHO/FAO).

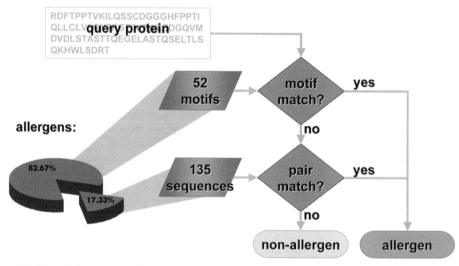

Figure 3. Motif-based allergenicity prediction.

Among the known autoantigens tropomyosin is an important allergen occurring in insects and shellfish, but also in bacteria. The vertebrate tropomyosin has been associated with various autoimmune diseases, e.g., ulcerative colitis [6]. Amino acid sequence alignments between the invertebrate and vertebrate tropomyosins allowed the identification of a protein region sharing over 60% identity. Interestingly one region has already been identified both as an allergenic IgE-binding and an autoantigenic epitope. In order to investigate whether this epitope represents an antigenic structure corresponding to the original tropomyosin protein, two consensus sequences derived from either the invertebrate or the vertebrate sequences were designed. Both artificially constructed peptides representing the IgE binding and autoantigenic epitopes were recognized by patients' sera from either an allergic or autoimmune background. Even though both epitopes were overlapping, only the allergenic construct was recognized by IgE from shellfish-allergic patients to the same degree as the tropomyosin in commercial UNI-CAP assays.

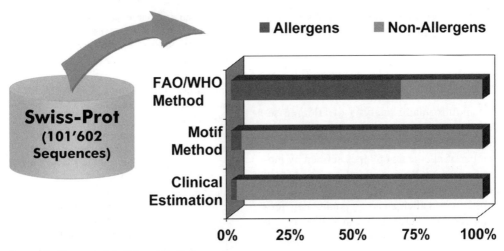

Figure 4. Performance of prediction: Swiss-Prot sequences.

Sequence alignment

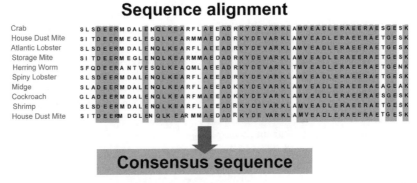

Consensus sequence

LLSDEERMDALENQLKEARMLAEEADRKYDEVARKLAMVEADLERAEERAESGESK

TropMot1

Figure 5. A consensus sequence for "allergenic" tropomyosin.

Pathophysiological Role of Crossreactive Allergens/Autoantigens

The question may be asked whether a typical response against an allergen with a structural homology to an autoantigen will induce allergy only or also an autoimmune response. Does the immune system have a way to preferentially choose the allergic or the autoimmune track and which of the two is actually the first response? We intend to address this question based on a crossreaction between Ves v 5, one of the three major allergens in wasp venom [7] and human autoantigens. Ves v 5 is the top ranking allergen in Motif 5 as defined by our bioinformatic ap-

proach. This motif can also be detected in the human testis-specific protein TPX-1 precursor and the Cysteine-rich secretory protein-1 and 3 precursors from the CRISP-family. These proteins are believed to be the target of anti-sperm antibodies that may lead to immune infertility resulting from the presence of antisperm antibodies (ASA) in the sera of sensitized individuals or in their genito-urinary milieu [8].

We produced recombinant Ves v 5 as a fusion protein in E. coli and could demonstrate that both ASA positive patient serum and sera from Ves v 5 allergic donors recognized the recombinant Ves v 5. As there exists a strong sequence homology between the murine and the human sperm proteins, we are currently investigating whether recombinant Ves v 5 can induce infertility in mice.

Conclusion

The bioinformatic analysis of allergen sequences suggests that the number of allergens may have to be redefined, namely as a small number of allergenic epitopes defined by motifs. Such a motif-based allergy prediction may not only be useful to characterize crossreactions between allergens or to predict new proteins as being allergenic, it can also be used to find new potential allergens.

Most interestingly the relation between autoantigens and allergens may be based on a structural similarity, thus, also allowing the study of the pathophysiological role of some allergens in the context of autoimmunity.

References

1. Valenta R, Kraft D: From allergen structure to new forms of allergen-specific immunotherapy. Curr Opin Immunol 2002; 14:718–727.
2. Mari A, Riccioli D: The allergome web site – a database of allergenic molecules: aim, structure, and data of a web-based resource. 60th Annual Meeting American Academy of Allergy, Asthma & Immunology. San Francisco, 2004. J Allergy Clin Immunol 2004; 113(2, part 2):301.
3. Stadler MB, Stadler BM: Allergenicity prediction by protein sequence. FASEB J 2003; 17:1141–1143.
4. Breiteneder H, Radauer C: A classification of plant food allergens. J Allergy Clin Immunol 2004; 113:821–830.
5. Valenta R, Natter S, Seiberler S, Roschanak M, Mothes N, Mahler V, Eibensteiner P: Autoallergy: a pathogenetic factor in atopic dermatitis? Curr Probl Dermatol 1999; 28:45–50.
6. Biancone L, Monteleone G, Marasco R, Pallone F: Autoimmunity to tropomyosin isoforms in ulcerative colitis (UC) patients and unaffected relatives. Clin Exp Immunol 1998; 113:198.
7. Henriksen A, King TP, Mirza O, Monsalve RI, Meno K, Ipsen H, Larsen JN, Gajhede M, Spangfort MD: Major venom allergen of yellow jackets, Ves v 5: structural characterization of a pathogenesis-related protein superfamily. Proteins 2001 Dec 1; 45(4):438–448.
8. Domagala A, Kurpisz M: Immunoprecipitation of sperm and somatic antigens with antibodies from sera of sperm-sensitized and antisperm antibody-free individuals. Am J Reprod Immunol 2004; 51:226–234.

Beda M. Stadler

Institute of Immunology Bern, Inselspital, Sahli-Haus 2, CH-3010 Bern, Switzerland, E-mail beda.stadler@iib.unibe.ch

Dendritic Cells and Regulatory T-Cells in the Allergic Immune Response and its Modulation

I. Bellinghausen, B. Klostermann, I. Böttcher, J. Knop, and J. Saloga

Department of Dermatology, SFB 548, Joh. Gutenberg University, Mainz, Germany

Summary: *Background:* Dendritic cells (DC) and T-cells play key roles in the initiation and regulation of adaptive immune responses. We investigated their functions in the human allergic immune response and its modulation. *Methods and results:* Exposure of immature blood/monocyte-derived DC to allergens leads to their activation initiating distinct signals like phosphorylation of STAT6 and subsequent (low) production of IL-13. IL-13 enhances IL-4 but not IFN-γ production of allergen-specific T-cells cocultured with autologous allergen-pulsed mature DC. Treatment of DC with IL-10 arrests them in an immature state and results in the induction of "anergy" in cocultured allergen-specific T-cells, which can be broken by addition of external high doses of IL-2. "Anergic" T-cells do not proliferate or produce cytokines normally (except of IL-10) even after restimulation with allergen-pulsed mature DC, and suppress the proliferation and cytokine production of peripheral allergen-specific T-cells. A more profound suppression of proliferation and Th1-cytokine production of allergen-specific T-cells can be achieved by coculture with autologous CD25$^+$ CD4$^+$ regulatory T-cell (T$_{reg}$). In most cases these cells can also suppress the production of Th2 cytokines, however this suppression is dependent on allergen concentration and the type of allergen. An additional way to modify the allergic immune response is the use of allergen-DNA, which can be transfected into DC very efficiently using adenoviral vectors. The induced response of autologous T-cells by such cells is much more dominated by CD8$^+$ T-cells and type 1 cytokine production. *Conclusions:* These findings underline the important roles of DC and Treg in allergic immune responses and provide promising therapeutic perspectives.

Keywords: allergy, dendritic cells, human regulatory T cells (T$_{reg}$), CD25, Th1/Th2

Allergic/atopic diseases such as allergic rhinitis, bronchial asthma, and atopic dermatitis are mainly mediated by Th2 cells. However, the immunologic mechanisms that protect against these diseases are poorly understood. Suppressor T-cells play an important role in the regulation of immune responses and the mediation of immunologic tolerance [1]. DC are also involved in the initiation and regulation of immune responses. The presented data summarize the function of DC in the human allergic immune response and its modulation by Treg, IL-10-treated DC, and allergen DNA-transfected DC.

Allergen-pulsed DC (generated from peripheral blood monocytes from atopic donors by culture in GM-CSF and IL-4 and matured with IL 1β, TNF-α, and prostaglandin E$_2$) are able to initiate Th1 as well as Th2 immune responses [2–4]. While DC-derived IL-12 and IL-18 are responsible for IFN-γ production [5, 6], the increased secretion of IL-4 with increased allergen concentrations is difficult to explain. We investigated the activation of the transcription factor STAT6, an early signal transduction event induced in Th2 cells [7], and also in DC. Time course studies revealed the activation/phosphoryla-

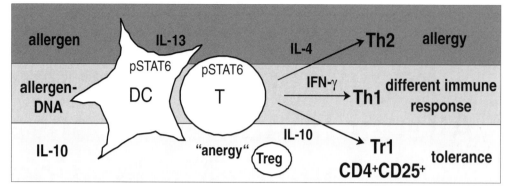

Figure 1. Function of DC in the human allergic immune response and its modulation by allergen DNA-transfected DC, IL-10-treated DC, and T$_{reg}$.

tion of this transcription factor in immature DC 10 min after stimulation with allergen [8]. The addition of increasing amounts of allergen to immature monocyte-derived DC not only induced increased activation of STAT6, but also the production of IL-13 as detected by ELISpot. Allergen concentrations of 10 µg/ml were able to induce similar IL-13 spot counts as the known inductor of IL-13 in DC, PMA/ionomycin [9], while LPS had no effect on the number of IL-13 secreting cells. To investigate the functional role of IL-13 produced by DC, an IL-13 neutralizing Ab was added together with allergen and cytokine cocktail during DC maturation. STAT6 phosphorylation was decreased under these conditions resulting in a reduced production of the Th2 cytokine IL-4 by T-cells, while IFN-γ production was not affected. Conversely, the addition of IL-13 to the cocultures led to an increase of IL-4 secretion probably due to the down-regulation of IL-12 [8, 10].

DC pretreated with the anti-inflammatory cytokine IL-10, which was added during their maturation phase, inhibited the production of Th1 as well as of Th2 cytokines [11]. "Anergic" T-cells induced by IL-10-treated DC did not proliferate and produced low cytokine levels (except of IL-10) after restimulation with mature allergen-pulsed DC. Only the addition of IL-2 could restore the cytokine levels of T-cells previously inhibited by coculture with IL-10-treated DC [11]. Additionally, "anergic" T-cells behaved as Treg as they were

able to suppress activation and function of T-cells in an antigen-specific manner [12].

A population of CD4+ T-cells expressing the IL-2 receptor α chain (CD25) has been demonstrated to play an important role in the inhibition of autoreactive T-cells and the maintenance of self-tolerance [13]. As CD4+ CD25+ Treg with regulatory properties were also found in human peripheral blood [14], we investigated the role of these Treg in allergic immune response. We demonstrated that in comparison with nonatopic donors, atopic or allergic patients also possess CD4+ CD25+ Treg, which show little or no proliferative activity and cytokine production and suppress the proliferative, as well as Th1 and Th2 cytokine, responses of peripheral CD4+ CD25− T-cells [15]. However, CD4+ CD25+ Treg-mediated suppression of proliferation of CD4+ CD25− T-cells from grass-pollen allergic patients but not from nonatopic donors was impaired at high allergen doses, while Th1 and Th2 cytokine production was inhibited at all allergen concentrations. The finding that responder T-cells from healthy donors did not escape CD4+ CD25+ Treg-mediated suppression at high allergen concentrations is in line with one recent report by Ling et al. who demonstrated that inhibition of allergen-driven proliferation and IL-5 production by CD4+ CD25+ Treg from allergic donors was less pronounced than that in healthy individuals especially during the pollen season [16].

The modification of the allergic immune response can also be achieved by allergen-gene vaccines. Vaccination of mice with replication-defective adenovirus encoding βgalactosidase with CMV-promoter prevents the development of specific IgE responses, shifting the immune response from Th2 to Th1 domination and generating IFN-γ-producing CD8+ T-cells [17]. According to these results in the murine system, allergen transfected human DC preferentially induced type-1-cytokine production in human autologous CD4+ and CD8+ T-cells [18].

Taken together, our data indicate the importance of Treg and DC in the prevention and therapy of human allergic immune responses (summarized in Figure 1). The fact that Treg are able to suppress allergen-specific responses and the production of Th2 cytokines might open new possibilities for therapeutic interventions. Adenoviral transfection of human DC with allergen-DNA or direct application of allergen-DNA may represent a potential new form of immunotherapy in severe cases of atopic-allergic diseases.

References

1. Umetsu DT, Akbari O, DeKruyff RH: Regulatory T-cells control the development of allergic disease and asthma. J Allergy Clin Immunol 2003; 112:480–487.

2. Bellinghausen I, Brand U, Knop J, Saloga J: Comparison of allergen-stimulated dendritic cells from atopic and nonatopic donors dissecting their effect on autologous naive and memory Th cells of such donors. J Allergy Clin Immunol 2000; 105:988–996.

3. Lambrecht BN: The dendritic cell in allergic airway diseases: a new player to the game. Clin Exp Allergy 2001; 31:206–218.

4. Kalinski P, Hilkens CM, Snijders A, Snijdewint FG, Kapsenberg ML: IL-12-deficient dendritic cells, generated in the presence of prostaglandin E2, promote type 2 cytokine production in maturing human naive Th cells. J Immunol 1997; 159:28–35.

5. Trinchieri G: Interleukin-12 and its role in the generation of TH1 cells. Immunol Today 1993; 14:335–338.

6. Stoll S, Jonuleit H, Schmitt E, Muller G, Yamauchi H, Kurimoto M et al.: Production of function-

al IL-18 by different subtypes of murine and human dendritic cells (DC): DC-derived IL-18 enhances IL-12-dependent Th1 development. Eur J Immunol 1998; 28:3231–3239.

7. Christodoulopoulos P, Cameron L, Nakamura Y, Lemiere C, Muro S, Dugas M et al.: Th2 cytokine-associated transcription factors in atopic and nonatopic asthma: evidence for differential signal transducer and activator of transcription 6 expression. J Allergy Clin Immunol 2001; 107:586–591.

8. Bellinghausen I, Brand P, Bottcher I, Klostermann B, Knop J, Saloga J: Production of IL-13 by human dendritic cells after stimulation with protein allergens is a key factor for induction of Th2 cytokines and is associated with activation of STAT-6. Immunology 2003; 108:167–176.

9. de Saint Vis B, Fugier Vivier I, Massacrier C, Gaillard C, Vanbervliet B, Ait Yahia S et al.: The cytokine profile expressed by human dendritic cells is dependent on cell subtype and mode of activation. J Immunol 1998; 160:1666–1676.

10. Wills-Karp M: IL-12/IL-13 axis in allergic asthma. J Allergy Clin Immunol 2001; 107:9–18.

11. Bellinghausen I, Brand U, Steinbrink K, Enk AH, Knop J, Saloga J: Inhibition of human allergic T-cell responses by IL-10-treated dendritic cells: differences from hydrocortisone-treated dendritic cells. J Allergy Clin Immunol 2001; 108:242–249.

12. Steinbrink K, Graulich E, Kubsch S, Knop J, Enk AH: CD4+ and CD8+ anergic T-cells induced by IL-10-treated human dendritic cells display antigen-specific suppressor activity. Blood 2002; 99:2468–2476.

13. Sakaguchi S: Naturally arising CD4+ regulatory T-cells for immunologic self-tolerance and negative control of immune responses. Annu Rev Immunol 2004; 22:531–562.

14. Jonuleit H, Schmitt E, Stassen M, Tuettenberg A, Knop J, Enk AH: Identification and functional characterization of human CD4+ CD25+ T-cells with regulatory properties isolated from peripheral blood. J Exp Med 2001; 193:1285–1294.

15. Bellinghausen I, Klostermann B, Knop J, Saloga J: Human CD4+ CD25+ T-cells derived from the majority of atopic donors are able to suppress Th1 and Th2 cytokine production. J Allergy Clin Immunol 2003; 111:862–868.

16. Ling EM, Smith T, Nguyen XD, Pridgeon C, Dallman M, Arbery J et al.: Relation of CD4+ CD25+ regulatory T-cell suppression of allergen-driven T-cell activation to atopic status and expression of allergic disease. Lancet 2004; 363:608–615.

17. Sudowe S, Montermann E, Steitz J, Tuting T, Knop J, Reske-Kunz AB: Efficacy of recombinant adenovirus as vector for allergen gene therapy in a mouse model of type I allergy. Gene Ther 2002; 9:147–156.

18. Klostermann B, Bellinghausen I, Bottcher I, Petersen A, Becker WM, Knop J et al.: Modification of the human allergic immune response by allergen-DNA-transfected dendritic cells *in vitro*. J Allergy Clin Immunol 2004; 113:327–333.

Iris Bellinghausen

Universitäts-Hautklinik, Langenbeckstraße 1, D-55131 Mainz, Germany, Tel. +49 6131 172298, Fax +49 6131 175505, E-mail bellinghausen@hautklinik.klinik.uni-mainz.de

Expression of High Affinity IgE Receptors on Skin- and Blood-Derived Plasmacytoid Dendritic Cells in Inflammatory Skin Diseases

A. Wollenberg[1], T. Pavicic[1], S. Wetzel[1], and G. Hartmann[2]

[1]Department of Dermatology and Allergy, Ludwig Maximilians University, Munich, Germany,
[2]Division of Clinical Pharmacology, Department of Internal Medicine, Ludwig Maximilians University, Munich, Germany

Summary: *Background:* High affinity IgE receptors (FcεRI) have been described on Langerhans cells (LC) of normal and inflamed skin and on inflammatory dendritic epidermal cells (IDEC) of inflamed skin by us and others. Another dendritic cells (DC) subset are plasmacytoid dendritic cells (PDC), which produce large amounts of type-I interferon upon viral infection. Using flow cytometry for simultaneous enumeration of LC, IDEC, and PDC, we recently identified PDC in lupus erythematosus, psoriasis, contact dermatitis, and atopic dermatitis (AD) lesions. Many IDEC but very few PDC were detected in AD, whereas lupus erythematosus contained many PDC but few IDEC. We hypothesized a role for FcεRI on PDC in inflamed skin. *Methods:* Freshly isolated, cultured, or CPG-stimulated PDC from lesional skin or peripheral blood were analyzed by four-color immunophenotyping and flow cytometry, immuno-electronmicroscopy, real-time RT-PCR, Calcium influx assays, and cytokine ELISA. *Results:* The IgE-binding FcεRIα chain was expressed on PDC isolated from peripheral blood and inflamed skin. The expression depended on the underlying diagnosis. The receptor consisted of FcεRIα and FcεRIγ but no FcεRIβ chains. A strong but transient calcium influx was induced by FcεRIα ligation in PDC. The CPG-induced type-I interferon production of PDC was downregulated by FcεRIα ligation. *Conclusions:* PDC are selectively recruited to inflamed skin depending on the skin disease. PDC express non-mediator-releasing FcεRIαγγ identical to LC and monocyets but different from basophils and mast cells. This FcεRIαγγ is functionally active and may alter the immunobiological contribution of PDC to atopic skin disease. Functional alteration and depletion of PDC may predispose AD patients to viral infections such as eczema herpeticum.

Keywords: Langerhans cells, inflammatory dendritic epidermal cells, plasmacytoid dendritic cells, high-affinity IgE receptor, atopic dermatitis, lupus erythematosus, calcium influx, toll-like receptor, CPG oligonucleotide, eczema herpeticum

DC link innate and adoptive immunity by their ability to induce appropriate immune responses upon recognition of invading pathogens. Two distinct myeloid DC populations have been identified in the inflamed epidermis – the classical LC which contain Birbeck granules (CD1a[+++], HLA-DR[+++], CD11b[-]) and are also present in normal human skin, and the IDEC, which lack Birbeck granules (CD1a[+], HLA-DR[+++], CD11b[+++]) and are exclusively present in inflamed skin [1]. Epidermal dendritic cell phenotyping of these LC and IDEC has already been used as a diagnostic tool for inflammatory skin diseases [2].

Another DC subset is the PDC, which was first described in the peripheral blood (CD123^{+++}, BDCA-2$^+$, HLA-DR). Originally this cell type was termed DC-2 based on its intrinsic activity to induce Th2 responses [3] and regulatory T-cells [4]. Later it became evident that PDC produce large amounts of type I interferon (INF-α and INF-β) upon viral infection [5].

The presence of PDC in human skin has been demonstrated first in cutaneous lupus erythematosus [6]. Shortly thereafter, we showed that PDC are also present in skin lesions of psoriasis, contact dermatitis, and AD, but that the number of PDC varies strongly with the underlying diagnosis [7]. Lesional skin samples from patients with psoriasis vulgaris, contact dermatitis, and especially lupus erythematosus contained relatively high numbers of PDC, whereas only few PDC could be detected in AD lesions [7]. This selective lack of PDC in AD lesions is regarded as one of the reasons for the high susceptibility of AD patients to viral skin infections [8].

In addition to the impact of the microbial molecules detected, the type of immune response is determined by the type of the Fc receptor that is used by the DC for internalization of antigen-antibody complexes [9]. The uptake, procession, and presentation of IgE-bound antigens by high affinity IgE receptors (FcϵRI) expressed on LC [10] and IDEC [1] is considered an essential event in the pathogenesis of AD [11]. We hypothesized that FcϵRI on PDC might be involved in the pathogenesis of different inflammatory skin diseases and designed a number of experiments to address this issue.

We performed immuno-electronmicroscopy of peripheral blood mononuclear cells and of epidermal cell suspensions with monoclonal antibodies. In the peripheral blood, we identified basophils as well as PDC with anti-CD123-coated gold grains, whereas only PDC were detected with the PDC-specific BDCA-2 antibody. Morphologically identical cells were labeled with the FcϵRI-specific monoclonal antibody 22E7. Epidermal cell suspensions

prepared from inflamed skin revealed identical results, providing a first evidence for FcϵRI-expression in the skin.

To formally proof the expression of FcϵRI on skin PDC, we performed a flow cytometric analysis following our published four-color staining protocol for PDC [7] and confirmed the presence of the IgE-binding FcϵRIα chain on PDC isolated from skin lesions of patients with psoriasis vulgaris, contact dermatitis, and lupus erythematosus, as well as from the peripheral blood. We could confirm the depletion of PDC from AD skin lesions as well as the accumulation of these cells in lupus erythematosus lesions, which we had published 2 years ago [7]. The expression of the IgE-binding FcϵRIα chain on PDC varied strongly with the underlying diagnosis and was significantly higher in psoriasis lesions than in lupus erythematosus.

FcϵRI is expressed on basophils and mast cells as a tetramer of one α- (FcϵRIα), one β-(FcϵRIβ), and two γ-subunits (FcϵRIγ), whereas LC and monocytes do not express the β-chain [12]. We were, therefore, interested in the expression of the FcϵRI subunits on PDC. Quantitative real-time RT-PCR revealed the presence of FcϵRIα- and FcϵRIγ-subunits, but no β-chain. Hence, the RNA data obtained from PDC correspond nicely to the expected $\alpha\gamma\gamma$ type described on monocytes and other DC, and is clearly different from the $\alpha\beta\gamma\gamma$ type expressed on effector cells of anaphylactic reactions [13].

The ligation of FcϵRI on effector cells is followed by a transient calcium influx witnessing the cell activation, whereas this activation sign may or may not be present on epidermal DC depending on the level of FcϵRI expression [14]. Therefore, we measured the calcium influx in PDC by flow cytometry in order to determine the functional activity of FcϵRI. A ligation of FcϵRI by cross-linking of the preloaded surface-bound IgE with an anti-human-IgE antibody induced a strong and transient calcium influx in PDC, indicating that FcϵRI on PDC is indeed functionally active.

The early initiation of an effective antiviral T-cell response by Toll-like receptor stimulated production of type-I interferon is a hallmark of PDC function [15]. As AD patients are highly susceptible to disseminated viral infections such as eczema herpeticum [16], we hypothesized for immunosuppressive mechanisms in AD, which may be relevant in addition to the published lack of PDC in AD lesions [7]. Consequently, we investigated the effect of FcεRI ligation on Toll-like receptor stimulated interferon production of PDC. Ligation of FcεRI prior to stimulation of PDC with CPG oligonucleotides diminished the production of interferon, thus, demonstrating an important functional consequence of PDC ligation.

Considering these observations, the functionally important role of PDC in cutaneous defense mechanisms may be altered by ligation of the FcεRI expressed on these cells. A better understanding of the cellular events linked to the allergen binding to FcεRI on PDC and their activation via crosslinking may provide the basis for new therapeutic or prophylactic strategies for cutaneous inflammation and skin diseases.

References

1. Wollenberg A, Kraft S, Hanau D, Bieber T: Immunomorphological and ultrastructural characterization of Langerhans cells and a novel, inflammatory dendritic epidermal cell (IDEC) population in lesional skin of atopic eczema. J Invest Dermatol 1996; 106:446–453.
2. Wollenberg A, Wen S, Bieber T: Phenotyping of epidermal dendritic cells – clinical applications of a flow cytometric micromethod. Cytometry 1999; 37:147–155.
3. Rissoan MC, Soumelis V, Kadowaki N, Grouard G, Briere F, de Waal Malefyt R, et al.: Reciprocal control of T helper cell and dendritic cell differentiation. Science 1999; 283:1183–1186.
4. Gilliet M, Liu YJ: Human plasmacytoid-derived dendritic cells and the induction of T-regulatory cells. Hum Immunol 2002; 63:1149–1155.
5. Krug A, Luker GD, Barchet W, Leib DA, Akira S, Colonna M: Herpes Simplex Virus type 1 activates murine natural interferon-producing cells through toll-like receptor 9. Blood 2004; 103: 1433–1437.
6. Farkas L, Beiske K, Lund-Johansen F, Brandtzaeg P, Jahnsen FL: Plasmacytoid dendritic cells (natural interferon-α/β-producing cells) accumulate in cutaneous lupus erythematosus lesions. Am J Pathol 2001; 159:237–243.
7. Wollenberg A, Wagner M, Günther S, Towarowski A, Tuma E, Moderer M, et al.: Plasmacytoid dendritic cells: a new cutaneous dendritic cell subset with distinct role in inflammatory skin diseases. J Invest Dermatol 2002; 119:1096–1102.
8. Wollenberg A, Wetzel S, Burgdorf WHC, Haas J: Viral infections in atopic dermatitis: pathogenic aspects and clinical management. J Allergy Clin Immunol 2003; 112:667–674.
9. Mahnke K, Knop J, Enk AH: Induction of tolerogenic DCs: "you are what you eat." Trends Immunol 2003; 24:646–651.
10. Bieber T, de la Salle H, Wollenberg A, Hakimi J, Chizzonite R, Ring J, et al.: Human epidermal Langerhans cells express the high affinity receptor for IgE (FcεRI). J Exp Med 1992; 175:1285–1290.
11. Leung DY, Bieber T: Atopic dermatitis. Lancet 2003; 361:151–160.
12. Kraft S, Weßendorf JHM, Hanau D, Bieber T: Regulation of the high affinity receptor for IgE on human epidermal Langerhans cells. J Immunol 1998; 161:1000–1006.
13. von Bubnoff D, Koch S, Bieber T: Dendritic cells and atopic eczema/dermatitis syndrome. Curr Opin Allergy Clin Immunol 2003; 3:353–358.
14. Jürgens M, Wollenberg A, Hanau D, de la Salle H, Bieber T: Activation of human epidermal Langerhans cells by engagement of the high affinity receptor for IgE, FcεRI. J Immunol 1995; 155:5184–5189.
15. Krug A, Luker GD, Barchet W, Leib DA, Akira S, Colonna M: Herpes simplex virus type 1 activates murine natural interferon-producing cells through Toll-like receptor 9. Blood 2004; 103: 1433–1437.
16. Wollenberg A, Zoch C, Wetzel S, Plewig G, Przybilla B: Predisposing factors and clinical features of eczema Herpeticum – a retrospective analysis of 100 cases. J Am Acad Dermatol 2003; 49:198–205.

Andreas Wollenberg

Department of Dermatology and Allergy, Ludwig Maximilians University, Frauenlobstr. 9–11, D-80337 Munich, Germany, Tel. +49 89 5160-6251, Fax +49 89 5160-6252, E-mail wollenberg@lrz.uni-muenchen.de

M-DC8+ Dendritic Cells as Potent Inducers of Th1 Polarized Immune Responses

K. Schäkel[1,2], M. von Kietzell[1], L. Schulze[1], and E.P. Rieber[1]

[1]Institute of Immunology, [2]Department of Dermatology, Medical Faculty,
Technical University of Dresden, Germany

Summary: *Background:* The immunoregulatory potential of dendritic cells (DC) critically depends on their state of maturation. With the help of the mAb M-DC8 we previously identified a new population of high level TNF-α producing proinflammatory human blood DC. Here, we demonstrate the IL-12 production and T-cell programming capacity of M-DC8+ DC. *Methods:* An *ex vivo* time kinetic analysis of the phenotype and the lipopolysaccharide- (LPS) induced intracellular IL-12p40/p70 production was done on purified M-DC8+ DC. The Th1/Th2 programming capacity of M-DC8+ DC was studied in cocultures with allogenic CD4+ naïve cord blood T-cells. *Results:* Immature freshly isolated M-DC8+ DC lacked CD83 expression and failed to produce IL-12 after LPS stimulation. After 3 h of culture without stimulation a marked upregulation of CD83 was noticed. In parallel to the phenotypic changes, M-DC8+ DC acquired the capacity to produce IL-12. In addition, a strong capacity of M-DC8+ DC to program IFN-γ dominated Th1 responses in an IL-12-dependent fashion was noted. *Conclusion:* These data indicate a remarkable functional plasticity of M-DC8+ DC, which warrants future studies on their relevance for the progression of acute Th2 biased into chronic Th1-dominated forms of the allergic inflammation observed in atopic dermatitis and allergic asthma.

Keywords: M-DC8, dendritic cells, IL-12, Th1, human

Dendritic cells(DC) are equipped with a unique capacity to initiate and to program the quality of primary immune responses [1]. The aberrant programming of IL-4, IL-5, and IL-13-producing T-cells (Th2) specific for allergens is held responsible for the development of Type 1 allergies, while Th1 cells are shown to contribute to the pathology of late stages of the allergic inflammatory response such as chronic lesions of atopic dermatitis and chronic allergic asthma [2]. Understanding the regulatory role of human DC in health and disease critically requires a better understanding of the functional heterogeneity among DC in terms of cytokine production and T-cell programming. With the help of the mAb M-DC8 we recently described a novel proinflammatory population of human blood DC best documented by their strong TNF-α production, the expression of anaphylatoxin receptors, and FcγRIII (CD16) [3, 4]. We here describe the strong IL-12-producing and Th1-programming capacity of M-DC8+ DC.

Material and Methods

The cell medium was RPMI 1640 medium containing 10% human AB serum (CCPRO, Neustadt, Germany). LPS (Escherichia coli

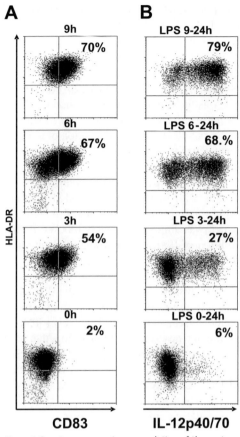

Figure 1. Spontaneous *ex vivo* upregulation of the maturation marker CD83 by M-DC8⁺ DC is paralleled by the capacity to produce IL-12 in response to LPS. Purified M-DC8⁺ DC were cultured for different lengths of time before expression of CD83, and HLA-DR expression was studied by flow cytometric analysis (A) or stimulation with 100 ng/ml LPS in the presence of brefeldin A was initiated (B). Stimulated cells were cultured for a total of 24 h before staining for the intracytoplasmatic production of IL-12p40/70 and expression of HLA-DR was done.

026:B6, 100 ng/ml) was from Sigma (Deisenhofen, Germany). MAbs specific for CD83, HLA-DR, and IL-12 p40/70 (clone C11.5) were all from BD Pharmingen (La Jolla, CA, USA). M-DC8⁺ DC were isolated by magnetic cell sorting from the blood of healthy donors as described previously [5]. CD4⁺ CD45RA⁺ T-cells were prepared from cord blood by using a CD4-T-cell isolation kit (Miltenyi, Bergisch Gladbach, Germany). Intracytoplasmatic staining of M-DC8⁺ DC for IL-12 p40/70 production was done after 24 h of culture as outlined previously [3]. To determine the T-cell programming by M-DC8⁺ DC cocultures with naive allogenic T-cells at a ratio of 1:10 were restimulated after 10–14 days of culture with ionomycin 1 µg/ml and PMA 10 ng/ml, and secreted cytokines were quantified in 24 h cell culture supernatants by ELISA (BD Pharmingen).

Results

When freshly isolated from blood, M-DC8⁺ DC have the phenotype of immature DC [5], they express FcγRIII, CD86, CD40, and HLA-DR but lack CD80 and CD83. When cultured, marked phenotypic changes became evident. Within 6 h of culture in the absence of overt stimulation, the majority of cells became positive for maturation marker CD83 (Figure 1A).

When freshly isolated M-DC8⁺ DC were stimulated with 100 ng/ml of the TLR4-ligand LPS no intracellular IL-12p40/70 expression was observed. However, upon culture M-DC8⁺ DC cells spontaneously gained a strong

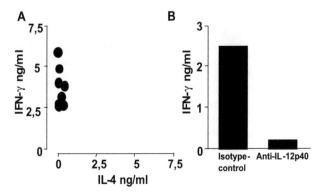

Figure 2. IL-12-dependent Th1-programming by M-DC8⁺ DC. Cocultures of M-DC8⁺ DC and allogenic CD4⁺ cord blood T-cells were restimulated with ionomycin and PMA and the IFN-γ and IL-4 production quantified by ELISA. Results of eight different experiments are given in (A). In (B) anti-IL-12p40 blocking antibodies were added as indicated. Results are the mean of duplicate values.

capacity to respond to LPS-stimulation with intracellular IL-12-p40/70 expression (Figure 1B). The Th1/Th2 T-cell programming capacity of M-DC8$^+$ DC has not been defined so far. To this end, M-DC8$^+$ DC were cocultured with allogenic CD4$^+$ naïve cord blood T-cells. After restimulation of the cultures with PMA and ionomycin a high level production of the Th1 cytokine IFN-γ was evident in all donors tested (Figure 2A), while the Th2-cytokine IL-4 was hardly detectable. In the presence of an IL-12p40 blocking mAb a substantial reduction of the Th1-inducing capacity became evident (Figure 2B).

Discussion

The human immune system harbors functionally distinct types of DC. Initially two DC populations were defined in human blood, a "myeloid" DC population referred to as DC1 (CD11c$^+$, CD16$^-$, CD123 lo) and a "lymphoid" DC population also called DC2 or plasmacytoid DC (CD11c$^-$, CD16$^-$, CD123 hi) [1]. An additional DC population, representing the majority of blood DC was identified by our group with the help of the mAb M-DC8 (CD11c$^+$, CD16$^+$, CD123 lo) [3,4]. The epitope identified by the three mAbs M-DC8, DD1, and DD2 is 6-sulfoLacNAc, a carbohydrate decoration of the P-selectin-binding protein-1 which fails to bind P- or E-selectin. While the endothelial ligand of 6-sulfoLacNAc remains to be found, this DC type can be rapidly recruited by C5a in an *in vivo* model. Furthermore, M-DC8$^+$ DC have a remarkable capacity to produce TNF-α when stimulated with the bacterial endotoxin LPS but not with herpes simplex virus. According to these functional characteristics M-DC8$^+$ DC appear as a new population of proinflammatory DC.

We here demonstrate the functional plasticity of M-DC8$^+$ DC. Although immature when circulating in blood M-DC8$^+$ DC spontaneously undergo rapid phenotypical changes *in vitro*. After 3 h of culture the cell surface expression of the maturation marker CD83 is already detectable on half of the M-DC8$^+$ DC. CD83 is a member of the immunoglobulin superfamily proteins, which can be found preformed intracellularly in M-DC8$^+$ DC and other DC types (data not shown, [6]). In most instances CD83 cell surface expression is accompanied by the capacity of monocytes-derived DC to produce IL-12 [7]. Similarly, in our kinetic analysis the spontaneous expression of CD83 by native M-DC8$^+$ blood DC *in vitro* was directly paralleled by the acquisition of a prominent capacity to produce IL-12 in response to LPS.

Coculture experiments of naive cord blood T-cells with M-DC8$^+$ DC revealed a strong programming of Th1-dominated responses, which was almost completely blocked by the addition of IL-12p40 neutralizing antibodies. *In vivo* M-DC8$^+$ DC are mainly found in inflamed tonsils, gut mucosa of patients with Crohn's disease, as well as in the dermis of lesional atopic dermatitis ([8], and unpublished observation). The high level TNF-α production described previously, together with the strong IL-12-producing and Th1-inducing capacity documented here, give evidence that M-DC8$^+$ DC may be of importance for the progression of acute Th2- into chronic Th1-dominated allergic inflammatory responses.

References

1. Steinman RM: Some interfaces of dendritic cell biology. APMIS 2003; 111:675–697.
2. Akdis CA, Akdis M, Trautmann A, Blaser K: Immune regulation in atopic dermatitis. Curr Opin Immunol 2000; 12:641–646.
3. Schäkel K, Kannagi R, Kniep B, Goto Y, Mitsuoka C, Zwirner J, et al.: 6-Sulfo LacNAc, a novel carbohydrate modification of PSGL-1, defines an inflammatory type of human dendritic cells. Immunity 2002; 17:289–301.
4. Schäkel K, Poppe C, Mayer E, Federle C, Riethmuller G, Rieber EP: M-DC8$^+$ leukocytes – a novel human dendritic cell population. Pathobiology 1999; 67(5–6):287–290.
5. Schäkel K, Mayer E, Federle C, Schmitz M, Riethmuller G, Rieber EP: A novel dendritic cell population in human blood: one-step immunomagnetic isolation by a specific mAb (M-DC8) and *in vitro* priming of cytotoxic T lymphocytes. Eur J Immunol 1998; 28:4084–4093.
6. Cao W, Lee SH, Lu J: CD83 is preformed inside

monocytes, macrophages, and dendritic cells but it is only stably expressed on activated dendritic cells. Biochem J 2005; 385:85–93.

7. Jonuleit H, Kuhn U, Muller G, Steinbrink K, Paragnik L, Schmitt E, et al.: Proinflammatory cytokines and prostaglandins induce maturation of potent immunostimulatory dendritic cells under fetal calf-serum-free conditions. Eur J Immunol 1997; 27:3135–3142.

8. de Baey A, Mende I, Baretton G, Greiner A, Hartl WH, Baeuerle PA, et al.: A subset of human dendritic cells in the T-cell area of mucosa-associated lymphoid tissue with a high potential to produce TNF-α. J Immunol 2003; 170:5089–5094.

Knut Schäkel

Institute of Immunology, Medical Faculty, Technical University of Dresden, Fiedlerstr. 42, D-01307 Dresden, Germany, Tel. +49 351 458-6502, Fax +49 351 458-6316, E-Mail schaekel@rcs.urz.tu-dresden.de

Characteristics of Plasmacytoid Dendritic Cells in Patients with Atopic Dermatitis

N. Novak and T. Bieber

Department of Dermatology, University of Bonn, Germany

Summary: *Background:* The high affinity receptor for IgE (FcεRI) on myeloid dendritic cells has been shown to play a major role in atopic dermatitis (AD). Plasmacytoid dendritic cells (pDC), which are instrumental in the defense against viral infections are present in reduced amounts in the skin of AD patients, which are characterized by a high susceptibility to viral infections. *Objective:* We explored phenotypical and functional characteristics of pDC in the peripheral blood of patients with AD and of healthy individuals. *Methods:* Blood dendritic cell antigen (BDCA)2⁺ CD123⁺ pDC were enriched from the peripheral blood of patients with AD and studied in functional assays. *Results:* Skin-homing molecules such as cutaneous lymphocyte antigen (CLA) and L-selectin CD62L were expressed in lower levels on pDC of patients with AD. PDC expressed high amounts of IgE-occupied FcεRI. Further, FcεRI-aggregation on pDC impaired the surface expression of MHC I and II, induced the production of IL-10, and enhanced the apoptosis of pDC. Importantly, FcεRI preactivated pDC produced less IFN-α and IFN-β after stimulation with CpG motifs and enhanced the outcome of immune responses of the Th2 type. *Conclusion:* From these data we conclude that (1) FcεRI-bearing pDC from patients with AD are different from pDC of healthy individuals, (2) might be important in the pathophysiology of AD, and (3) contribute to the enhanced susceptibility of AD patients to viral infections.

Keywords: plasmacytoid dendritic cells, atopic dermatitis, IgE receptor

Patients with AD display a higher susceptibility to viral infections. The rapid spreading of *Herpes simplex virus* or *Poxvirus*-induced skin lesions may develop into Eczema herpeticum or Eczema molluscatum in these patients.

The reason for this high susceptibility to viral infections and the underlying deficiency on the cellular level is completely unknown.

In the human immune system, two major dendritic cells subtypes can be distinguished: Myeloid dendritic cells (mDC) and pDC, which are negative for CD1a but positive for the BDCA2 and the α-chain of the IL-3 receptor (CD123) [1]. PDC play a crucial role in the defense against virus infections in the immune system. A few years ago it was shown that in inflammatory skin diseases such as psoriasis, allergic contact dermatitis, or lupus erythematosus pDC are detectable in the eczematous skin lesions. In contrast, the number of pDC in acute and chronic skin lesions of AD patients is low [2,3].

Therefore, it was the aim of our study to evaluate the characteristic phenotypical and functional features of pDC in the peripheral blood of patients with AD.

We found a lower expression of the costimulatory molecule CD80 and MHC I on pDC of the peripheral blood of patients with AD in comparison to pDC of healthy control donors [4].

It has recently been established that in the effector phase of allergic contact dermatitis pDC are recruited from the blood into the skin and that skin-homing molecules such as L-Selectin (CD62L) and CLA seem to be crucial in this process [5,6].

Therefore, we analyzed the expression of skin-homing molecules in patients with AD by flow cytometric staining. We found a reduced expression of both CLA and CD62L on pDC isolated from the peripheral blood of patients with AD in comparison to healthy, nonatopic control donors.

Further, an enhanced expression of the trimeric variant of the high affinity receptor for IgE (FcεRI) has been detected on pDC from patients with AD [7]. Most of the IgE binding sites of the FcεRI-α chain were occupied with IgE molecules and the surface expression of FcεRI positively correlated with the IgE serum level of these patients. Additionally, we could show that FcεRI-bearing pDC were able to take up allergens and present these allergens to naïve T-cells inducing the priming of T-cells of the Th2 type.

In addition, aggregation of FcεRI on the surface of pDC led to the downregulation of the MHC I, MCH II molecule and the costimulatory molecule CD40 and cross-linking of FcεRI leads to the release of IL-10 and induces IL-10-mediated apoptosis of pDC [8].

Since the production of IFN-α and IFN-β by pDC is important for the defense against virus infections [9], we next investigated the capacity of pDC from patients with AD to release IFN-α and INF-β in response to viral stimuli after preactivation of FcεRI via allergen challenge [10].

We found a reduced capacity of pDC to produce both IFN-α and IFN-β after FcεRI-activation.

In view of these data a picture emerges that pDC of patients with AD differs phenotypically and functionally from pDC of healthy volunteers and might be responsible for the higher susceptibility of these patients to viral infections. The reduced expression of CLA and CD62L might lead to a lower recruitment of pDC into the skin in the case of inflammation. Further, the high FcεRI-surface expression

and IgE binding in combination with their capacity to take up and present allergens to T-cells might indicate a role of pDC in the amplification of allergic immune responses of the Th2 type, which direct the course of AD.

Frequent allergen challenge and FcεRI activation of pDC in AD may lead to the release of IL-10 and induce endogenously an enhanced apoptosis and reduced capacity to produce IFN-α and IFN-β of these cells. Together, these characteristic features might lead to a deficiency of pDC in the defense against viral infections and underlie the higher susceptibility of AD patients to viral infections.

References

1. Rissoan MC, Soumelis V, Kadowaki N, Grouard G, Briere F, de Waal Malefyt R et al.: Reciprocal control of T helper cell and dendritic cell differentiation. Science 1999; 283:1183–1186.
2. Wollenberg A, Wagner M, Gunther S, Towarowski A, Tuma E, Moderer M et al.: Plasmacytoid dendritic cells: a new cutaneous dendritic cell subset with distinct role in inflammatory skin diseases. J Invest Dermatol 2002; 119:1096–1102.
3. Farkas L, Beiske K, Lund-Johansen F, Brandtzaeg P, Jahnsen FL: Plasmacytoid dendritic cells (natural interferon-α/β-producing cells) accumulate in cutaneous lupus erythematosus lesions. Am J Pathol 2001; 159(1):237–243.
4. Novak N, Allam JP, Hagemann T, Jenneck C, Laffer S, Valenta R et al.: Characterization of FcεRI-bearing CD123 blood dendritic cell antigen-2 plasmacytoid dendritic cells in atopic dermatitis. J Allergy Clin Immunol 2004; 114:364–370.
5. Bangert C, Friedl J, Stary G, Stingl G, Kopp T: Immunopathologic features of allergic contact dermatitis in humans: participation of plasmacytoid dendritic cells in the pathogenesis of the disease? J Invest Dermatol 2003; 121:1409–1418.
6. Jahnsen FL, Lund-Johansen F, Dunne JF, Farkas L, Haye R, Brandtzaeg P: Experimentally induced recruitment of plasmacytoid (CD123high) dendritic cells in human nasal allergy. J Immunol 2000; 165:4062–4068.
7. Prussin C, Griffith DT, Boesel KM, Lin H, Foster B, Casale TB: Omalizumab treatment downregulates dendritic cell FcεRI expression. J Allergy Clin Immunol 2003; 112:1147–1154.

8. Nolan KF, Strong V, Soler D, Fairchild PJ, Cobbold SP, Croxton R et al.: IL-10-conditioned dendritic cells, decommissioned for recruitment of adaptive immunity, elicit innate inflammatory gene products in response to danger signals. J Immunol 2004; 172:2201–2209.

9. Cella M, Jarrossay D, Facchetti F, Alebardi O, Nakajima H, Lanzavecchia A et al.: Plasmacytoid monocytes migrate to inflamed lymph nodes and produce large amounts of type I interferon. Nat Med 1999; 5:919–923.

10. Krug A, Rothenfusser S, Hornung V, Jahrsdorfer B, Blackwell S, Ballas ZK et al.: Identification of CpG oligonucleotide sequences with high induction of IFN-α/β in plasmacytoid dendritic cells. Eur J Immunol 2001; 31:2154–2163.

Natalija Novak

Department of Dermatology, University of Bonn, Sigmund-Freud-Str. 25, D-53105 Bonn, Germany, Tel. +49 228 287-4420, Fax +49 228 287-4883, E-mail natalija.novak@ukb.uni-bonn.de

Activation of SPHK 1 in Mast Cells by Tyrosine Kinase Lyn

T. Baumruker[1], A. Billich[1], A. Olivera[2], E. Bofill-Cardona[1], J. Rivera[2], and N. Urtz[1]

[1]*Novartis Institute for BioMedical Research, Vienna, Austria,* [2]*National Institutes of Health, Molecular Immunology and Inflammation Branch, Bethesda, MD, USA*

Summary: Sphingosine kinase (SPHK) has lately been recognized as a key enzyme in the generation of a new class of sphingolipid "second messenger molecules" and extracellular mediators. These include primarily, but are not limited to, ceramide (Cer; as a mediator of apoptosis), sphingosine (S; an inhibitor of effector functions – the substrate for SPHK) and sphingosine-1-phosphate (S1P; a mediator of proliferation and cell activation – the product of SPHK). Activation of SPHK after a variety of stimuli, including triggering of the FcεRI on mast cells, has been shown; however, any clear assignment to a particular signaling cascade or the link to a cellular readout is still unknown. Here we report that SPHK interacts directly with the tyrosine kinase Lyn and that this interaction not only stimulates the enzymatic activity of both molecules, but also leads to a recruitment of SPHK to the γ-chain of the FcεRI and further into rafts after IgE plus antigen (IgE/Ag) stimulation.

Keywords: allergy, protein/protein interaction, lipid kinase, sphingolipids, tyrosine kinase

Sphingolipids, and especially the products of the sphingomyelin pathway (Cer, S, and S1P), have lately been recognized as a new class of the important "second messenger" type of signaling molecules [1, 2]. As a specific feature of their role in signaling, the relative concentration of two or more of these lipids rather than the absolute concentration of any particular lipid alone determines processes such as differentiation, apoptosis, and allergic excitability [1]. This hypothesis has been termed the "rheostat concept" and is exemplified in particular in the regulation of apoptosis by the ratio of Cer:S1P and of mast cell/allergic excitability by the ratio of S:S1P [3, 4, 5]. As SPHKs are induced by a variety of cellular stimuli [6, 7, 8], including the IgE/Ag trigger of the FcεRI on mast cells, and as S1P overcomes not only the proapoptotic effect of Cer but also the inhibitory effect of S on mast cell activation, SPHK(s) seem to have a pivotal

role in determining cell fate. One facet of understanding the complex regulation by these lipids is to determine how SPHK(s) are regulated and induced, and in which signaling cascades they are placed. Here we report a direct interaction of the tyrosine kinase Lyn with SPHK1 in mast cells that leads to both an enhanced lipid and protein kinase activity [9].

Results and Discussion

In the last 2 years, several SPHK interacting proteins (see, i.e., TRAF2, AKAP-related protein, RPK 118) were identified by using the yeast two hybrid system [10, 11, 12]. The nature of these proteins, many being adaptor molecules and insufficiently characterized, has so far prevented these findings from profoundly impacting on our understanding of the function and regulation/induction of SPHK(s). Experi-

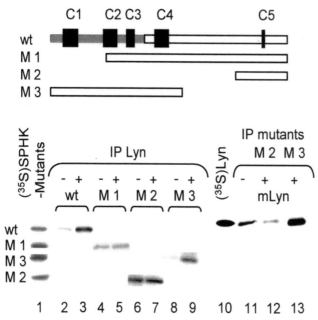

Figure 1. SPHK interacts with Lyn tyrosine kinase by its NH₂ terminus. Coimmunoprecipitation of mLyn and various deletion mutants of mSPHK1. Top: Schematic map of mSPHK1 and the deletion mutant proteins. Bottom: Lane 1, starting material radiolabeled mSPHK1 and corresponding deletion mutants (M 1–M 3), as indicated to the left. Lanes 2–9, coimmunoprecipitations of radiolabeled mSPHK1 and mutants (indicated above the lanes by wt, M 1–M 3) with an Ab directed to Lyn in the absence (even lane numbers, –) and presence (uneven lane numbers, +) of unlabeled Lyn protein (indicated by IP Lyn). Lane 10, starting material radiolabeled mLyn. Lanes 11–13, coimmunoprecipitations of radiolabeled mLyn with a mAb to myc-tagged mSPHK1 mutants in the absence (lane 11, –) and presence (+) of two mutant unlabeled mSPHK1 proteins (indicated by IP mutants M 2, M 3, see lanes 12 and 13).

mentally, we approached the identification of interacting proteins from mast cells by using an antibody array with 500 defined monoclonal antibodies to a variety of signaling molecules, which was reacted with *in vitro* transcribed and translated, radiolabeled murine SPHK and whole cell extracts from bone marrow-derived mast cells (BMMC) whole cell extracts. This identified an interaction with tyrosine kinase Lyn (but not Syk) that was confirmed using co-IPs with *in vitro* transcribed and translated molecules as well as purified recombinant Lyn and SPHK 1 proteins (indicating a direct interaction of both molecules). A further confirmation of the specificity of this interaction comes from inverse IP experiments, using 5' and 3' successive deletion constructs of SPHK 1 and "full length" Lyn protein, designed to map the interaction site more closely. These experiments showed that the NH₂-terminus of SPHK 1, up to the middle of the conserved sequence stretch C2, is essential for the interaction with Lyn, while the COOH-terminal half of the molecule is dispensable (see Figure 1).

Measurement of the (lipid and protein) kinase activities in complexes of highly purified recombinant Lyn and SPHK 1 showed enhancement of the enzymatic activity for both molecules in the complex as compared to the single components. Furthermore, S stimulated the tyrosine kinase activity of Lyn in the complexes even further – in line with "lipid interaction blottings" that identified Lyn as an S-binding protein [9]. Phosphorylation of SPHK 1 by Lyn was not detectable. We conclude that conformational changes induced by formation of a SPHK 1/Lyn complex, and further by S binding to the substrate site(s), result in the activation of both kinases; in fact, additional substrate or pseudosubstrate sites are known to positively or negatively regulate enzymes.

These *in vitro* findings are relevant in the context of closing a gap between earlier studies demonstrating that the activity of FcεRI-associated Lyn kinase is unchanged prior to and after IgE/Ag stimulation [13, 14] and findings by Young and colleagues, which showed increased Lyn kinase activity in the raft domains and changes in the phosphorylation of the regulatory tyrosines of Lyn [15]. As most experiments measuring Lyn activity are *in vitro* kinase assays, where SPHK or S are not added, or may not have been present in the IP material, the influence of the latter (the raft environment and SPHK) on Lyn activation in triggered mast cells has most likely been overlooked. This assigns an important role to the raft compartment (and SPHK), not only in terms of proper localization of the activating receptor/tyrosine kinase(s), but also to the direct activation of Lyn. In line with this assumption, we found that Lyn recruits SPHK 1 to FcεRI (as determined by anti-γ chain IP) in mast cells. This results in enhanced SPHK activity – immediately after activation – in the rafts.

From our data we deduce the following model: After IgE/Ag triggering of mast cells, SPHK 1 and Lyn interact, stimulating a "first round" of Lyn activation. This complex (with an enhanced tyrosine kinase activity) is then recruited to FcεRI that either already is in the rafts or migrates to these microdomains. Here, the Lyn/SPHK/FcεRI complex is exposed to high concentrations of S that further stimulates the tyrosine kinase activity of Lyn, which now amplifies the phosphorylation of the β- and γ-chains of the FcεRI. Interestingly, we also showed that, contrary to S, S1P has a negative effect on the activity of Lyn that is dominant over the S/SPHK stimulatory effect. Therefore, one may assume that SPHK 1 converts S into S1P in the microenvironment of (S and SPHK) activated Lyn, which then acts as a negative "feedback" loop, to shut down this kinase activity. As it was recently shown that Lyn also has a negative regulatory effect in the activation of mast cells [16], these findings demonstrate that multiple mechanisms are required for control of Lyn activity and, in part, explain the mechanism of the S/S1P rheostat in the activation of this cell type by IgE/Ag.

Acknowledgment
We are grateful to all our colleagues at the Novartis Research Institute Vienna who have supported our work over the years.

References

1. Baumruker T, Prieschl EE: Sphingolipids and the regulation of the immune response. Semin Immunol 2002; 14:57–63.
2. Prieschl EE, Baumruker T: Sphingolipids: second messengers, mediators and raft constituents in signaling. Immunol Today 2000; 21:555–560.
3. Olivera A, Kohama T, Edsall L, Nava V, Cuvillier O, Poulton S, Spiegel S: Sphingosine kinase expression increases intracellular sphingosine-1-phosphate and promotes cell growth and survival. J Cell Biol 1999; 147:545–558.
4. Prieschl EE, Csonga R, Novotny V, Kikuchi GE, Baumruker T: The balance between sphingosine and sphingosine-1-phosphate is decisive for mast cell activation after FcεRI triggering. J Exp Med 1999; 190:1–8.
5. Spiegel S, Cuvillier O, Edsall LC, Kohama T, Menzeleev R, Olah Z, Olivera A, Pirianov G, Thomas DM, Tu Z, Van Brocklyn JR, Wang F: Sphingosine-1-phosphate in cell growth and cell death. Ann NY Acad Sci 1998; 845:11–18.
6. Olivera A, Spiegel S: Sphingosine-1-phosphate as second messenger in cell proliferation induced by PDGF and FCS mitogens. Nature 1993; 365:557–560.
7. Xia P, Gamble JR, Rye KA, Wang L, Hii CS, Cockerill P, Khew-Goodall Y, Bert AG, Barter PJ, Vadas MA: Tumor necrosis factor-α induces adhesion molecule expression through the sphingosine kinase pathway. Proc Natl Acad Sci USA 1998; 95:14196–14201.
8. Meyer zu Heringsdorf HD, Lass H, Alemany R, Laser KT, Neumann E, Zhang C, Schmidt M, Rauen U, Jakobs KH, van Koppen CJ: Sphingosine kinase-mediated Ca^{2+} signalling by G-protein-coupled receptors. EMBO J 1998; 17:2830–2837.
9. Urtz N, Olivera A, Bofill-Cardona E, Csonga R, Billich A, Mechtcheriakova D, Bornancin F, Woisetschläger M, Rivera J, Baumruker T: Early activation of Sphingosine kinase in mast cells and recruitment to FcεRI is mediated by its interaction with Lyn kinase. Mol Cell Biol 2004; 24:8765–8777.
10. Xia P, Wang L, Moretti PA, Albanese N, Chai F, Pitson SM, D'Andrea RJ, Gamble JR, Vadas MA: Sphingosine kinase interacts with TRAF2 and dissects tumor necrosis factor-α signaling. J Biol Chem 2002; 277:7996–8003.
11. Lacana E, Maceyka M, Milstien S, Spiegel S: Cloning and characterization of a protein kinase A anchoring protein (AKAP)-related protein that interacts with and regulates sphingosine kinase 1 activity. J Biol Chem 2002; 277:32947–32953.
12. Hayashi S, Okada T, Igarashi N, Fujita T, Jahangeer S, Nakamura S: Identification and characterization of RPK118, a novel sphingosine kinase-1-binding protein. J Biol Chem 2002; 277:33319–33324.
13. Pribluda VS, Pribluda C, Metzger H: Transphosphorylation as the mechanism by which the high-affinity receptor for IgE is phosphorylated upon

aggregation. Proc Natl Acad Sci USA 1994; 91: 11246–11250.

14. Yamashita T, Mao SY, Metzger H: Aggregation of the high-affinity IgE receptor and enhanced activity of p53/56 lyn protein-tyrosine kinase. Proc Natl Acad Sci USA 1994; 91:11251–11255.

15. Young RM, Holowka D, Baird B: A lipid raft environment enhances Lyn kinase activity by protecting the active site tyrosine from dephosphorylation. J Biol Chem 2003; 278:20746– 20752.

16. Odom S, Gomez G, Kovarova M, Furumoto Y, Ryan JJ, Wright HV, Gonzales-Espinosa C, Hibbs ML, Harder KW, Rivera J: Negative regulation of IgE-dependent allergic responses by Lyn kinase. J Exp Med 2004; 199:1491–1502.

Thomas Baumruker

Novartis Institute for Biomedical Research Vienna, Brunner Straße 59, A-1235 Vienna, Austria, Tel. +43 1 86634 527, Fax +43 1 86634 582, E-mail thomas.baumruker@novartis.com

Comparative Database for Transcriptomes of Human and Mouse Inflammatory Cells

H. Saito[1,2], T. Yamamoto[3], K. Aoshima[3], T. Nakajima[1], K. Matsumoto[1,2], and H. Nagai[4]

[1]Department of Allergy & Immunology, National Research Institute for Child Health & Development, Tokyo, Japan, [2]Research Unit for Allergy Transcriptome, RIKEN Research Center for Allergy & Immunology, Yokohama, Japan, [3]R&D Department, Bioscience Division, Mitsui Knowledge Industry Co., Ltd., Tokyo, Japan, [4]Department of Pharmacology, Gifu Pharmaceutical University, Gifu, Japan

Summary: *Background:* It has become possible to see all the expressed genes present in a cell (transcriptome) at once using microarray. At present, microarray technology is applied in two different strategies. One is aimed at the discovery of a novel molecule crucially involved in the pathogenesis of a disease, and another is the trial for "system biology." *Methods:* We have constructed an interspecies comparison database, which deals mainly with human and mouse mast cell (MC) transcriptomes. We have also constructed a database for transcriptomes expressed by various cell types. *Results:* Using the interspecies comparative database, we found that the transcriptional levels of several CC chemokines were markedly increased both in human and mouse MCs after stimulation via high-affinity IgE receptor. Using the comparative database for various cell types, we identified several orphan G-protein coupled receptors selectively expressed by MCs and other inflammatory cell types. *Conclusion:* Mouse disease models will not be used any longer where key orthologous genes function differently than in humans. The safety of any candidate drug must be evaluated by comparing its efficacy with its toxicity to physiologically important organs. Analysis of cell-type-selective transcripts from database searches is expected to minimize the efforts required for drug discovery. In the future, we expect to use computational modeling to analyze integrative biological function without performing any *in vivo* or *in vitro* experimentation.

Keywords: basophils, mast cells, microarray, system biology, transcriptome

After completion of human genome sequencing, it became possible to see all the expressed genes present in a cell (transcriptome) at once using microarray. At present, microarray technology is being applied in two different strategies. One is the discovery of a novel molecule crucially involved in the pathogenesis of a disease, and another is the trial for "system biology." Using a high density oligonucletotide microarray (GeneChip, Affymetrix, Santa Clara, CA.), we have recently discovered and reported several critical molecules or new insights involved in the pathogenesis of allergic diseases [1].

Comprehension of the genome is accelerating the understanding of all the functional elements in a cell. Utilizing such a comprehensive array, we will not miss unexpected adverse effects induced by a new therapy. As such, the sequencing of the human genome is offering unprecedented system biology, with the intent to comprehend the total function of a cell, an organ, or in the near future, the human body. Here, we introduce a few examples of studies dealing with system biology by examining our transcriptome database based on two recently published papers dealing with comparisons between human and mouse mast cells (MCs) [2] and comparisons between various cell types [3].

Materials and Methods

Recombinant human IL-3, IL-6, and stem cell factor (SCF) for human MC culture were purchased from Intergen (Purchase, NY). CD34+ cells were positively selected from cord blood-derived MNCs[please define] using a CD34+ cell isolation kit and a magnetic separation column and were applied to human MC culture (MACS II, Miltenyi Biotec, Bergisch Gladbach, Germany) as previously reported [2]. Human CD34+ cells were then cultured in serum-free Iscove's methylcellulose medium (Stem Cell Technologies Inc., Vancouver, BC, Canada), which contained stem cell factor (SCF) at 200 ng/ml, IL-6 at 50 ng/ml, and IL-3 at 1 ng/ml as previously described. [2]. On day 42

of culture, methylcellulose was dissolved in PBS and the cells were suspended and cultured in Iscove's modified Dulbecco's medium (IMDM; Life Technologies, Rockville, MD, USA) supplemented with 1% insulin-transferrin-selenium supplement (Life Technologies), 50 μM 2-ME (Life Technologies), 100 units/ml penicillin (Life Technologies), 100 μg/ml streptomycin (Life Technologies) and 0.1% endotoxin-free bovine serum albumin (BSA) (Sigma Co., Ltd., St. Louis, MO, USA). The purification of seven types of leukocytes (basophils, eosinophils, neutrophils, CD4+ cells, CD8+ cells, CD14+ cells, and CD19+ cells), platelets, and fibroblasts was done by the methods previously described [3]. Mouse MCs were cultured with the methods described elsewhere [2]. GeneChip (U133A; Affymetrix, Santa Clara, CA, USA) expression analysis was done by the methods previously reported [2, 3].

Results

Interspecies Comparison

Animal disease models have been used as surrogates for human and have been informative.

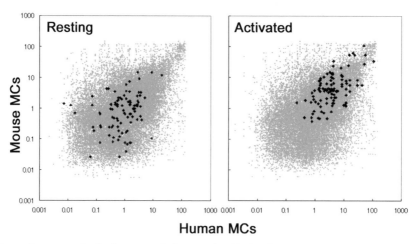

Figure 1. Genes whose expression levels were markedly upregulated both in human and mouse MCs after stimulation via FcεRI. Human and mouse cultured MCs were stimulated via FcεRI aggregation and were applied for GeneChip. The expression levels were normalized against the median value of each GeneChip. The vertical axis and horizontal axis respectively stand for mouse and human MCs' gene expression levels. Grey small dots represent > 10,000 orthologous genes' expression and black large dots represent genes whose expression levels were markedly upregulated both in human and mouse MCs after stimulation via FcεRI.

The use of mouse models for diseases related to allergy and immunology has increased because of the rapidly developing technologies to selectively knock out genes contributing to the pathogenesis of the disease. Regarding the relevance of these models of allergic diseases such as asthma, however, controversy still exists. Recently, many human and mouse orthologous genes have become available at a genome-wide level in electronic format, which facilitates interspecies comparisons. However, it had not been proven whether these structure-based orthologs are similarly regulated. Thus, we constructed and published online an interspecies comparison database (http://bio.mki. co.jp/en/results/_notes/comparativeDB_inde x.html), which deals mainly with human and mouse MC transcriptomes.

After stimulation via high-affinity IgE receptor (FcεRI), genes whose expression levels were markedly upregulated both in human and mouse MCs (Figure 1) were *CCL4* (macrophage inflammatory protein-1; MIP-1β), *CCL1*(I-309), *NFKBIA*, *CCL3* (MIP-1α), *CSF2* (GM-CSF), *SPP1*, *FYN*, *CD9*, *SERPINE1* (plasminogen activator inhibitor-1), *ICAM1*, *HMGN1*, *LBH*, *PTGS2*, *IL7R*, *PTPRE*, *CRTAM*, *IL3*, *EMP1*, *TNFAIP3*, *GADD45B*, *FYN*, *EMP1*, *PHLDA1*, *TNFRSF9* (4–1BB), *ITGAV*, *ITGAV*, *MAN1A1*, *FHL2*, *TNFAIP3*, *EGR2*, *CSF1*, *HSPC111*, *ELL2*, *UPP1*, *METTL1*, *IL1RN*, *TNF*, *GNAI1*, *ABCE1*, *TNFRSF1B*, *WSX1*, *WSX1*, *YKT6*, and *IRF4*, suggesting that FcεRI-mediated induction of these genes is highly conserved between human and mouse. Among these orthologous genes, we found that *PRG2* (major basic protein) mRNA levels were abundantly expressed by human MCs but not by mouse MCs. *AREG* (amphiregulin) was markedly upregulated only in human MCs after stimulation via FcεRI.

"Druggable" Genes for Allergic Diseases

We have also constructed the database for transcriptomes expressed by various cell types (http://www.nch.go.jp/imal/GeneChip/JACI. htm). The safety of any candidate drug must be evaluated by comparing its efficacy with its toxicity to physiologically important organs. We used GeneChip to examine the cell type-selective transcriptome expression of seven types of leukocytes (basophils, eosinophils, neutrophils, CD4+ cells, CD8+ cells, CD14+ cells, and CD19+ cells), platelets, MCs, and fibroblasts. Approximately 400 genes are selectively expressed by MCs, eosinophils, and basophils among all genes present in the human genome.

Granulocyte degranulation pathway is Ca^{2+}-dependent or G protein-dependent. Thus, ion channels and G protein-coupled receptors (GPCR) both play essential roles in degranulation as well as other cellular functions important for granulocytes, and are thought to be good targets of drug development. Receptor genes and ion channel genes are found only in 5% and 1.3% of all genes present in the human genome, respectively. However, receptors and ion channels are respectively found in 45% and 5% of the molecular targets of all known drugs [3]. Thus, after filtering with MC-, basophil-, and eosinophil-selective transcripts from transcriptomes, we focused on the expression of granulocyte-selective genes for ion channels, GPCR, and other receptors. It was estimated that approximately 50 "druggable" genes are selectively expressed by MCs, eosinophils, and basophils among all genes present in the human genome. We identified GPCR genes that were selectively expressed by MCs, basophils, and/or eosinophils under the conditions described previously [3]. They were *HRH4* (histamine H4 receptor), *PTGER3* (prostaglandin E receptor type 3a2), *ADORA3* (adenosine A3 receptor), *P2RY2* (purinergic receptor), *GPR44* (chemoattractant receptor-homologous molecule expressed on Th2 cells; CRTH2), *EMR1* (egf-like module containing, mucin-like, hormone receptor-like sequence 1), *CCR3* (chemokine receptor 3), *C3AR1* (C3a receptor), and *GPR34* (orphan GPCR).

Discussion

We succeeded in constructing a comparative database of human and mouse cells. In the near future, we propose to use computational modeling to analyze integrative biological function and to test hypotheses without performing any *in vivo* or *in vitro* testing. Although the transcriptome assay is considered to be merely a first-screening tool, it will be possible to select the information obtained from animal models only where the orthologous genes are functioning similarly. To simulate the human body in computational models, we still have to use many animal models. Differently regulated orthologous genes in mice may also be compared with human information in the future.

We also presented the comparative database of various inflammatory cell types. The safety of any candidate drug must be evaluated by comparing its efficacy with its toxicity to physiologically important organs. By using the database, analysis of cell type-selective transcripts is now possible to minimize the efforts required for drug discovery.

References

1. Saito H: Translation of the human genome into clinical allergy. Allergol Int 2003; 52:65–70.
2. Nakajima T, Inagaki N, Tanaka H, Tanaka A, Yoshikawa M, Tamari M, Hasegawa K, Matsumoto K, Tachimoto H, Ebisawa M, Tsujimoto G, Matsuda H, Nagai H, Saito H: Marked increase in CC chemokine gene expression in both human and mouse mast cell transcriptomes following Fcε receptor I cross-linking: an interspecies comparison. Blood 2002; 100:3861–3868.
3. Nakajima T, Iikura M, Okayama Y, Matsumoto K, Uchiyama C, Shirakawa T, Yang X, Adra CN, Hirai K, Saito H: Identification of granulocyte subtype-selective receptors and ion channels by high-density oligonucleotide probe array. J Allergy Clin Immunol 2004; 113:528–535.

Hirohisa Saito

Department of Allergy & Immunology, National Research Institute for Child Health & Development, 2–10–1 Okura, Setagaya-ku, Tokyo 157-8535, Japan, E-mail hsaito@nch.go.jp

Mast Cell Inhibition by β2-Adrenoceptor Agonists

T. Gebhardt[1] and S.C. Bischoff[2]

[1]Department of Gastroenterology, Hepatology, and Endocrinology, University Medical School of Hannover, Germany, [2]Department of Clinical Nutrition, Prevention and Immunology, University of Hohenheim, Stuttgart, Germany

Summary: *Background:* Previous studies have indicated potent inhibitory effects mediated by the β2 subtype of adrenoceptors (β2AR) on the immunological mediator release of mast cells (MC). Here, we studied the effects of β2AR activation on human intestinal MC. In particular, we were interested, apart from effects on mediator release, in other MC functions such as proliferation, adhesion, and migration that might be modulated by β2AR ligands. *Methods:* MC were isolated from human intestinal surgery tissue specimen, purified up to 95%, and subsequently cultured for up to 3 weeks in the presence of stem cell factor (SCF). Thereafter, MC mediator release, growth, adhesion, as well as SCF-induced migration was studied in purified MC preparations. In addition, cellular F-actin content was measured by flow cytometry. *Results:* β2AR activation by epinephrine, norepinephrine, and salbutamol (all at 1 μM) clearly inhibited the release of histamine, lipid mediators, and TNF-α as well as the SCF-dependent proliferation and migration of cultured human intestinal MC. Moreover, pretreatment with β2AR agonists suppressed the activation-induced adhesion of MC to fibronectin, as well as the interaction of MC with cocultured human endothelial cells. The inhibitory effects of β2AR ligands seem to be related to a drop in the cellular F-actin content caused by β2AR activation. *Conclusion:* β2AR agonists negatively regulate MC functions such as mediator release, proliferation, migration, and adhesion. The findings support the concept of neuroimmune interactions involved in the pathophysiology of gastrointestinal inflammation and allergy.

Keywords: mast cells, human, mucosa, adrenoceptor, epinephrine

In order to prevent uncontrolled release of potentially harmful mediators, MC are equipped with several receptors that negatively regulate their activation. These inhibitory pathways include surface receptors bearing immunotyrosine-based inhibitory motifs, such as FcγRIIb and gp49B1, and receptors for the immunoregulatory cytokines IL-10 and TGF-β1 [1]. Another means to quickly and effectively control MC activation is mediated by the β2AR found to be expressed in different murine and human MC populations [2]. Activation of these receptors by either synthetic or endogenous agonists, e.g., salbutamol or epinephrine, respectively, results in the rapid accumulation of intracellular 3',5'-adenosine monophosphate (cAMP), which is associated with a profound suppression of the IgE-dependent release of histamine, lipid mediators, and cytokines from

MC [2–4]. In the present study, we confirmed these previous findings for human intestinal MC and extended them by raising the question of whether activation of β2AR might also affect SCF-dependent MC functions such as proliferation, adhesion, and migration.

Material and Methods

In order to generate homogeneous human MC populations we isolated cells from the human intestinal mucosa, purified the *c-kit* positive MC using the MACS system, and subsequently cultured them for up to 3 weeks in the presence of SCF (50 ng/ml). After overnight culture in the absence of SCF, the MC were used in different *in vitro* assays carried out to analyse MC mediator release (IgER crosslinking

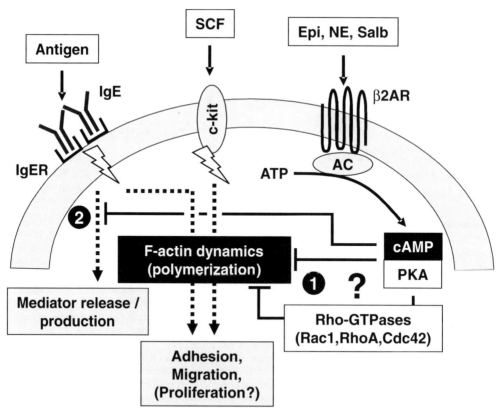

Figure 1. Anticipated mechanism of MC inhibition by β2AR agonists. Binding of epinephrine (Epi), norepinephrine (NE), or salbutamol (Salb) to the β2AR activates the adenyl cyclase (AC) triggering a rise in intracellular cAMP and subsequent activation of the proteinkinase A (PKA). Subsequently, either through members of the Rho family of GTPases or other yet undefined regulatory factors, rise in cAMP or PKA activity causes a direct inhibition of F-actin polymerization and, thus, of MC adhesion, migration, and proliferation (1). In parallel, rise in cAMP causes inhibition of IgE receptor signaling leading to inhibition of mediator release (2).

by mAb22E7), growth ([³H]-thymidine uptake, Ki67 staining), adhesion, and SCF-induced migration (48 well Boyden chamber). Prior to the activation by SCF or IgE receptor crosslinking or prior to the coculture with human umbilical vein endothelial cells (HU-VEC), respectively, the MC were incubated with epinephrine, norepinephrine, and salbutamol for 5 min (all at 1 μM).

Results

In accordance with several previous reports we found that all β2AR agonists at 1 μM nearly totally abolished the release of histamine, cysteinyl leukotrienes, prostaglandin D2, and TNF-α from MC triggered by IgER crosslink-

ing (n = 3–8). Furthermore, β2AR activation by epinephrine, norepinephrine, and salbutamol, respectively, strongly reduced the adhesion of MC to fibronectin-coated wells to about half of control conditions following activation by SCF (n = 6). Interestingly, pretreatment with either of the β2AR agonists also negatively affected other SCF-triggered MC functions. For example, MC recovery was reduced to less than half of control conditions (n = 5), an effect that was mainly attributable to an inhibition of MC proliferation as measured by [³H] thymidine uptake and Ki67 immunostaining. The SCF-induced migration of human intestinal MC was also clearly impaired following β2AR activation. Finally, β2AR activation was found to interfere with the interaction between MC and cocultured human umbilical vein endothelial cells that normally leads to a strong adhesion of both cell types to each other even in the absence of any exogenous stimuli [5].

Adhesion, migration, and possibly also proliferation of cells are dependent on highly dynamic cytoskeletal structures such as the F-actin network. Therefore, we monitored changes in the overall F-actin content following MC activation with or without prior β2AR activation. Stimulation of the MC by SCF caused a long-lasting increase in the amount of intracellular F-actin. In contrast, activation of the β2AR caused a rapid decline in F-actin levels, and, most interestingly, abolished the F-actin response toward SCF-stimulation. Similar results were also obtained regarding F-actin accumulation induced by IgER crosslinking. These preliminary data suggest that β2AR ligand-induced MC inhibition is closely associated with changes of intracellular F-actin polymerization.

Discussion

Previous studies indicated a correlation between the inhibition of MC mediator release and the intracellular rise in cAMP following activation of the β2AR-coupled adenyl cyclase [2–4]. However, the precise mechanism of how cAMP interferes with IgER-dependent mediator production and subsequent release remained elusive. A disruption of the F-actin network by β2AR activation, as we described here, does not seem to be critical in this respect, because disassembly of the F-actin cytoskeleton rather facilitates than inhibits MC degranulation [6]. In contrast, this effect might be of particular importance for the β2AR-mediated inhibition of adhesion, migration, and proliferation, because these cellular functions are known to involve the dynamic rearrangement of the F-actin network. Accordingly, our experiments using cytochalasin D and latrunculin B as inhibitors of actin polymerization confirmed the requirement of dynamic F-actin rearrangements for migration and adhesion in human intestinal MC (data not shown). Thus, two distinct inhibitory pathways employed by

the β2AR that operate in MC might be anticipated (Fure 1). First, β2AR activation induces an elevation of intracellular cAMP that occurs independently of its effect on F-actin, and that interferes via an as yet unknown mechanism with the signaling pathways of the IgER [2–4]. Alternatively, β2AR activation directly interferes with the F-actin turnover, decreasing the overall amount of F-actin in resting MC and causing unresponsiveness of the F-actin network toward stimulation by IgER crosslinking and SCF challenge in activated MC.

Elevation of cAMP levels and the consecutive activation of protein kinase A (PKA) have been shown to exert strong regulatory effects on the cytoskeleton in a number of different cell types; therefore, it is likely that the effect of β2AR activation on the cytoskeleton in human MC is also mediated via the cAMP/PKA pathway [7]. Among others, the members of the Rho family GTPases (e.g., Rho, Rac1, Cdc42) acting as major regulators of the F-actin cytoskeleton were shown to represent downstream targets of cAMP/PKA in different cell lines [7]. The question of whether these small GTPases are also involved in the β2AR-dependent inhibition of F-actin dynamics in human MC is currently being addressed in ongoing experiments.

The potent suppression of major MC functions by β2AR activation strengthens the concept of a functional interplay between the sympathetic nervous system and intestinal MC. According to our *in vitro* data, circulating and nerve-derived catecholamines are potent regulators of humoral MC functions, and also of MC distribution and expansion in tissue.

In cases of physical or psychological stress characterized by the rapid increase of blood and tissue catecholamine levels, the inhibition of MC might lead to an impairment of both functions of visceral organs dependent on normal smooth muscle functions regulated by MC and functions of the innate immune system required for host defence against infection. On the other hand, chronic inflammation that frequently results in the progressive loss of sympathetic tissue innervation might perpetuate by the loss of inhibition of inflammatory cells such as MC. These hypotheses illustrate the potential impact of our findings for the under-standing of mast cell-nerve cell-interactions *in vivo*, but also of the mechanisms of antiallergic drugs like β2AR agonists exerting not only bronchodilator functions but also potent anti-inflammatory effects.

References

1. Katz HR: Inhibitory receptors and allergy. Curr Opin Immunol 2002; 14:698–704.
2. Johnson M: Effects of β2-agonists on resident and infiltrating inflammatory cells. J Allergy Clin Immunol 2002; 110:282–290.
3. Peachell PT, MacGlashan Jr. DW, Lichtenstein LM, Schleimer RP: Regulation of human baso-phil and lung mast cell function by cyclic adeno-sine monophosphate. J Immunol 1988; 140:571–579.
4. Shichijo M, Inagaki N, Kimata M, Serizawa I, Saito H, Nagai H: Role of cyclic 3',5'-adenosine monophosphate in the regulation of chemical me-diator release and cytokine production from cul-tured human mast cells. J Allergy Clin Immunol 1999; 103:421–428.
5. Mierke C, Ballmeier M, Werner U, Manns MP, Welte K, Bischoff SC: Human endothelial cells regulate survival and proliferation of human mast cells. J Exp Med 2000; 192:801–811.
6. Frigeri L, Apgar JR: The role of actin microfila-ments in the down-regulation of the degranula-tion response in RBL-2H3 mast cells. J Immunol 1999; 162:2243–2250.
7. Howe AK: Regulation of actin-based cell migra-tion by cAMP/PKA. Biochim Biophys Acta 2004; 1692:159–174.

Stephan C. Bischoff

Chair of Clinical Nutrition, Prevention and Immunology, Uni-versity of Hohenheim, Fruwirthstr. 12, D-70593 Stuttgart, Germany, Tel. +49 711 459-4101, Fax +49 711 459-4343, E-mail bischoff.stephan@uni-hohenheim.de

Effects of Cannabinoid Agonists on Histamine Release from Activated Human Skin Mast Cells

S. Guhl, K. Grunow, M. Babina, P. Welker, B.M. Henz, and T. Zuberbier

Department of Dermatology and Allergy, Allergy Center Charité,
Charité – Universitätsmedizin Berlin, Germany

Summary: *Background:* Mast cells (MC) have been reported to express cannabinoid receptors that are utilized by endocannabinoids and cannabimimetics to alter their secretory functions. Data published are, however, in part contradictory, and normal human MC have not yet been studied. *Methods:* We have, therefore, examined isolated human cutaneous MC for their responsiveness to the endocannabinoid palmitoylethanolamide (PEA) and the synthetic cannabinoid WIN55,212–2 during cell activation. *Results:* Both agonists suppressed histamine release elicited by cross-linking of high-affinity IgE receptor in a dose-dependent fashion, with significant inhibition starting at 4 μM (PEA) and 2 μM (WIN55,212–2), respectively. Pertussis toxin (PTX) fully abolished the effect of PEA, suggesting an involvement of G proteins G_i/G_o. In order to explore whether this effect was receptor mediated, skin MC preparations from several donors, along with appropriate control cells, were assayed for the expression of two known cannabinoid receptors, CB1 and CB2, by RT-PCR. Transcripts for both receptors were detected in skin MC, with a consistently preferential expression of brain-type CB1. CB1 was also detected at lower levels in other immune cells, suggesting that its participation in immunomodulation is greater than hitherto suspected. *Conclusions:* The present data demonstrate a cannabinoid-dependent system of communication between MC and nerves and provide further evidence for an antiinflammatory and immunomodulatory function of the endocannabinoid system.

Keywords: mast cells, CB1, CB2, palmitoylethanolamide, WIN55,212–2

MC are specialized myeloid cells involved in allergic reactions and other inflammatory conditions, due in particular to the constitutively high expression of high-affinity receptors for IgE and the responsiveness of the cells to several immunologic and nonimmunologic stimuli. As a result of MC activation, the cells rapidly produce and release a broad spectrum of mediators, including histamine, leukotrienes, and a number of cytokines that are responsible for allergic and inflammatory symptoms [1, 2]. There is also recent evidence suggesting an important role for MC in establishing innate immunity toward intruding pathogens [3].

MC are of bone marrow origin, but complete their maturation in peripheral tissues where they are predominantly localized in close proximity to blood/lymph vessels or nerves. In fact, a bidirectional communication between MC and nerves seems to consist in a network made up of both stimulatory and repressive functions of nerves on MC and vice versa [4–6]. This is also illustrated by the fact that cutaneous MC degranulate in response to the potent neuropeptide substance P, a key interplayer in stress-activated MC degranulation [6–8].

Endocannabinoids that are produced by var-

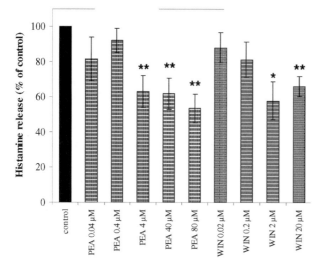

Figure 1. Cannabinoids dose-dependently inhibit histamine release from activated human skin MC. Cells were isolated from human breast skin and preincubated with the indicated doses of palmitoylethanolamide (PEA) or WIN55,212–2 (WIN) for 1 h at 37 °C prior to FCεRI crosslinking (by the addition of mouse or rabbit anti-human IgE), as described [23, 24]. Histamine release was assessed with a histamine analyzer, with the release observed in the absence of cannabinoid agonists being set at 100%. Values obtained in the presence of PEA and WIN are given as percentage of the respective control. Results are the mean ± SEM of 5–8 independent tests. *$p < 0.05$; **$p < 0.01$ significantly lower than control.

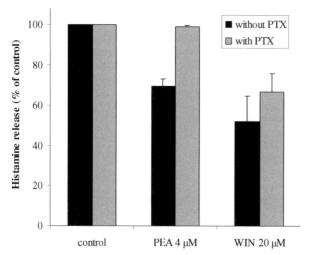

Figure 2. PEA mediated suppression of MC activation is sensitive to pertussis toxin. Skin MC were prepared and activated, as described in Figure 1. Pretreatment with pertussis toxin (PTX) at 2 µg/ml was performed for 30 min at 37 °C. Cells were then washed, before addition of the cannabinoid (for a further 1 h), followed by anti-IgE-induced FcεRI crosslinking for 30 min (as in Figure 1). Results are the mean ± SEM of 5–8 independent tests. Effects of Ptx on PEA mediated suppression were highly significant ($p < 0.001$), but not with WIN55,212–2.

ious cell types, most prominently by nerves, represent a class of fatty acid derivatives that act as endogenous agonists of cannabinoid receptors and mimic several pharmacological effects of delta 9-tetrahydrocannabinol, the active principle of hashish and marijuana [9, 10]. Endocannabinoid effects *in vivo* span a wide spectrum of functions, including not only to those associated with nervous system, but also selective aspects of immunological defense and inflammation [11, 12].

MC have early on been recognized as potentially significant targets of the endocannabinoid system [13]. However, depending on the organism, the tissue, and the state of cellular maturation, opposing effects have been documented in the literature as to the expression pattern of cannabinoid receptors (CB) in these cells. The same holds for their responsiveness toward naturally occurring or synthetic cannabinomimetics. For instance, MC secretion has been reported by different groups to be either inhibited, to remain unaffected, or even to be induced *de novo* by cannabinoid agonists [13–16]. However, primary human tissue MC have not yet been investigated for their responsiveness toward cannabinoids or with regard to the expression of CB receptors.

As a first step to understand the possible impact of this important substance class on untransformed MC in the human body, we employed MC isolated from human skin tissue and studied effects of cannabinoid agonists on the cells' secretory function. As illustrated in Figure 1, histamine release triggered by cross-linking of the high-affinity receptor for IgE (FcεRI) was inhibited by pretreatment of skin MC with both cannabinoid agonists employed. The effects were dose-dependent and reached statistical significance at 4 μM of PEA and 2 μM of WIN55,212–2. Maximal inhibition of 46% was achieved with 80 μM PEA, and this molecule also significantly suppressed MC degranulation induced by the neuropeptide substance P (data not shown), pointing toward a cannabinoid-mediated suppression of neuronally (in addition to immunologically) activated MC.

So far, two major cannabinoid receptor species, designated CB1 and CB2, have been described [10, 12]. CB1 is the dominant receptor in the central nervous system (with some expression also reported for splenocytes and other immune cells [16–19]), while CB2 is regarded as the peripheral cannabinoid receptor that is particularly active in cells of the immune system. As a further contribution to the controversy observed with cannabinoid-mediated effects in terms of MC activation (see above), normal animal or leukemic MC have also been shown to express either only CB2, both CB1 and CB2, or none of the two major receptor subtypes [13,15,16,20]. PEA is preferentially active at the CB2 receptor, whereas WIN55,212–2 represents a synthetic agonist of both receptor subtypes [12]. CB1 and CB2 both represent classical heptahelical G protein coupled receptors, and an involvement of Gi/Go as the signal-transducing principle appears relevant to both these receptors [10,21]. Nonreceptor mediated effects of cannabinoids, in part resulting from the hydrophobicity of the substance class, reportedly occur as well [10,22].

In order to explore the possible involvement of cannabinoid receptors in the signal transduction pathway that ultimately culminates in the inhibition of skin MC degranulation, we first investigated the effects of PTX on the suppression of histamine secretion in normal human skin MC. As shown in Figure 2, PTX was in fact able to fully re-

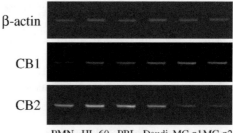

β-actin

CB1

CB2

PMN   HL-60   PBL   Daudi   MC-p1 MC-p2

Figure 3. Human skin MC express transcripts for both CB1 and CB2. mRNA was obtained from different preparations of human skin MC ($n = 6$), and subjected to reverse transcription and PCR, essentially as described [24], using 500 ng of total mRNA per 20 μl of cDNA. PCR was run under the following conditions, using appropriately diluted cDNA: 94 °C / 5 min (1 cycle); 94 °C / 45 s, 62 °C / 45 s, 72 °C / 1 min (40 cycles); 72 °C / 10 min (1 cycle). Primers for CB1 were: 5'-GTTCACGGTGGAGTTCAGCA; 5'-GCCCCTGGCCTATAAGAGGA and those for CB2: 5'-TGTGGGTAGCCTCCTGCTGA; 5'-CTGACCCAAGGCCCCTCACA. Different cell lines and primary cells isolated from the peripheral blood of healthy volunteers served as controls and for semiquantitation, all preparations were first adjusted to equivalent amounts of β-actin (5'-AATCTCATCTTGTTTTC TGCG; 5'-CCTTCCTGGGCATGGA GTCCT). PMN, polymorphonuclear cells; PBL, peripheral blood lymphocytes; MC-p1/p2, skin mast cells, preparation 1/2. Results are representative for at least 4 separate experiments. Results were confirmed with a second primer pair for CB1 and CB2, respectively.

verse the suppression of histamine secretion mediated by PEA, such that Gi/Go activation and, thus, a receptor-mediated mechanism of action presumably underlie the PEA-driven effect. A lower effect of PTX was, however, noted when WIN55,212–2 was used to suppress anti-IgE triggered histamine release, so that receptor-independent mechanisms cannot be excluded in the inhibitory effects mediated by this synthetic compound.

To help resolve the existing controversy as to whether MC express cannabinoid receptors or not, we next tested the expression pattern of the two receptor subtypes in a variety of hematopoietic lineages, including several preparations of skin MC. As illustrated in Figure 3, virtually all of the cell lines tested expressed low, yet detectable transcript levels for CB1. However, of all primary leukocytes tested (PMN, PBL, monocytes and MC, Figure 3 and data not shown), skin MC consistently expressed the highest level of CB1 transcript.

This rather unexpected result was confirmed with a second primer pair (data not shown). CB2 was also detectable in MC, albeit at lower level, compared to other leukocytes. Considering the fact that PEA is a preferential CB2 agonist and that very low receptor copies appear to suffice for signal transduction [12], it appears likely that CB2 is involved in this process. However, since a recent report clearly demonstrated the participation of the brain-type CB1 receptor as the major principle in suppression of secretory responses in a rat MC line [16], a mechanism that is shared by both receptor subtypes (both coupled to Gi/Go, as indicated above) seems quite feasible in skin MC. The expression of functional CB1 on skin MC is, furthermore, underlined by our data that anandamide (a CB1 active endocannabinoid agonist) had a substantial inhibitory effect on TNF-α production from skin MC, whereas PEA remained without such effect (data not shown). Most interestingly, however, the ratio of CB1/CB2 is clearly enhanced in skin MC over that in other haematopoietic cells, and MC, thus, appear to be attractive candidates to clarify the poorly understood function of CB1 receptor specific function in cells outside the nervous system.

In conclusion, cutaneous MC seem to clearly constitute targets of the cannabinoid system by expressing CB receptors and by displaying divergent and selective responses toward different agonists. Our data add to the recently established view of a modulation of MC function via both CB2 and CB1 [16], but importantly, extend this observation to nonleukemic primary human MC. Cannabinoids might, thus, work as locally acting suppressors of MC-induced inflammation by reducing the activation of MC in human skin. Our data furthermore corroborate an antiinflammatory and immunomodulatory function of the endocannabinoid system. Of note, although not the primary issue of the present work, the presence of CB1 in leukocyte subsets other than MC indicates that immune regulation may in fact also proceed through the brain-type cannabinoid receptor.

Acknowledgments

This work was supported by a grant from the German Federal Ministry of Education and Research for the Clinical Study Group Allergy (BMBF, Klinische Forschergruppe Allergologie, TP VII, 01 GC 0002) and Schering AG, Berlin.

References

1. Metcalfe DD, Baram D, Mekori YA: Mast cells. Physiol Rev 1997; 77:1033–1079.
2. Artuc M, Hermes B, Steckelings UM, Grützkau A, Henz BM: Mast cells and their mediators in cutaneous wound healing – active participants or innocent bystanders? Exp Dermatol 1999; 8:1–16.
3. Maurer M, Theoharides T, Granstein RD, Bischoff SC, Bienenstock J, Henz B, Kovanen P, Piliponsky AM, Kambe N, Vliagoftis H, Levi-Schaffer F, Metz M, Miyachi Y, Befus D, Forsythe P, Kitamura Y, Galli S: What is the physiological function of mast cells? Exp Dermatol 2003; 12:886–910.
4. McKay DM, Bienenstock J: The interaction between mast cells and nerves in the gastrointestinal tract. Immunol Today 1994; 15:533–538.
5. Gottwald T, Coerper S, Schaffer M, Koveker G, Stead RH: The mast cell-nerve axis in wound healing: a hypothesis. Wound Repair Regen 1998; 6:8–20.
6. Suzuki R, Furuno T, McKay DM, Wolvers D, Teshima R, Nakanishi M, Bienenstock J: Direct neurite-mast cell communication in vitro occurs via the neuropeptide substance P. J Immunol 1999; 163:2410–2415.
7. Columbo M, Horowitz EM, Kagey-Sobotka A, Lichtenstein LM: Substance P activates the release of histamine from human skin mast cells through a pertussis toxin-sensitive and protein kinase C-dependent mechanism. Clin Immunol Immunopathol 1996; 81:68–73.
8. Singh LK, Pang X, Alexacos N, Letourneau R, Theoharides TC: Acute immobilization stress triggers skin mast cell degranulation via corticotropin releasing hormone, neurotensin, and substance P: A link to neurogenic skin disorders. Brain Behav Immun 1999; 13:225–239.
9. Maccarrone M, Finazzi-Agro A: Endocannabinoids and their actions. Vitam Horm 2000; 65:225–255.
10. Piomelli D: The molecular logic of endocanna-

binoid signaling. Nat Rev Neurosci 2003; 4:873–884.

11. Parolaro D, Massi P, Rubino T, Monti E: Endocannabinoids in the immune system and cancer. Prostaglandins Leukot Essent Fatty Acids 2002; 66:319–332.

12. Klein TW, Newton C, Larsen K, Lu L, Perkins I, Nong L, Friedman H: The cannabinoid system and immune modulation. J Leukoc Biol 2003; 74:486–496.

13. Facci L, Dal Toso R, Romanello S, Buriani A, Skaper SD, Leon A: Mast cells express a peripheral cannabinoid receptor with differential sensitivity to anandamide and palmitoylethanolamide. Proc Natl Acad Sci USA 1995; 92:3376–3380.

14. Mazzari S, Canella R, Petrelli L, Marcolongo G, Leon A: N-(2-hydroxyethyl)hexadecanamide is orally active in reducing edema formation and inflammatory hyperalgesia by down-modulating mast cell activation. Eur J Pharmacol 1996; 300:227–236.

15. Lau AH, Chow SS: Effects of cannabinoid receptor agonists on immunologically induced histamine release from rat peritoneal mast cells. Eur J Pharmacol 2003; 464:229–235.

16. Samson MT, Small-Howard A, Shimoda LM, Koblan-Huberson M, Stokes AJ, Turner H: Differential roles of CB1 and CB2 cannabinoid receptors in mast cells. J Immunol 2003; 170:4953–4962.

17. Schatz AR, Lee M, Condie RB, Pulaski JT, Kaminski NE: Cannabinoid receptors CB1 and CB2: a characterization of expression and adenylate cyclase modulation within the immune system. Toxicol Appl Pharmacol 1997; 142:278–287.

18. Sacerdote P, Massi P, Panerai AE, Parolaro D: In vivo and in vitro treatment with the synthetic cannabinoid CP55, 940 decreases the in vitro migration of macrophages in the rat: involvement of both CB1 and CB2 receptors. J Neuroimmunol 2000; 109:155–163.

19. Matias I, Pochard P, Orlando P, Salzet M, Pestel J, Di Marzo V: Presence and regulation of the endocannabinoid system in human dendritic cells. Eur J Biochem 2002; 269:3771–3778.

20. Maccarrone M, Fiorucci L, Erba F, Bari M, Finazzi-Agro A, Ascoli F: Human mast cells take up and hydrolyze anandamide under the control of 5-lipoxygenase and do not express cannabinoid receptors. FEBS Lett 2000; 468:176–180.

21. Sugiura T, Kondo S, Kishimoto S, Miyashita T, Nakane S, Kodaka T, Suhara Y, Takayama H, Waku K: Evidence that 2-arachidonoylglycerol but not N-palmitoylethanolamine or anandamide is the physiological ligand for the cannabinoid CB2 receptor. Comparison of the agonistic activities of various cannabinoid receptor ligands in HL-60 cells. J Biol Chem 2000; 275:605–612.

22. Kaplan BL, Rockwell CE, Kaminski NE: Evidence for cannabinoid receptor-dependent and -independent mechanisms of action in leukocytes. J Pharmacol Exp Ther 2003; 306:1077–w1085.

23. Zuberbier T, Chong, SU, Grunow K, Guhl S, Welker P, Grassberger M, Henz BM: The ascomycin macrolactam pimecrolimus (Elidel, SDZ ASM 981) is a potent inhibitor of mediator release from human dermal mast cells and peripheral blood basophils. J Allergy Clin Immunol 2001; 108:275–280.

24. Bamina M, Guhl S, Starke A, Kirchhof L, Zuberbier T, Henz BM: Comparative cytokine profile of human skin mast cells from two compartments – strong resemblance with monocytes at baseline but induction of IL-5 by IL-4 priming. J Leukoc Biol 2004; 75:244–252.

Prof. Dr. Torsten Zuberbier

Department of Dermatology and Allergy, Charité – Universitätsmedizin Berlin, Campus Mitte, Schumannstr. 20/21, D-10117 Berlin, Germany, Tel. +49 30 450-518135, Fax +49 30 450-518919, E-mail torsten.zuberbier@charite.de

Expression and Function of Inhibitory and Activatory Receptors on Mast Cells and Eosinophils

New Mechanisms in Mast Cell-Eosinophil Crosstalk

A. Munitz, I. Bachelet, and F. Levi-Schaffer

Department of Pharmacology, School of Pharmacy, Faculty of Medicine,
Hebrew University of Jerusalem, Israel

Summary: *Background:* Evidence has emerged indicating that a cross-talk between mast cells (MC) and eosinophils (EOS) exists that might perpetuate and aggravate the allergic inflammatory response. Both MC and EOS express several cell surface activatory and/or inhibitory receptors but their expression and function on human MC and human EOS has not been addressed thoroughly, and not at all in the context of MC-EOS interactions. *Methods:* MC from cord blood mononuclear cells (CBMC) and from human lung were obtained using standard procedures. Human peripheral blood EOS were purified from mildly atopics/normals (MACS). Expression of IRp60 or CD2-subfamily receptors on MC or EOS, respectively, was assessed (FACS). CBMC and EOS were activated by cross-linking IRp60 or CD2-subfamily receptors, respectively. As activation markers β-hexosaminidase, tryptase for MC, and eosinophil-peroxidase (EPO) for EOS, were determined using enzymatic-colorimetric assays. IFN-γ and IL-4 were determined by ELISA. *Results:* CBMC and human lung MC express IRp60. EOS display various CD2-subfamily receptors. Cross-linking of IRp60 with FcϵRI inhibited β-hexosaminidase, tryptase, and IL-4 release from CBMC. Cross-linking of 2B4, CD48, or NTB-A caused EPO release. Crosslinking of 2B4 on EOS induced IFN-γ and IL-4 release and ERK 1/2 phosphorylation. Coculture of EOS and MC induced MC activation while neutralization of 2B4 on EOS or CD48 on CBMC abrogated the activatory effect. In addition, EOS major basic protein (MBP) downregulated the expression of IRp60 on the MC. *Conclusions:* The demonstration that activatory receptors expressed on EOS play a role in MC-EOS cross-talk, and that MBP can downregulate inhibitory receptors on MC, suggests a new pathway to regulate the inflammatory responses coordinated by these cells.

Keywords: Ig-superfamily cell surface receptors, CD2-subfamily, 2B4, CD48, IRp60, Mast cell-eosinophil cross-talk

EOS "encounter" MC in the tissue during the late phase of the allergic inflammatory process. Recently, evidence has emerged indicating that an important cross-talk between these two cells exists.It has been demonstrated *in vitro* that EOS intracellular calcium is elevated upon incubation with the MC products histamine and PGD$_2$ [1]. Moreover we have demonstrated that EOS survival is enhanced by MC-derived TNF-α by binding to TNFαRI and TNFαRII receptors [2]. In addition, preformed MC-neutral protease tryptase induces IL-6 and IL-8 cytokine production and release by binding to PAR II receptors, which initiates the mitogen-activated protein kinase/AP-1 pathway [3].

On the MC side, it has been shown that GM-CSF (produced by IgE-activated MCs) induces EOS survival and ECP release [4]. We have provided further evidence for MC/EOS cross-talk by demonstrating that human lung-derived MCs become responsive to EOS-derived MBP when cocultured with fibroblasts, by a process dependent upon membrane SCF [5]. Notably, EOS also synthesize SCF and NGF [6,7], two factors critical for MC survival and activation.

Over the past several years it has become increasingly apparent that both MCs and EOS express several inhibitory receptors belonging either to the Ig receptor superfamily or to the c-type (calcium dependent) lectin superfamily [8].

IRp60 is an inhibitory receptor belonging to the Ig superfamily. It is expressed on many cell types such as T-cells, NK cells and granulocytes. Cross-linking of IRp60 on NK cells, results in down-regulation of NK cytolytic activity [9]. In addition treatment of IRp60 with sodium pervanadate leads to marked IRp60 tyrosine phosphorylation and association with both SHP-1 and SHP-2. IRp60 cross-linking also inhibited the cytolytic activity of T-cell clones in redirected killing assays using anti-CD3 mAb [9].

In opposition to the inhibitory receptor families, there are several activatory receptor/coreceptor subfamilies. Of these, CD2 has largely grown into a distinctive subfamily of activating receptors/coreceptors belonging to the immunoglobulin superfamily (Ig-SF), which includes CD2, CD48 (Blast-1, BCM-1), CD58 (LFA-3), CD84 (Ly9B), CD150 (SLAM), CD229 (Ly9), 2B4 (CD244), BLAME (BCM-like membrane protein), SF2001 (CD2F-10), NTB-A (SF2000, Ly108), and CS1 (CRACC) [10–12]. Interestingly, several of the CD2-subfamily members interact with themselves or with other members of the CD2 family. In fact CD58 is a high affinity ligand for CD2, whereas CD48 is a low affinity ligand for CD2 [13] but a high affinity ligand for 2B4 [14].

Therefore our aim was to examine the expression and function of these specific inhibitory or activatory receptors/coreceptors and to evaluate whether they may play a role in MC-EOS interactions.

To investigate this possibility, human cord blood-derived mast cells (CBMC), human lung MCs and human peripheral blood EOS were first examined by FACS for the presence of IRp60 or CD2 subfamily receptors, respectively. IRp60 was expressed on both CBMC and human lung MCs ($n = 5, 3$, respectively). Cross-linking of IRp60 with FcεRI inhibited IgE-mediated β-hexosaminidase release ($59.28 \pm 9.55\%$ inhibition, $n = 4, p < 0.01$) and IL-4 release ($64.43 \pm 2.91\%$ inhibition, $n = 3$, $p < 0.01$) from CBMC. The expression level of IRp60 remained constant in the presence of various cytokines (IL-4, IL-13, IL-2 and IFN-γ). However, incubation of CBMC with 10nM EOS MBP specifically downregulated the expression of IRp60 in comparison to untreated cells or cells treated with 25–100 nM of Poly-L-Arginine (ΔMFI = 12 MBP treated cells vs. ΔMFI = 0 Poly-L-Arginine treated cells). Importantly other cell surface molecules on CBMC such as c-kit and CD48 were not affected by MBP.

Freshly isolated EOS expressed CD48, CD58, CD84, 2B4, and NTB-A but not CD2 or CD150 ($n = 15$). Cross-linking of 2B4, CD48 and NTB-A on the surface of EOS caused EOS peroxidase release, respectively (0.650 ± 0.98, $1.872 \pm 0.402, 0.522 \pm 0.047$ O.D units activated vs. $0.156 \pm 0.04, 0.294 \pm 0.022, 0.357 \pm 0.004$ O.D units isotype incubated cells, $n = 5, 3, 3$ respectively, $p < 0.001$,). Furthermore, cross-linking of 2B4 induced INF-γ release (53.7–502.9 pg/ml 2B4 vs. 0–97.5 pg/ml isotype, $p < 0.001, n = 9$), IL-4 release (16.5–67.3 pg/ml 2B4 vs. 10.48–51.7 pg/ml isotype, $p < 0.05, n = 4$). Cross-linking of 2B4 induced phosphorylation of ERK1/2 as soon as 2 min after the cross-linking process and peaked at 4–6 min.

In order to assess whether 2B4-CD48 receptor-ligand interactions can play a role in MC-EOS cross-talk we cocultured CBMC (CD48$^+$) with freshly isolated EOS (2B4$^+$) in the presence or absence of neutralizing antibodies recognizing CD48 on the surface of CBMC and 2B4 on the surface of EOS. The culture supernatant was collected and assessed for tryptase release. Freshly isolated EOS caused significant tryptase release from CBMC (0.322 ± 0.05 O.D units coculture vs. 0.032 ± 0.003 O.D units CBCMC alone $n = 3, p < 0.01$). The activatory effect was abrogated by neutralizing CD48 on MCs (0.006 ± 0.07 O.D units $n = 3, p < 0.001$) or 2B4 on EOS (0.025 ± 0.11 $n = 3, p < 0.05$). Interestingly coculture of CBMC with EOS did not elicit any EOS activation.

In summary, we have demonstrated that IRp60 is expressed and functional on CBMC and modulated by MBP. Furthermore we have shown that human EOS express functional CD2-subfamily receptors and that CD48–2B4 interactions are an additional component of the cross-talk between MC and EOS.

In conclusion the richness of functional activatory and inhibitory receptors on human MC and EOS indicate to us a tuning of the allergic inflammatory response that is much richer than the one conceived till now.

References

1. Takafuji S, Tadokoro K, Ito K, Nakagawa T: Release of granule proteins from human eosinophils stimulated with mast cell mediators. Allergy 1998; 53:951–956.
2. Temkin V, Levi-Schaffer F: Mechanism of tumor necrosis factor α mediated eosinophil survival. Cytokine 2001; 15:20–26.
3. Temkin V, Kantor B, Weg V, Hartman ML, Levi-Schaffer F: Tryptase activates the mitogen-activated protein kinase/activator protein-1 pathway in human peripheral blood eosinophils, causing cytokine production and release. J Immunol 2002; 169:2662–2669.
4. Simon HU, Weber M, Becker E, Zilberman Y, Blaser K, Levi-Schaffer F: Eosinophils maintain their capacity to signal and release eosinophil cationic protein upon repetitive stimulation with the same agonist. J Immunol 2000; 165:4069–4075.
5. Piliponsky AM, Gleich GJ, Nagler A, Bar I, Levi-Schaffer F: Non-IgE-dependent activation of human lung- and cord blood-derived mast cells is induced by eosinophil major basic protein and modulated by the membrane form of stem cell factor. Blood 2003; 101:1898–1904.
6. Hartman M, Piliponsky AM, Temkin V, Levi-Schaffer F: Human peripheral blood eosinophils express stem cell factor. Blood 2001; 97:1086–1091.
7. Micera A, Puxxedu I, Aloe L, Levi-Schaffer F: New insights on the involvement of Nerve Growth Factor in allergic inflammation and fibrosis. Cytokine Growth Factor Rev 2003; 14:369–374.
8. Katz HR: Inhibitory receptors and allergy. Curr Opin Immunol 2002; 14:698–704.
9. Cantoni C, Bottino C, Augugliaro R, Morelli L, Marcenaro E, Castriconi R, Vitale M, Pende D, Sivori S, Millo R, Biassoni R, Moretta L, Moretta A: Molecular and functional characterization of IRp60, a member of the immunoglobulin superfamily that functions as an inhibitory receptor in human NK cells. Eur J Immunol 1999; 29: 3148–3159.
10. Cocks BG, Chang CC, Carballido JM, Yassel H, de Vries JE, Aversa G: A novel receptor involved in T-cell activation. Nature 1995; 376:260–263.
11. Bottino C, Falco M, Parolini S, Marcenaro E, Augugliaro R, Sivori S, Landi E, Biassoni R, Notarangelo LD, Moretta L, Moretta A: NTB-A a novel SH2D1A-associated surface molecule contributing to the inability of natural killer cells to kill Epstein-Barr virus-infected B-cells in X-linked lymphoproliferative disease. J Exp Med 2001; 194:235–246.
12. Bouchon A, Cella M, Grierson HL, Cohen JI, Colonna M: Activation of NK cell-mediated cytotoxicity by a SAP-independent receptor of the CD2 family. J Immunol 2001; 167:5517–5521.
13. Sidorenko SP, Clark EA: The dual-function CD150 receptor subfamily: The viral attraction. Nat Immunol 2003; 4:19–24.
14. Brown MH, Boles K, van der Merwe PA, Kumar V, Mathew PA, Barclay AN: 2B4, the natural killer and T-cell immunoglobulin superfamily surface protein, is a ligand for CD48. J Exp Med 1998; 188:2083–2090.

Francesca Levi-Schaffer

Department of Pharmacology, School of Pharmacy, Faculty of Medicine, The Hebrew University of Jerusalem, POB 12065, Jerusalem 91120, Israel, Tel. +972 2 675-7512, Fax +972 2 675-8144, E-mail fls@cc.huji.ac.il

Relaxin Inhibits Activation of Human Neutrophils *in vitro* by a Nitric-Oxide-Dependent Mechanism

E. Masini, S. Nistri, A. Vannacci, C. Marzocca, P.F. Mannaioni, and D. Bani

Department of Preclinical and Clinical Pharmacology, Department of Anatomy, Histology, & Forensic Medicine, University of Florence, Florence, Italy

Summary: The pregnancy hormone relaxin (RLX) has been shown to reduce the recruitment of leukocytes, especially neutrophils, in inflamed tissues in animal models of inflammation. The current study was designed to clarify whether RLX could inhibit activation of isolated human neutrophils challenged with N-formyl-Met-Leu-Phe (fMLP) and, if so, whether the nitric oxide (NO) biosynthetic pathway is involved, as occurs in other RLX targets. Human neutrophils were preincubated with 1, 10, and 100 nmol/l porcine relaxin for 1 h before activation with fMLP (10 mmol/l). In selected experiments, the NO synthase inhibitor L-NMMA (100 µmol/l) and the guanylate cyclase inhibitor ODQ (100 µmol/l) were added to the samples 30 min before RLX. In other experiments, chemically inactivated relaxin (iRLX,10 nmol/l) was substituted for authentic RLX. Untreated, unactivated neutrophils were the controls. The stimulation of human neutrophils with fMLP (10 µmol/l) significantly increased the production of superoxide anion, which was barely detectable in the unstimulated cells. This effect was paralleled with an increase in the intracellular calcium and in a decrease of cGMP concentrations. RLX reduced significantly and in a concentration-dependent fashion the generation of superoxide anion, and the rise of intracellular calcium, while the cGMP levels were significantly increased. These RLX effects were blunted by pretreating the cells with L-NMMA or ODQ and could not be reproduced by iRLX. This study provides evidence that RLX inhibits the activation of human neutrophils stimulated by proinflammatory agents, through the stimulation of the generation of endogenous NO production, and a cGMP-dependent mechanism. This novel property of RLX could be of relevance in toning down maternal neutrophil activation during pregnancy, counteracting the occurrence of pregnancy-related disorders.

Keywords: human neutrophils, relaxin, chemotactic peptide, reactive oxygen species, NO pathway, cGMP

Relaxin (RLX) ia a peptide hormone produced mainly by the corpus luteum during pregnancy with well-established effects on the female organs and mammary glands [1]. There is increasing evidence that RLX is more than a pregnancy hormone, especially considering its ability to influence the cardiovascular system [2]. Recent evidence has shown that RLX has a prompt, potent, protective action against tissue injury in an animal model of inflammatory

diseases. In rats undergoing cardiac ischemia-reperfusion *in vivo*, RLX reduces neutrophil extravasation into the tissue and protects against peroxidative damage because of the generation of reactive oxygen species [3]. Similarly, RLX has been shown to strongly reduce histamine and mast cell degranulation [4] and decrease the severity of asthma-like reaction in sensitized guinea pigs subjected to inhalation of allergen, an effect which is paralleled by a significant reduction in leukocyte infiltration in the lung [5]. Our group has shown that RLX is a potent stimulator of endogenous nitric oxide (NO) biosynthesis in mast cells [4], platelets [6] and basophils [7]. On this basis, it appears that RLX could exert an antiinflammatory effect by interfering with neutrophil activation. The current study was designed to further investigate the intracellular mechanisms by which RLX can modulate human neutrophil activation.

Methods

20 ml of venous blood anticoagulated with sodium heparin (500 IU/ml) were collected from adult male volunteers who had not taken any drugs in the previous 4 weeks and gave their informed consent before enrolling in this study. Neutrophils were obtained by dextran sedimentation followed by Ficoll-Paque density gradient centrifugation and hypotonic lysis for residual erythrocytes. The final pellet was resuspended in Sorensen phosphate buffer containing 138 mM NaCl; 2.7 mM KCl; 1 mm $MgCl_2$ to a final concentration of 2.5×10^5 cells/ml. Neutrophils were preincubated with different concentrations of porcine RLX for 1 h before activation with chemotactic peptide N-formyl-Met-Leu-Phe (10 µmol/l, fMLP). Relaxin was inactivated by blocking functional arginine residue with cyclohexanedione and was used in control experiments [5]. The NO synthase competitive inhibitor N^G-monomethyl-L-arginine (L-NMMA, 10 µmol/l) or the guanylate cyclase inhibitor 1H-[1,2,4]oxadiazolo[4,3-a]quinoxalin-1-one (ODQ, 10 mmol/l) were added to the samples 30 min before RLX. Human neutrophil activation was evaluated by measuring superoxide anion generation monitored with a spectrophotometric method as previously reported [8]. Cyclic GMP levels were determined with a radioimmunological method (RIA) using a commercial kit (Amersham, Bucks, UK). Cytosolic free calcium concentrations were determined fluorimetrically using a Shimadzu DR 15 spectrofluorimeter in fura -2 AM-loaded neutrophils activated with fMLP [4, 7].

The reagents used were from Sigma Chemical Co. (St. Louis, MO), while purified porcine RLX, prepared according to Sherwood and O'Byrne [9] was a generous gift of Dr. O.D. Sherwood (University of Illinois at Urbana-Champaign, Urbana, IL, USA).

Results and Discussion

The stimulation of human neutrophils with fMLP (10 µmol/l) significantly increased the production of superoxide anion, which was barely detectable in the unstimulated cells. This effect was paralleled by an increase in the intracellular calcium and a decrease in cGMP concentrations. The pretreatment of neutrophils with RLX caused a dose-dependent inhibition of superoxide anion production, as well as a rise in intracellular calcium, while the levels of cGMP were significantly and dose-dependently increased (Figure 1). These effects were blunted by the pretreatment of the cells with L-NMMA (100 µmol/l) and with ODQ (100 µmol/l). These results provide evidence that RLX inhibits the activation of human neutrophils stimulated with the chemotactic peptide. Moreover, human neutrophils appear to be a specific target for RLX as evidenced by the dose-dependent effect of RLX on the inhibition of neutrophil activation and also by the fact that inactivated RLX had no effect (Figure 1). The present results could explain the reduction of neutrophil infiltration in the myocardial tissue of rats subjected to ischemia-reperfusion [3] and in the lung of sensitized guinea pigs undergoing an allergic asthma-like reaction [5]. This novel property of RLX could be of relevance during pregnancy by down-regulating maternal neutrophil activation to prevent pregnancy-related disorders such as preeclampsia, which is regarded as an excess of maternal inflammatory response to embryo implantation [10].

Acknowledgments

This work was supported by a grant from the Italian Ministry for Education, University and Research (MIUR), cofunding of Research Programs of National Interest, year 2000–2001.

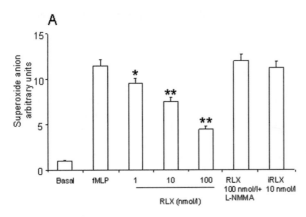

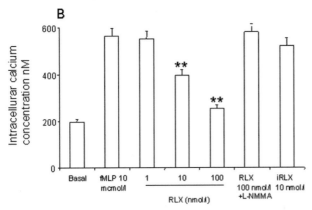

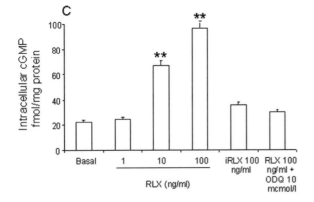

Figure 1. Effects of RLX on superoxide anion production (Panel A), intracellular calcium (PB) and cGMP levels (PCc) in human neutrophils under different experimental conditions. Pretreatment of the cells with RLX reduces the rise in superoxide anion generation and in calcium induced by fMLP (10 µmol/l) while it increases the cGMP levels. The effects of RLX are blunted by L-NMMA (100 µmol/l), and ODQ (100 µmol/l) and are not reproduced by iRLX (10 nmol/l).

References

1. Sherwood OD: Relaxin's physiological roles and other diverse actions. Endocr Rev 2004; 25:205–234.
2. Bani D: Relaxin, a pleiotropic hormone. Gen Pharmacol 1997; 28:13–22.
3. Bani D, Masini E, Bello MG, Bigazzi M, Bani Sacchi T: Relaxin protects against myocardial injury caused by ischemia and reperfusion in rat heart. Am J Pathol 1998; 152:1367–1376.
4. Masini E, Bani D, Bigazzi M, Mannaioni PF, Bani Sacchi T: Effects of relaxin on mast cells. *In vitro* and *in vivo* studies in rats and guinea pigs. J Clin Invest 1994; 94:1974–1980.
5. Bani D, Ballati L, Masini E, Bigazzi M, Bani Sacchi T: Relaxin counteracts asthma-like reaction induced by inhaled antigen in sensitized

guinea pigs. Endocrinology 1997; 138:1909–1915.

6. Bani D, Bigazzi M, Masini E, Bani G, Bani Sacchi T: Relaxin depresses platelet aggregation. *In vitro* studies on isolated human and rabbit platelets. Lab Invest 1995; 73:709–713.

7. Bani D, Baronti R, Vannacci A, Bigazzi M, Bani Sacchi T, Mannaioni PF, Masini E: Inhibitory effects of relaxin on human basophils activated by stimulation of Fcε receptor: The role of nitric oxide. Int Immunopharmacol 2002; 2:1195–1204.

8. Masini E, Nistri S, Vannacci A, Bani Sacchi T, Novelli A, Bani D: Relaxin inhibits the activation of human neutrophils. Involvement of the nitric oxide pathway. Endocrinology 2004; 145:1106–1112.

9. Sherwood OD, O'Byrne EM: Purification and characterization of porcine relaxine. Arch Biochem Biophys 1974; 60:185–196.

10. Redman CW, Sacks GP, Sergent IL: Preeclampsia: an excessive maternal inflammatory response to pregnancy. Am J Obstet Gynecol 1999; 180:499–506.

Emanuela Masini

Department of Preclinical and Clinical Pharmacology, Viale Pieraccini, I-50139 Firenze, Italy, Tel. +39 055 4271233, Fax +39 055 4271280, E-mail emanuela.masini@unifi.it

Cloning, Expression, Characterization, and Skin Prick Testing of NADPH-Dependent Mannitol Dehydrogenase

A New Major Allergen of *Cladosporium herbarum*

M. Breitenbach[1], B. Simon-Nobbe[1], U. Denk[1], P. Schneider[1], K. Richter[1], M. Teige[2], C. Radauer[3], C. Ebner[3], S. Nobbe[4], P. Schmid-Grendelmeier[4], and R. Crameri[5]

[1]*Department of Cell Biology, University of Salzburg, Austria,* [2]*Department of Biochemistry, Vienna Biocenter, University of Vienna, Austria,* [3]*Department of Pathophysiology, Medical University of Vienna, Austria,* [4]*Dermatologische Klinik und Poliklinik, Universitätsspital Zürich, Switzerland,* [5]*SIAF, Davos, Switzerland*

Summary: *C. herbarum* represents one of the most prominent fungal sources causing Type-I allergy. In the last years several minor allergens, as are enolase, Aldehyde Dehydrogenase, ribosomal protein P1 and P2, YCP4-homolog protein and hsp70 have been cloned by screening *C. herbarum* cDNA expression libraries with the sera of *C. herbarum* allergic patients. In order to isolate the major allergen of about 30kD, the respective protein was purified by standard chromatographic methods and subjected to protein sequencing. From the partial protein sequences degenerated oligonucleotide primers were deduced and used for PCR. A full-length clone was isolated showing homology to the NADPH-dependent Mannitol-Dehydrogenase from *C. fulvum*. The biological activity of the enzyme was confirmed by enzymatic measurement. The 28,3kD protein is recognized by 52% of *C. herbarum* sensitized patients and thus the first major allergen of *C. herbarum*.

Keywords: *Cladosporium herbarum*, allergens, recombinant, mannitol dehydrogenase, skin test

The worldwide occurring mold, *Cladosporium herbarum* (C.h.), is among the most important causes of fungal allergy. In regions with a hot and humid climate, up to 30% of the allergic population may be sensitized to molds. However, in central Europe the number of mold-sensitized patients is lower and may be between 2 and 5%. The molds are indoor as well as outdoor allergens with seasonal peaks in late summer and autumn. C. h. is not usually an infectious agent. Most of the mold-allergic patients are simultaneously sensitized to other allergen sources like pollens and house dust mites. Surprisingly, research into the molecular nature of the allergens of C.h. has been comparatively slow. On the other hand, molecular information is needed because the reproducibility and the negative, as well as pos-

Allergy Clin Immunol Int: J World Allergy Org, Supplement 2 (2005)

itive, predictability of commercially available mold extracts for skin prick testing is poor and hyposensitization with C.h. extracts has rarely been attempted. Here we present the cloning and characterization of mannitol dehydrogenase (MtDH) from C.h. and show that it is a major allergen of 28 KD. About 52% of the ImmunoCAP (Pharmacia Diagnostics, Uppsala, Sweden) positive *Cladosporium*-sensitized patients react to recombinant non-fusion (rnf) mannitol dehydrogenase (MtDH). Functional homologs of this enzyme occur in plant and fungal species and are stress-inducible pathogenesis-related (PR) proteins [1].

We prepared a cDNA expression library from a C.h. strain in the lambda-derived vector Uni-ZAP XR (Stratagene, La Jolla, CA, USA). The starting material was carefully chosen to contain both spores and hyphae and was grown on solid media containing 2% glucose, 1% yeast extract, and 2% peptone (YPD). As a control, the aqueous extract from this material ("in-house extract" [2]) was blotted and decorated with patients' IgE. At least 20 well-defined bands were visible, the most prominent being a 28 KD band, which was recognized by about two thirds of the patients. No other bands were recognized by such a high percentage of the patients. Several attempts to clone the cDNA corresponding to the 28 KD allergen by immunological screening with appropriate patients' sera completely failed. We, therefore, set out to purify the 28 KD allergen to homogeneity. This goal was achieved by sequentially applying three purification steps and rechecking the purity by SDS-PAGE and the immunological reactivity by IgE immune blots after each step. The soluble fraction after cell lysis (in-house extract) was precipitated with 50% ammonium sulphate and the soluble fraction was applied to a hydrophobic interaction chromatographic (HIC) column. The low salt eluted fraction that contained the allergen was then rechromatographed by anion exchange chromatography and proved to be free of contaminating proteins and immunologically reactive toward patients' IgE. The pure protein was now sequenced by solid phase Edman degradation both at the N-terminus of the protein and internally after digestion with trypsin. All sequences obtained showed a very high degree of identity with the published protein sequence of MtDH from *Cladosporium fulvum* [3]. We, therefore, tested the purified natural protein and found that it catalyzed the conversion of D-fructose to mannitol in a strictly NADPH-dependent manner. NADH was inactive as a cofactor and fructose-6-phosphate was a weak inhibitor of the reaction. The Michaelis constant for D-fructose was 735 mM. Two-dimensional protein analysis and immune blotting of the in-house extract showed that MtDH is an abundant protein of the soluble extract under the growth conditions used by us. Based on the known physiological function [4] of MtDH in plants, we suggest that the probable biological role of MtDH in C.h. is the production of the osmoprotectant, mannitol, from fructose under osmotic stress and other stress conditions.

Degenerate oligonucleotide primers were constructed using the known peptide sequences of C.h. MtDH and a radioactively labeled PCR product of 636 nt was isolated. Subsequently, this was used to perform a hybridization screen after plaque lifting of the C.h. cDNA library mentioned above. Four different cDNA clones were isolated and after plaque purification were excised *in vivo* to produce plasmid clones of the corresponding cDNAs using the Uni-ZAP XR Vector Kit according to manufacturer's instructions). These clones were sequenced using the ABI capillary electrophoresis method (Applied Biosystems, Vienna, Austria) and shown to be identical in the coding region. Both this result and the fact that MtDH produces a single spot in 2D immune blotting point to the conclusion that MtDH may be a single copy gene and may produce a single gene product. The coding sequence obtained was compared with the molecular mass of the natural protein and of the subsequently obtained rnf protein showing exact identity of the predicted and measured mass (ion spray MS/MS measurements). The open reading frame (ORF) did not show any N-terminal targeting sequence. Together with the mass determination this excludes a secreted protein or any postsynthetic modifications like glycosylation. The molecular mass is 28.3 kD and the pI is 5.8. The reaction equation of MtDH is

$$D\text{-fructose} + NADPH + H^+ =$$
$$D\text{-mannitol} + NADP^+$$

PCR cloning of the ORF coding for MtDH and insertion into the expression vector pMW172 [5] via directed insertion (NdeI/EcoRI) and IPTG induction in E. coli led to high level expression of the rnfMtDH. This protein was purified to homogeneity from the soluble E. coli extract in four steps similar to the procedure described above for the natural protein. The rnfMtDH displayed the same specific enzyme activity and immunological reactivity that was found for the natural MtDH. The purified rnf-MtDH allowed us to determine the exact incidence of sensitization to MtDH among C.h. positive (CAP-test positive) patients to be 52%. This was based on 35 patients' sera from outpatient clinics in Vienna, Salzburg, and Zürich. Conventional skin prick tests showed that at a concentration of $100\,\mu g/ml$ a very strong skin reaction occurred that was more pronounced than the one obtained with a commercial extract or with 0.1% histamine.

In conclusion, we identified, cloned, and produced as a highly purified rnf protein a new major allergen of C.h. which shows a higher incidence of sensitization among C.h. positive patients than any other previously cloned and characterized C.h. allergen. This allergen is MtDH, a protein which was previously identified in some fungal and plant species as a stress or pathogenesis-related enzyme.

References

1. Stoop JMH, Mooibroek H: Cloning and characterization of NADP-mannitol dehydrogenase cDNA from the button mushroom, Agaricus bisporus, and its expression in response to NaCl stress. Appl Environ Microbiol 1998; 64:4689–4696.
2. Achatz G, Oberkofler H, Lechenauer E, Simon B, Unger A, Kandler D, Ebner C, Prillinger H, Kraft D, Breitenbach M: Molecular cloning af major and minor allergens of Alternaria alternata and Cladosporium herbarum. Mol Immunol 1995; 32:213–227.
3. Noeldner PDM, Coleman MJ, Faulks R, Oliver PR: Purification and characterization of mannitol dehydrogenase from the fungal tomato pathogen Cladosporium fulvum (syn. Fulvia fulva). Physiol Mol Plant Pathol 1994; 45:281–289.
4. Jennings DB, Ehrenshaft M, Pharr DM, Williamson JD: Roles for mannitol and mannitol dehydrogenase in active oxygen-mediated plant defence. Proc Natl Acad Sci USA 1998; 5:15129–15133.
5. Susani M, Jertschin P, Dolecek C, Sperr WR, Valent P, Ebner C, Kraft D, Valenta R, Scheiner O: High level expression of birch pollen profilin (Bet v 2) in E. coli: purification and characterization of the recombinant allergen. Biochem Biophys Res Commun 1995; 215:250–263.

Dr. Michael Breitenbach

University of Salzburg, Department of Cell Biology, Hellbrunnerstr. 34, A-5020 Salzburg, Austria, Tel. +43 662 8044-5786, Fax +43 662 6389-5787, E-mail michael.breitenbach@sbg.ac.at

Cosensitization to Cockroach and Mite Is Not Explained by Tropomyosin Cross-Reactivity

S. Satinover[1], A. Reefer[1], N. Custis[1], T.A.E. Platts-Mills[1], K. Arruda[2], A. Pomes[3], M. Chapman[3], and J. Woodfolk[1]

[1]Asthma and Allergic Diseases Center, University of Virginia, Charlottesville, VA, USA,
[2]Department of Pediatrics, School of Medicine of Ribeirao Preto, University of Sao Paulo, Brazil,
[3]Indoor Biotechnologies Inc., Charlottesville, VA, USA

Summary: *Background:* Tropomyosins derived from mite species (Der p 10 and Der f 10) and German or American cockroach (CR) species (Bla g 7 and Per a 7, respectively) have the potential to elicit cross-reactivity. This could explain the high prevalence of cosensitization to mite among CR-sensitized subjects. *Methods:* Cross-reactivity to tropomyosins was tested using 131 sera with IgE ab to CR extract (CAP assay, Pharmacia). IgE ab to mite extract was measured by CAP assay while specific IgE ab to recombinant Der p 10 (rDer p 10) and rPer a 7 were measured using a novel Streptavidin CAP assay. *Results:* The frequency of sensitization to mite extract (either *D. pteronyssinus* or *D. farinae* or both species) was 82% (108/131). Among mite-sensitized subjects, there was no quantitative correlation between IgE ab to either *D. pteronyssinus* ($r = 0.08$, $p = 0.366$) or *D. farinae* ($r = -0.019$, $p = 0.828$) and CR. Only 19% (21/108) of subjects with IgE ab to mite had IgE ab to rPer a 7; however, mite and CR anti-tropomyosin IgE ab titers were highly correlated ($r = 0.899$, $p < 0.001$). No anti-tropomyosin IgE ab were measurable in mite-negative sera. Finally, patients without anti-Per a 7 IgE ab showed variable patterns of IgE ab responsiveness to other CR allergens. *Conclusions:* Cosensitization to CR and mite only partially reflects tropomyosin cross-reactivity. Instead, consistent with climatic and social issues, concomitant exposure to mite and CR allergens with potent IgE ab-inducing properties is a more likely explanation.

Keywords: cockroach, tropomyosin, allergy, IgE antibodies, IgG antibodies, house dust mite

In the urban environment, an important role for both CR and house dust mite (HDM) antigens in the etiology of house dust allergy and asthma is well recognized [1–3]. A high prevalence of cosensitization to HDM and CR has also been widely reported [4–6]. Despite this association, it is unclear whether cosensitization arises by virtue of coexposure, antigenic cross-reactivity, or both [5–8]. Several allergens derived from the principal domiciliary CR species, *Blatella germanica* and *Periplaneta americana*, have

been well characterized [9]. These include the CR tropomyosins (Bla g 7 and Per a 7), which are potential targets for cross-reactive IgE antibodies (ab) based on their high sequence identity (> 80%) with HDM tropomyosins (Der p 10 and Der f 10) [6,7,9,10]. However, data regarding whether CR tropomyosins constitute major allergens is conflicting [6, 10, 11]. The present study was designed to examine whether tropomyosin cross-reactivity contributes to cosensitization to CR and HDM.

Material and Methods

Serum Samples

Serum samples were obtained from: (1) Atlanta, Georgia ($n = 57$); (2) Wilmington, Delaware ($n = 36$); (3) Charlottesville, Virginia ($n = 23$); (4) New Zealand ($n = 9$); and (5) Brazil ($n = 6$). Studies were approved by the University of Virginia Human Investigation Committee.

CR and HDM allergens

Recombinant tropomyosins were generously provided by Karla Arruda (Per a 7) and Wayne Thomas (Der p 10). Other recombinant allergens (Bla g 1, Bla g 2, Bla g 4, and Bla g 5) were obtained from Indoor Biotechnologies, Inc., (Charlottesville, VA).

Measurement of Serum IgE ab

IgE ab to extracts of *B. germanica, D. pteronyssinus,* and *D. farinae* were measured by CAP assay (Pharmacia Biotech, Uppsala, Sweden). Specific IgE ab to purified recombinant CR (rBla g 1, rBla g 2, rBla g 4, rBla g 5, rPer a 7) and dust mite (rDer p 10) allergens were measured by Streptavidin CAP assay [12] using biotin-labeled purified allergen linked to Streptavidin CAPs. Sera were incubated with allergen-bound Streptavidin CAPs at room temperature (1 h) and the assay developed using standard techniques (Pharmacia CAP system). IgG ab to rPer a 7 and rDer p 10 were measured by antigen binding radioimmunoprecipitation assay [13].

Statistical Analysis

The relationship between variables was analyzed by linear regression. All statistical tests were 2-tailed and p values < 0.05 were considered statistically significant. Data were analyzed with SPSS for Windows (version 10.0, SPSS Inc., Chicago, ILL.).

Results

The prevalence of IgE ab to HDM allergens (either *D. farinae* or *D. pteronyssinus,* or both) was high (82%) among CR-sensitized subjects. Titers of IgE ab to *D. farinae* or *D. pteronyssinus* were not correlated with IgE ab titers to CR ($r < 0.1, p > 0.3$). Furthermore, only a minority of subjects (19%) with IgE ab to HDM had IgE ab to rPer a 7 (Figure 1). Though there was a strong quantitative correlation for IgE ab to HDM and CR tropomyosins ($r = 0.899, p < 0.001$), titers of IgG ab to the tropomyosins showed a weaker relationship ($r = 0.46, p < 0.001$). Similar patterns of IgE ab responsiveness to other purified CR allergens were observed among subjects cosensitized to HDM and CR with and without tropomyosin sensitivity; however, the prevalence of IgE ab to purified CR allergens was moderately decreased among CR-sensitized subjects who were not sensitized to HDM (data not shown).

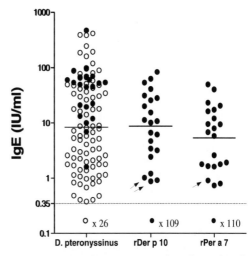

Figure 1. Tropomyosin sensitization and IgE ab to cockroach allergens. A. IgE ab to *D. pteronyssinus,* rDer p 10 and rPer a 7 among CR-sensitized subjects ($n = 131$). Black circles in left column denote subjects with IgE ab to rDer p 10. Three sera had low titer IgE ab to either rDer p 10 or rPer a 7, but not both (arrows). No IgE ab to rDer p 10 were measurable among CR-sensitized subjects with no IgE ab to dust mite allergen *(D. farinae* or *D. pteronyssinus).*

Discussion

Tropomyosins derived from HDM and CR exhibit antigenic cross-reactivity as judged by IgE ab binding. Nevertheless, CR tropomyosin is a minor allergen. Thus, the high prevalence of cosensitization to HDM and CR is only partially explained by tropomyosin cross-reactivity. Instead, this may arise from parallel exposure to allergens of HDM and CR with potent IgE-inducing properties. The apparent diminished IgE ab responsiveness to purified CR allergens among CR-sensitized subjects without IgE ab to HDM or tropomyosins could be explained by reduced allergen exposure, a less atopic phenotype, or a combination of both factors.

References

1. Gelber LE, Seltzer LH, Bouzoukis JK, Pollart SM, Chapman MD, Platts-Mills TAE: Sensitization and exposure to indoor allergens as risk factors for asthma among patients presenting to hospital. Am Rev Respir Dis 1993; 147:573–578.
2. Call RS, Smith TF, Morris E, Chapman MD, Platts-Mills TA: Risk factors for asthma in inner city children. J Pediatr 1992; 121:862–866.
3. Huss K, Adkinson NF, Eggleston PA, Dawson C, Van Natta ML, Hamilton RG: House dust mite and cockroach exposure are strong risk factors for positive allergy skin test responses in the Childhood Asthma Management Program. J Allergy Clin Immunol 2001; 107:48–54.
4. Hulett AC, Dockhorn RJ: House dust mite (D. farinae) and cockroach allergy in a midwestern population. Ann Allergy 1979; 42:160–165.
5. van Wijnen JH, Verhoeff AP, Mulder-Folkerts DK, Brachel HJ, Schou C: Cockroach allergen in house dust. Allergy 1997; 52:460–464.
6. Beatriz A, Santos R, Chapman MD, Aalberse RC, Vailes LD, Ferriani PL, Oiver C, Rizzo C, Naspitz CK, Arruda LK: Cockroach allergens and asthma in Brazil: Identification of tropomyosin as a major allergen with potential cross-reactivity with mite and shrimp allergens. J Allergy Clin Immunol 1999; 104:329–337.
7. Fernandes J, Reshef A, Patton L, Ayuso R, Reese G, Lehrer SB: IgE antibody reactivity to the major shrimp allergen, tropomyosin, in unexposed Orthodox Jews. Clin Exp Allergy 2003; 33:956–961.
8. Leaderer BP, Belanger K, Triche E, Hoford T, Gold DR, Kim Y, Jankun T, Ren P, McSharry J-E, Platts-Mills TAE, Chapman MD, Bracken MB: Dust mite, cockroach, cat, and dog allergen concentrations in homes of asthmatic children in the Northeastern United States: Impact of socioeconomic factors and population density. Environ Health Perspect 2002; 110:419–425.
9. Arruda LK, Vailes LD, Ferriani VP, Santos AB, Pomes A, Chapman MD: Cockroach allergens and asthma. J Allergy Clin Immunol 2001; 107:419–428.
10. Jeong KY, Lee J, Lee IY, Ree HI, Hong CS, Yong TS: Allergenicity of recombinant Bla g 7, German cockroach tropomyosin. Allergy 2003; 58:1059–1063.
11. Jeong KY, Hwang H, Lee J, Lee IY, Kim DS, Hong CS, Ree HI, Yong TS: Allergenic characterization of tropomyosin from the dusky brown cockroach, Periplaneta fuliginosa. Clin Diagn Lab Immunol 2004; 11:680–685.
12. Erwin EA, Custis NJ, Satinover SM, Perzanowski MS, Woodfolk JA, Crane J, Wickens K, Platts-Mills TA. Quantitative measurement of IgE antibodies to purified allergens using streptavidin linked to a high-capacity solid phase. Allergy Clin Immunol 2005; 115:1029–1035.
13. Platts-Mills T, Vaughan J, Squillace S, Woodfolk J, Sporik R: Sensitization, asthma, and a modified Th2 response in children exposed to cat allergen: a population-based cross-sectional study. Lancet 2001; 357:752–756.

Judith A. Woodfolk

UVA Asthma & Allergic Diseases Center, PO Box 801355, Charlottesville, VA 22908-1355, USA, Tel. +1 434 924-1293, Fax +1 434 924-5779, E-mail jaw4m@virginia.edu

Can Chinese Elm Pollen Cause Asthma?

M.M. Glovsky[1,2], A.G. Miguel[1], R. Flagan[1], R. Esch[3], J. House[1], and P.E. Taylor[1]

[1]*Division of Chemistry and Chemical Engineering, California Institute of Technology,
Pasadena, CA, USA,* [2]*Asthma and Allergy Center, Huntington Medical Research Institute,
Pasadena, CA, USA,* [3]*Greer laboratories, Lenoir, NC, USA*

Summary: Chinese elm trees produce copious amounts of pollen in the fall and are a major cause of allergic rhinitis in Pasadena. Many studies over the past 20 years have shown that episodes of pollen-induced asthma occur especially after periods of rainfall or thunderstorm. In addition, combustion particles from automobile exhaust are known to act as catalysts in the allergic response. We investigated whether Chinese elm pollen allergens contribute to the respirable aerosol as well as their mechanism of release from flowers. Outdoor air sampling was performed with a liquid impinger with a 2.5 µm size cut. Immunological analysis showed levels of up to 260 ng of Chinese elm allergen per cubic meter of air. The mechanism of release of respirable allergens from fragmented elm pollen was found to be similar to the process recently described for flowering grasses [1] and birch trees [2]. In all cases, pollen remains on the open anthers in the absence of wind or other disturbances. If wetted, pollen can rupture within minutes. Fragmented cytoplasm is emitted through the pore region of the pollen grain. Drying winds release this cytoplasmic debris of allergen-loaded particles in the size range of 30 nm to 4.5 µm. The small size of these particles, combined with their abundance in the air, suggests that they can readily deposit in the lower airways and may trigger asthmatic reactions in susceptible people in cities with high levels of combustion pollutants.

Keywords: Chinese elm pollen, pollen fragments, asthma

Chinese elm is the most abundant pollen in the months of September and October in Pasadena (CA, USA). At peak levels, the pollen count has been recorded up to 650 counts/m³. It is highly allergenic and ~30% of atopic patients show positive skin tests. The pollen readily fragments upon exposure to high humidity. Recent results from our laboratory showing avid binding of proteins to filters have stimulated a search for other methods for collecting respirable aerosols. Like the Burkard spore trap, an AGI-30 liquid impinger is half-century old technology that predates modern instrument characterization and calibration methods, but it has provided a convenient test of alternate approaches to sample collection and analysis.

Methods

Since we seek to determine concentrations of respirable allergens, two stages of a well-characterized Marple impactor (Sierra Instruments) was installed upstream of the impinger to provide a well-defined 2.5 µm size cut and eliminate whole pollen grains and large spores from the samples. The AGI-30 was operated on ice at a flow rate of 11 lpm to collect airborne particles and pollen fragments directly into liquid. Samples were collected in Pasadena, CA during the Chinese elm pollination period in the fall of 2003.

Chinese elm pollen proteins immunoblots were analyzed by applying aliquots of the impinger liquid to a nitrocellulose mem-

Table 1. Chinese elm concentrations in the ambient atmosphere and in an emission chamber.

Sample Dates	Sample Location	Sample Time (h)	Sampled Air Volume (m³)	Final Liquid Volume (ml)	Chines Elm Concentration (ng/m³)
September 22/23, 2003	Ambient	10.5	6.9	2	13.8
September 24, 2003	Ambient	7	4.6	10	266
September 25, 2003	Field, Disturbed trees	2.5	1.65	15	2045
September 26/27, 2003	Field, Ambient	16.5	10.9	6	74.5
October 5, 2003	Indoor Controlled Chamber	0.66	0.44	7.5	2897

brane using a dot microfiltration apparatus (Bio-Rad Laboratories). Serial dilutions of a Chinese elm pollen extract, for which protein had been quantified, were applied in duplicate as a standard. The Chinese elm proteins were detected by the addition of polyclonal rabbit IgG raised against American elm pollen extract (Greer Laboratories, Lenoir NC). The membrane was further treated with an anti-rabbit IgG-alkaline phosphatase conjugate and developed with the alkaline phosphatase substrate mixture BCIP/NBT, 5-bromo-4-3-indolyl-1-phosphate and nitro blue tetrazolium. The relative color development was quantified by densitometry using a camera imaging system (Alpha Innotech gel documentation and analysis system).

Results and Discussion

The dot blot detection protocol applied to airborne particle samples collected with the AGI-30 liquid impinger successfully detected pollen proteins and allergens in the respirable particle size range. The levels of Chinese elm pollen protein from airborne particles, compared with a standard Chinese elm pollen extract are presented in Table 1. Chinese elm pollen proteins were detected in the five samples tested, while no background was observed in the negative control to which no primary antibody was added. Ambient atmospheric concentrations ranged from 14–266 ng m^{-3} and the highest levels were recorded from sites nearby and downwind from the trees. A 10-fold higher level was observed for a sample collected in the field where the trees were disturbed (shaken) compared with a sample collected from an indoor controlled chamber containing a freshly picked tree branch housing pollen. The long periods required for the ambient sampling were inconvenient because the impinger collection solution evaporated over time and liquid had to be added back occasionally. More practical sampling times, on the order of 1.5 to 5 h, could be employed if the sample liquid were concentrated before the dotblot assay. The present limit of detection for Chinese elm pollen proteins using the dotblot is about 6 ng, equivalent to about 15 ng m^{-3} when 0.4 ml of impinger liquid is applied per dot well. More robust sampling procedures will be needed to facilitate routine measurements of ambient respirable allergens.

Acknowledgments
The research described in this article was supported by Philip Morris USA Inc. and by Philip Morris International. We also thank the Ayrshire Foundation, Pasadena, for its support.

References

1. Taylor PE, Flagan R, Valenta R, Glovsky MM: Release of allergens in respirable aerosols: a link between grass pollen and asthma. J Allergy Clin Immunol 2002; 109:51–56.
2. Taylor PE, Flagan R, Miguel AG, Valenta R, Glovsky MM: Birch pollen rupture and the release of aerosols of respirable allergens. Clin Exp Allergy 2004, in press.

M. Michael Glovsky

Huntington Memorial Hospital, Asthma and Allergy Center, 39 Congress Street, Suite 301, Pasadena, CA 91105, USA, Tel. +1 626 397-3383, Fax +1 626 795-0982, E-mail yksvolg@caltech.edu

Inhalation Allergy and Desensitization to a Cysteine Protease Allergen

J.C. Lenzo, A.G. Jarnicki, S.R. Gunn, P.G. Holt, and W.R. Thomas

*Centre for Child Health Research, Telethon Institute for Child Health Research,
The University of Western Australia*

Summary: *Background:* It has been difficult to develop mouse models of respiratory sensitization. The sensitizing ability of papain, a homologue of the mite allergen Der p 1, was, therefore, examined. *Methods:* Papain was administered intranasally and IgE measured by passive cutaneous anaphylaxis (PCA) and immunoassay. BAL were examined for eosinophils and cytokines. E64 was used to inhibit the proteolytic activity. Vaccination was performed by subcutaneous (s.c.) injections of papain and intranasal treatment with a peptide containing a T-cell epitope.
Results: Papain induced boostable Th2 sensitization. The IgE was unaffected by blocking protease activity but eosinophilia was reduced. Vaccination by injection of allergen ameliorated respiratory sensitization while intranasal peptide was ineffective.
Conclusions: Papain induces respiratory sensitization that can be blocked by vaccination.

Keywords: respiratory sensitization, mice, mouse papain, vaccination, desensitization, intranasal

The high and increasing prevalence of allergic disease highlights the need for new strategies of allergy vaccination and desensitization [1]. Mice provide a good immunological model but it is difficult to induce respiratory sensitization in this species. Aerosols or intranasal installations of the nominal allergen OVA induce transient IgE titres that wane [2]. Thus, sensitization has usually been initiated by the injection of soluble or alum absorbed OVA [3]. Others have studied the initial transient response to intranasal administration [4]. Two recent studies have reported sustained Th2 responses with intranasal OVA [5,6] so the balance between sensitization and tolerance can be perturbated. Hoyne et al. [7] showed that intranasal Der p 1 peptide induced boostable transient sensitization, even when the mice were tolerant to parenteral immunization. The intranasal peptide also induced delayed hypersensitivity that could only be boosted intranasally [8]. Allergen extracts can induce respiratory sensitization [9] but they are variable mixtures and humans are not exposed to extracts. It could, however, be possible to harness an adjuvant-activity of pure allergen. The mite allergen Der p 1 is a cysteine protease homologous to papain and it has been shown that its proteolytic activity can enhance allergenicity [10]. The ability of papain, which is readily available in large quantities, to induce respiratory sensitization has, therefore, been studied.

Materials and Methods

C57BL/6 J mice and Sprague Dawley rats were used. Papain (2 × crystallized) and E64 were from Sigma-Aldrich, St Louis, MO, USA. Cytokine and antibody assays were conducted by dissociation-enhanced lanthanide fluorescence immunoassay (DELFIA™; Wallac, Turku, Finland) with europium-streptavidin. PCA in rats [11] was elicited by 2 mg papain. The IgE capture assay [11] was performed with a biotinylated antipapain monoclonal antibody. Cellular infiltrates and cytokines were measured from BAL [11] 24 h after three daily challenges with 100 µg of papain.

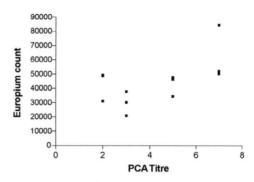

Figure 1. Papain-specific IgE levels measured by DELFIA and PCA. Serum samples from papain sensitized mice were measured for allergen-specific IgE by dissociation-enhanced lanthanide fluoroimmunoassay (DELFIA) and passive cutaneous anaphylaxis (PCA). Samples with high levels of IgE correlate well between the two methods of measurement.

Results

Intranasal papain induced IgE antibody detectable by PCA as measured 14 days after commencing sensitization. Mice receiving 5 daily doses (beginning Day 1) produced the highest titres followed by mice similarly receiving 3 and 1 daily doses. Doses of 1 µg induced higher titres than 100 µg doses. IgE was also measured by DELFIA™ (Figure 1). The binding of papain by antibody captured by anti-IgE was detected by biotinylated antipapain The IgE could be boosted by two more rounds of sensitization. The BAL had a prominent eosinophilia and Th2 cytokines. The protease inhibitor E64 did not affect the induction of IgE but the eosinophilia of mice sensitized by E64-treated papain was reduced. Vaccination by 6 × 100 µg s.c. injections of E64-treated papain reduced the sensitization. Intranasal administration of peptide p140–158 containing an H-2[b] T-cell epitope was ineffective.

Discussion

Low doses of papain reliably induced boostable IgE antibody and lung eosinophilia. A tested regimen is to sensitize mice with 5 daily administrations of 1 mg of papain and after a week's rest to repeat the daily cycle. The adjuvanticity of the proteolytic activity of the homologous cysteine protease Der p 1 has been extensively reported [10], although in investigations injecting allergen in alum. In contrast to the Der p 1 studies, the inhibitor E64 did not affect IgE responses although mice sensitized with E64-treated papain had reduced eosinophilia (when challenged with untreated papain). Other biochemical activities could be involved. Cysteine proteases have a varying range of proteolytic specificities and additional enzymatic activities such as esterase [12]. The reduction the allergic sensitization by vaccination provides a benchmark for strategies of vaccination and desensitization of respiratory sensitization. The inactivity of the intranasal peptide concurs with investigations with Der p 1. A Der p 1 peptide reduced IgE in mice immunized with Der p 1 in alum but not the responses induced by intranasal Der p 1 and enterotoxin adjuvant [11]. Intranasal vaccination with the Der p 1 peptide also induced boostable delayed hypersensitivity [8] so the possible side effects of intranasal peptides need to be considered. Clearly experiments on desensitization are a priority. The fact that the IgE response to papain could be boosted over 3 fortnightly cycles shows that the system can be used to monitor the boosting of already sensitized mice as well as the maintenance of sensitization.

Acknowledgment

The study was supported by ALK-Abello, Horsholm, Denmark.

References

1. Holt PG, Sly PD, Martinez FD, Weiss ST, Bjork-sten B, von Mutius E, Wahn U: Drug development strategies for asthma: in search of a new paradigm. Nat Immunol 2004; 5:695–598[**???**].
2. Holt PG, Batty JE, Turner KJ: Inhibition of specific IgE responses in mice by pre-exposure to inhaled antigen. Immunol 1981; 42:409–417.
3. Williams CM, Galli SJ: Mast cells can amplify airway reactivity and features of chronic inflammation in an asthma model in mice. J Exp Med 2000; 192:455–462.
4. Eisenbarth SC, Piggott DA, Huleatt JW, Visintin I, Herrick CA, Bottomly K: Lipopolysaccharide-enhanced, toll-like receptor 4-dependent T helper cell type 2 responses to inhaled antigen. J Exp Med 2002; 196:1645–1651.
5. McCusker C, Chicoine M, Hamid Q, Mazer B: Site-specific sensitization in a murine model of allergic rhinitis: role of the upper airway in lower airways disease. J Allergy Clin Immunol 2002; 110:891–898.
6. Hahn C, Teufel M, Herz U, Renz H, Erb KJ, Wohlleben G, Brocker EB, Duschl A, Sebald W, Grunewald SM: Inhibition of the IL-4/IL-13 receptor system prevents allergic sensitization without affecting established allergy in a mouse model for allergic asthma. J Allergy Clin Immunol 2003; 111:1361–1369.
7. Hoyne GF, Askonas BA, Hetzel C, Thomas WR, Lamb JR: Regulation of house dust mite responses by intranasally administered peptide: transient activation of CD4+ T-cells precedes the development of tolerance in vivo. Int Immunol 1996; 8:335–342.
8. Jarnicki AG, Tsuji T, Thomas WR: Hypersensitivity reactions after respiratory sensitization: effect of intranasal peptides containing T-cell epitopes. J Allergy Clin Immunol 2002; 110:610–616.
9. Johnson JR, Wiley RE, Fattouh R, Swirski FK, Gajewska BU, Coyle AJ, Gutierrez-Ramos JC, Ellis R, Inman MD, Jordana M: Continuous exposure to house dust mite elicits chronic airway inflammation and structural remodeling. Am J Resp Crit Care Med 2004; 169:378–385.
10. Gough L, Schulz O, Sewell HF, Shakib F: The cysteine protease activity of the major dust mite allergen Der p 1 selectively enhances the immunoglobulin E antibody response. J Exp Med 1999; 190:1897–1902.
11. Jarnicki AG, Tsuji T, Thomas WR: Inhibition of mucosal and systemic T(h)2-type immune responses by intranasal peptides containing a dominant T-cell epitope of the allergen Der p 1. Int Immunol 2001; 13:1223–1231.
12. Nagler DK, Tam W, Storer AC, Krupa JC, Mort JS, Menard R: Interdependency of sequence and positional specificities for cysteine proteases of the papain family. Biochemistry 1999; 38:4868–4874.

Professor Wayne Thomas

Telethon Institute for Child Health Research, PO Box 855, West Perth WA 6872, Australia, Tel. +61 8 9489 7777, Fax +61 8 9489 7700, E-mail wayne@ichr.uwa.edu.au

Apple Allergy

Different Patient Allergen Recognition Patterns Across Europe, Studied by Use of Recombinant Allergens

K. Hoffmann-Sommergruber[1], R. Asero[2], B. Bohle[1], S.T.H.P. Bolhaar[3], H. Breiteneder[1], M. Fernandez-Rivas[4], E. Gonzalez-Mancebo[4], A. Knulst[3], Y. Ma[1], R. van Ree[5], L. Zuidmeer[5]

[1]Dept. of Pathophysiology, Medical University of Vienna, Vienna, Austria, [2]Ambulatorio di Allergologia, Clinica San Carlo, Paderno Dugnano, Italy, [3]Dept. of Dermatology/Allergology, University Hospital Utrecht, The Netherlands, [4]Fundacion Hospital Alcorcon, Unidad de Allergia, Alcorcon, Spain, [5]Dept. of Allergy, Sanquin Blood Supply Foundation, Amsterdam, The Netherlands

Summary: Food allergy is defined as an IgE mediated reaction. However, the true prevalence of food allergy is still under discussion. This is in part caused by the lack of quality of diagnostic tools for food allergy. Using apple allergy as a model, a considerable number of allergic patients were recruited from four different locations in Europe and their IgE reactivity towards the already identified purified natural and recombinant apple allergens (Mal d 1–Mal d 4) determined by *in vitro* as well as *in vivo* assays. The use of individual allergens proved to be a valuable method compared to the total extracts. Moreover, different sensitization patterns in different apple-allergic patients' groups could be identified.

Keywords: recombinant allergens, apple, recognition pattern, allergy diagnosis

In industrialized countries the prevalence of allergies has significantly increased in the past decade [1, 2]. Allergic reactions to usually harmless proteins range from rhinitis, urticaria to asthma, diarrhea and even anaphylactic shock. In Europe apple allergy appears as two types: The pollen-fruit syndrome is common in areas where birch trees are growing and generally expressed in mild symptoms [3]. The second type is the food allergy against apples and related fruits such as peach and plum typical for Southern Europe and generally shows more severe reactivity [4]. The aim of the present study was to identify the allergen recognition patterns among a considerable number of apple-allergic patients derived from different geographical locations across Europe. Therefore individual, purified, natural and recombi- nant apple allergens (Mal d 1–Mal d 4) were used in various *in vitro* as well as *in vivo* assays.

Materials and Methods

Purified Apple Allergens

Mal d 1

The major birch pollen homolog, Mal d 1 (17 kDa; [5]), belongs to the group of pathogenesis related proteins (PR-proteins), family 10. The natural protein was purified from total protein extracts by immunoaffinity chromatography.

Recombinant Mal d 1 (EMBL Genbank database Access. no: AJ417551) was ex-

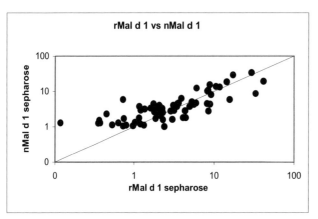

Figure 1. RAST data performed with purified natural Mal d 1 compared with purified recombinant Mal d 1.

pressed in *E. coli* and purified to homogeneity by anion exchange chromatography followed by hydrophobic interaction chromatography resulting in 80 mg purified recombinant Mal d 1 per liter culture.

Mal d 2

The thaumatin-like protein from apple is a member of family 5 of the PR-proteins [6]. Members of this protein family contain highly conserved cysteine residues (16) which form eight disulfide bridges. The recombinant protein (23 kDa) was transiently expressed in *Benthamiana tabacum* plants [7]. The heterologous protein was purified from leaf protein extracts by immunoaffinity chromatography.

Mal d 3

The nonspecific lipid transfer protein (ns LTP) is a member of another family (14) of plant PR-proteins [8]. Mal d 3 is a small protein (9 kDa) with a highly conserved structure (four disulfide bridges). Recombinant Mal d 3 was expressed in *Pichia pastoris* and purified as preprotein as well as mature protein by chromatographical methods.

Mal d 4

Apple profilin (13 kDa) is an actin-associated protein with allergenic properties [9]. The recombinant protein (EMBL Genbank access. No: AJ507459) was expressed in *E. coli* and purified by a single purification step on a poly-L-proline-sepharose column. Approximately

80 mg of pure allergen per liter of culture were obtained.

RAST

Purified apple allergens were coupled to CNBr-activated Sepharose (100 μg/100 mg, Amersham, Pharmacia Biotech, Uppsala, Sweden). Serum samples (50 μl per test) were incubated overnight with 0.5 mg Sepharose in a final volume of 300 μl PBS/0.3% BSA/0.1% Tween-20). After a washing step, Sepharose was incubated with ^{125}I-labeled sheep antibodies directed to human IgE (Sanquin, Amsterdam, The Netherlands) in 800 μl PBS-AT. After overnight incubation and washing, bound radioactivity was measured in a γ-counter (Figure 1).

Recruitment of Apple-Allergic Patients

Apple-allergic patients (n ~100 per center) were recruited according to standardized questionnaire, positive case history, positive RAST and SPT in four different clinical centers from Central and Southern Europe (Austria, Italy, The Netherlands, Spain).

Skin Prick Test (SPT)

SPTs were performed in apple allergic patients on the flexor surface of the forearm with fresh fruits (e.g., apple: Golden Delicious; peach), commercial pollen extracts (e.g., birch pollen

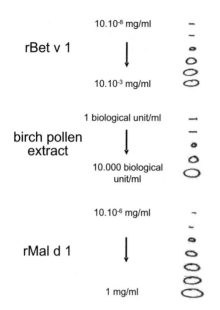

rBet v 1
10.10⁻⁸ mg/ml
10.10⁻³ mg/ml

birch pollen extract
1 biological unit/ml
10.000 biological unit/ml

rMal d 1
10.10⁻⁶ mg/ml
1 mg/ml

Figure 2. Skin prick tests: Titration of birch pollen extract, purified recombinant Bet v 1 (purchased by Biomay Comp, Austria) and purified recombinant Mal d 1.

extract), and purified recombinant allergens (rMal d 1 and rBet v 1). The SPT reactivity was measured after 15 min by copying the wheal reaction with transparent adhesive tape on to a record sheet for later comparison (Figure 2).

Results and Conclusions

Diagnostic tests for food allergy, particularly for fruit allergy, frequently have poor sensitivity and specificity [10]. Commercial skin test extracts for fruits usually have sensitivities under 50% due to ongoing endogenous enzymatic activity. For this reason most clinicians use the prick-to-prick method with fresh fruits for skin testing. Extracts for *in vitro* tests can be protected from enzymatic attack by addition of inhibitors that are not compatible with *in vivo* use. Therefore, the use of well-characterized purified individual allergens seems to be the method of choice. Purified allergens are protected against enzymatic attack and potentially facilitate distinction between clinically relevant and irrelevant IgE responses when used in various *in vitro* and *in vivo* assays. Their use in the diagnosis of food allergy can also help

elucidate the origins of sensitization. A considerable number of apple-allergic patients from Central and Southern Europe were tested for their IgE reactivity toward the four identified apple allergens Mal d 1, Mal d 2, Mal d 3, and Mal d 4. The allergenic potential of the individual apple allergens was found to be distinctly different: Mal d 1, Mal d 2, and Mal d 4-IgE reactivity was generally linked with mild allergic symptomatology – in contrast to Mal d 3-IgE recognition linked with severe symptomatology. In this study purified recombinant allergens were compared to purified natural allergens and proved to be valuable diagnostic tools identifying different sensitization patterns within a representative number of apple-allergic patients.

Acknowledgments

This work was sponsored by Grant from the EC Project: *SAFE, QLK1-CT-2000–01394*.

References

1. Worldwide variation in prevalence of symptoms of asthma, allergic rhinoconjunctivitis, and atopic eczema: ISAAC. The International Study of Asthma and Allergies in Childhood (ISAAC) Steering Committee. Lancet 1998; 351:1225–1232.

2. Grundy J, Matthews S, Bateman B, Dean T, Arshad SH: Rising prevalence of allergy to peanut in children: Data from two sequential cohorts. J Allergy Clin Immunol 2002; 110:784–789.

3. Van Ree R: The oral allergy syndrome. In S Amin, A Lahti, H Maibach (Eds.), Contact Urticaria Syndrome (pp. 289–299). Boca Raton: CRC Press 1997.

4. Fernandez-Rivas M, van Ree R, Cuevas M: Allergy to Rosaceae fruits without related pollinosis. J Allergy Clin Immunol 1997; 100:728–733.

5. Vanek-Krebitz M, Hoffmann-Sommergruber K, Laimer da Camara Machado M, et al.: Cloning and sequencing of Mal d 1, the major allergen from apple (*Malus domestica*), and its immunological relationship to Bet v 1, the major birch pollen allergen. Biochem Biophys Res Commun 1995; 214:538–551.

6. Hsieh LS, Moos M, Jr., Lin Y: Characterization of apple 18 and 31 kd allergens by microsequencing and evaluation of their content during

storage and ripening. J Allergy Clin Immunol 1995; 96:960–970.

7. Krebitz M, Wagner B, Ferreira F, et al.: Plant-based heterologous expression of Mal d 2, a thaumatin-like protein and allergen of apple (*Malus domestica*), and its characterization as an antifungal protein. J Mol Biol 2003; 329:721–730.

8. Garcia-Selles FJ, Diaz-Perales A, Sanchez-Monge R, et al.: Patterns of reactivity to lipid transfer proteins of plant foods and Artemisia pollen: an *in vivo* study. Int Arch Allergy Immunol 2002; 128:115–122.

9. Ebner C, Hirschwehr R, Bauer L, et al.: Identification of allergens in fruits and vegetables: IgE cross-reactivities with the important birch pollen allergens Bet v 1 and Bet v 2 (birch profilin). J Allergy Clin Immunol 1995; 95:962–969.

10. van Ree R, Akkerdaas J, van Leeuwen A: New perspectives for the diagnosis of food allergy. Allergy Clin Immunol Int 2000; 12:7–12.

Karin Hoffmann-Sommergruber

Department of Pathophysiology, Medical University of Vienna, AKH; EBO-3Q, Waehringer Guertel 18–20, A-1090 Vienna, Austria, Tel. +43 1 40400-5132, Fax +43 1 40400-5130, E-mail Karin.Hoffmann-Sommergruber@meduniwien.ac.at

Intracellular Targeting

A New Concept for the Development of Efficient Vaccines

R. Crameri[1], G. Schnetzler[2], I. Daigle[1], T. Kündig[2], and S. Flückiger[1]

[1]*Swiss Institute of Allergy and Asthma Research (SIAF), Davos, Switzerland*
[2]*University Hospital of Zürich, Zürich, Switzerland*

Summary: Current therapies for allergic diseases are usually not causative and merely treat the allergic symptoms with blockers of histamine, leukotrienes, or immunosuppressive agents. It would, however, be important to treat the underlying cause of allergy since common sensitization to environmental allergens may, over time, develop into life-threatening asthma. Allergen desensitization is the only curative therapy for allergy aiming to treat the underlying causes of the disease by modulation of the immune response. It is generally accepted that changing the allergen-specific immune response from a type 2 to a type 1 T-helper cell response, as well as the induction of protective IgG antibodies, are beneficial for the desensitization process. Although reasonably effective in many cases, allergen-specific immunotherapy suffers from bad compliance as a result of a long treatment period requiring 40 or more doctor's visits. Here we introduce the concept of modular antigen translocation molecules (MAT), which harnesses the optimization of antigen presentation by the MHC class II pathway through translocation of engineered molecules into the cytoplasm and subsequent targeting to the endoplasmic reticulum. The two mechanisms, translocation and intracellular targeting, lead to efficient uptake and presentation of exogenous proteins. Consequently, immunization with MAT should lead to preferential induction of type 1 T-helper cell responses.

Keywords: allergy, allergens, vaccine, immunotherapy, T-helper cell responses, modular antigen translocation molecules

According to present knowledge, antigens entering the body are taken up and processed by antigen presenting cells (APC) depending on the route of entry [1]. CD4+ T-cells recognize peptides bound to MHC class-II molecules on the surface of APC. Assembly of the α and β chains of MHC class-II complexes and their association with the invariant chain (Ii) begins in the endoplasmic reticulum (ER). The functional domains of Ii include a N-terminal cytoplasmic domain, a domain that occupies the peptide-binding groove of the MHC class-II complex, and a C-terminal trimerization motif. Ii is translocated into the ER where trimerization occurs, followed by association with the MHC class-II complex. Ii protected MHC class-II complexes are directed to lysosomes where the Ii chains are degraded, the complex loaded with antigenic peptides and directed to the APC surface [2]. A factor strongly affecting the development of type 1 versus type 2 T-helper cell response is the efficiency of antigen presentation. The more peptides presented, the more type 1 T-helper cells are induced [3]. Our approach to increasing MHC class-II-mediated antigen presentation was to generate MAT. MAT consists of a $[His]_6$ purification tag, an arginine rich peptide for protein delivery into cells [4], the Ii N-terminal domain, and a multiple cloning site allowing accommodation of any antigen. The Ii domain should assist specific targeting of cytoplasmatically delivered fusions to the ER through heterotrimerization with endogenous Ii. Incorporation of Ii-antigen fusions into MHC class-II complexes, thereafter selectively transported to lysosomes where antigen loading of MHC complexes with degraded antigen fragments occurs, should result in an increased presentation of selected antigen fragments on the APC surface. A combination of purification tag, translocation peptide, and the relevant domain of the Ii chain allows fast generation of pure fusion proteins easily convertible to cytoplasmic proteins by simple addition to cell cultures. The Ii N-terminal domain should potentially assist specific targeting of cytoplasmatically translocated fusion proteins to the endoplasmatic reticulum where MHC class II molecules are assembled. The assembly of Ii heterotrimers enhances the chance of the Ii-antigen fusion to be incorporated into the MHC class- II complex and, thus, to be selectively transported to lysosomes where antigen loading of the MHC complex with degraded antigen fragments occurs. Therefore, an increased presentation of the Ii fusion antigen in the MHC class-II context can be expected. We evaluated the utility of MAT in T-cell proliferation experiments using PBMC's isolated from allergic individuals by addition of different MAT fusions including Bet v 1, the major allergen of birch [5]; Der p 1, the major allergen of house dust mite [6]; and PLA_2 the major allergen of bee venom [7]. In all cases a stronger T-cell proliferation at 10–100 × lower antigen concentrations than the proliferation obtained with recombinant allergens was obtained, whereas control experiments with PBMC isolated from healthy individuals showed background proliferation. Immunization of CJ/2B mice with MAT-PLA_2 fusions showed a complete suppression of the IgE production paralleled with an increased production of IgG2a at concentrations where recombinant PLA_2 induces strong IgE responses. We conclude that MAT molecules represent potent allergy vaccines devoid of side effects because MAT proteins are produced as unfolded molecules and, thus, show a reduced IgE-binding capacity [8].

References

1. Lanzavecchia A: Mechanisms of antigen uptake for presentation. Curr Opin Immunol 1996; 8:348–354.
2. Pieters J: MHC class II-restricted antigen processing and presentation. Adv Immunol 2000; 75: 159–208.
3. Secrist H, DeKruyff RH, Umetsu DT: IL-4 production by CD4+ T-cells from allergic individuals is modulated by antigen concentration and antigen presenting cell type. J Exp Med 1995; 181: 1081–1089.
4. Morris MC, Depollier J, Mery J, Heitz F, Divita G: A peptide carrier for the delivery of biologically active proteins into mammalian cells. Nat Biotechnol 2001; 19:1173–1176.
5. Breiteneder H, Pettenburger K, Bito A, Valenta R, Kraft D, Rumpold H, Scheiner O, Breitenbach M: The gene coding for the major birch pollen allergen Bet v 1 is highly homologous to a pea disease resistance response gene. EMBO J 1989; 7:1935–1938.
6. Chua KY, Stewart GA, Thomas WR, Simpson RJ, Dilworth RJ, Plozza TM, Turner KJ: Sequence analysis of cDNA coding for a major house dust mite allergen Der p 1. Homology with cysteine proteases. J Exp Med 1988; 167:175–182.
7. Dudler T, Chen WQ, Wang S, Schneider T, Annand RR, Dempcy RO, Crameri R, Gmachl M, Suter M, Gelb MH: High-level expression in *Escherichia coli* and rapid purification of enzymatically active honey bee venom phospholipase A2. Biochim Biophys Acta 1992; 1005:201–210.
8. Crameri R: Correlating IgE reactivity with three-dimensional structure. Biochem J 2003; 376:e1–2.

Reto Crameri

Head Molecular Allergology, Swiss Institute of Allergy and Asthma Research (SIAF), Obere Strasse 22, CH-7270 Davos, Switzerland, Tel. +41 81 410 08 48, Fax +41 81 410 08 40, E-mail crameri@siaf.unizh.ch

The Molecular Requirements for Allergenicity

E. Jensen-Jarolim[1], E. Untersmayr[1], B. Hantusch[1], N. Kalkura[2], C. Betzel[2], W. Keller[3], S. Spitzauer[4], O. Scheiner[1], G. Boltz-Nitulescu[1], I. Schöll[1]

[1]Center of Physiology and Pathophysiology, Medical University of Vienna, Austria, [2]Dept. of Med. Biochemistry and Molecular Biology, University Clinics Hamburg-Eppendorf, Germany, [3]Dept. of Physical Chemistry, Karl-Franzens University, Graz, Austria, [4]Dept. of Clinical Chemistry and Laboratory Medicine, Medical University of Vienna, Austria

Summary: *Background:* The triggering phenomenon of FcεRI-bound IgE is today explained by multimeric allergens exposing several epitopes for crosslinking. The number of available epitopes on small allergens may, however, be limited to even a single epitope. We investigated whether di- or oligomerization could explain the crosslinking capability of allergens. *Methods:* Screening the literature we found that the number of reports on allergen dimers and higher oligomers is steadily increasing. We selected the major birch pollen allergen Bet v 1 as a model and analyzed it for the presence of di- or multimers in solid phase assays and in solution. *Results:* In our hands, this allergen represented a monomer only in rare experimental conditions, e.g., close to neutral pH and under the addition of glycerol. In this setting, it also did not elicit histamine release. *Conclusion:* From our data we conclude that allergens may acquire crosslinking capability upon dimerization. This opens a new perspective on common features of allergenic molecules.

Keywords: Bet v 1, allergens, crosslinking, IgE, dimer, oligomers

The question whether allergens have common features affects their potency to sensitize as well as their capacity to elicit an allergic response. We suggest that prerequisites of allergenic molecules are (1) conformational epitopes for IgE induction and triggering, and (2) effective presentation of epitopes for IgE crosslinking in a repetitive or multivalent fashion. Allergens possess conformational IgE epitopes that may even be of the discontinuous type, as revealed by our recent mimotope studies [1, 2] and crystallization experiments of other groups [3, 4]. Such conformational epitopes may be a precondition for primary IgE induction, whereas linear epitopes are targets of an antibody response after repetitive antigen exposure, such as in persistent milk and egg allergy [5, 6], hyposensitization therapy [7], or

during the production of monoclonal antibodies in animals [8, 9]. For example, a dietary protein is only able to sensitize and lead to IgE production when its B-cell epitopes are stabilized [10] or when they persist in the gastric transit [11, 12]. It is also a consideration that at least two allergen epitopes of the same type are needed to cross-link B-cell receptors, as the individual B-lymphocyte exposes membrane-bound immunoglobulins of a single specificity. Therefore, presentation of conformational epitopes in a repetitive manner is required for cross-linking and receptor aggregation before antibody production can occur. On the other hand, the effector phase of type I allergy is also dependent on the cross-linking of IgE that is passively bound to high affinity IgE receptors (FcεRI) on effector cells. To explain

Table 1. The number of reports on allergens forming dimers, trimers and oligomers is steadily increasing.

ABA 1	McGibbon et al. Mol Biochem Parasitol. 39: 163.	1990
Tropomyosin	Gimona et al. PNAS 92: 9776 .	1995
Phl p 1	Petersen et al. in: Progr. Allergy Clin Imm, 4: 139.	1997
Ara h 1	Shin et al. JBC 273: 13753.	1998
Tropomyosin	Reese et al. IAAI 119: 247.	1999
Equ c 1	Gregoire et al. Acta Cryst D Biol Cryst 55: 880.	1999
Equ c 1	Lascombe et al. JBC 275: 21572.	2000
ABA-1	Xia et al. Parasitology 120: 211.	2000
Ara h 1	Maleki et al. JI 164: 5844.	2000
Ves v 5	Suck et al. IAAI 121: 284.	2000
Profilin	Wopfner et al. Biol Chem. 383:1779–89	2002
Parvalbumin	Das Dores et al. Allergy 57, Suppl 72: 79;	2002
Ara h 2	Sen et al. JI 169: 882.	2002
Phl p 5b	Rajashankar et al. Acta Cryst D Biol Cryst 58: 1175;	2002
Phl p 7	Verdino et al. EMBO J 21: 5007.	2002
Fel d 1	Grönlund et al. J. Biol Chem 278 (41): 40144.	2003
Bet v 1	Schöll et al. (unpublished data)	2004

this mechanism, allergens in text books are routinely illustrated as multimeric oversized molecules, offering a panel of epitopes for interaction with IgE. In reality, IgE does by far exceed the size of allergens, making effective cross-linking less plausible. Moreover, some allergens are so small that they expose only single epitopes. Independent researchers (including ourselves) have claimed single predominant IgE epitopes of Bet v 1, the major birch pollen allergen, without discussing the impact of these findings on our understanding of IgE cross-linking [1, 4]. Interestingly, when we screened the literature we found several recent reports on repetitive epitopes on allergens (shrimp tropomyosin [13], Hev b 5 [14], Bla g 1 [15]) and an increasing number of studies reporting allergen dimers or higher oligomers (Table 1). This was our rational to investigate if our model allergen Bet v 1 possibly acquires cross-linking capacity because it forms di- or multimers.

Materials and Methods

Recombinant Bet v 1 was analyzed at a protein concentration of 4 mg/ml by dynamic light scattering (DLS) in a Spectroscatter 201 (RiNA GmbH, Berlin, Germany) at wavelength 680 nm. Samples were adjusted to different pH by mixing with 50 mM Tris-HCl, and were tested with or without addition of 4% glycerol. BALB/c mice were sensitized with rBet v 1 (permission number GZ 66.009/211-Pr/4/2001 of the Austrian Ministry of Science). For skin tests, mice were injected with Evans Blue and tested intradermally with compound 48/80, PBS, monomeric rBet v 1 (3 µg/ml Tris-HCl, pH. 6.2 + 4% glycerol), or dimeric rBet v 1 (3 µg/ml PBS).

Results

We found that birch pollen allergen Bet v 1 forms monomers, dimers, and oligomers not only in solid phase assays (SDS-PAGE and immunoblotting), but also in solution (dynamic light scattering analysis). However, using glycerol and nearly neutral pH (pH. 6.2) rendered a sole monomeric peak in these investigations. The cross-linking capacity of the different Bet v 1 samples was examined in a biological system. BALB/c mice were sensitized by intraperitoneal immunizations using rBet v 1 and

Al(OH)$_3$ as Th2-promoting adjuvants. These sensitized mice were then subjected to type I skin tests using Bet v 1 dimer, or the monomer in glycerol buffer, pH. 6.2. This experiment proved that only the dimeric allergen was capable of cross-linking cell bound IgE and, thus, leading to histamine release.

Discussion

Our data support the concept that Bet v 1 harbors a single IgE epitope. For these reasons, *in vivo* cross-linking of IgE can only be achieved when Bet v 1 forms at least dimers. In several experimental conditions, Bet v 1 indeed appeared as dimers and higher oligomers, and we found it difficult to achieve a Bet v 1 monomer. However, a condition (glycerol, pH. 6.2) could be defined where this allergen behaved as a monomer and did not show cross-linking capacity. Facing the fact that many allergens are very small molecules and that IgE has a relatively low flexibility caused by the absence of a hinge region, the concept of multimerization could make the cross-linking event much more plausible. Some authors have suggested that allergens may expose repetitive epitopes, such as shrimp tropomyosin, cockroach allergen Bla g 1 and latex allergen Hev b 5 [13–15]. Effective cross-linking of the B-cell receptor as well as of FcεRI-bound IgE are thereby facilitated. Similarly, multimerization of allergens would allow the presentation of identical epitopes in a repetitive manner. Evidence has been accumulating during recent years on important allergens representing di- or multimers (Table 1). In this study, we add the birch pollen allergen Bet v 1 to this list. We suggest that the presentation of several identical IgE epitopes might be a common feature of allergens, which explains their effectiveness in eliciting allergic symptoms. It is suggestive that the same features are preconditions for B-cell activation and IgE production in the sensitization phase.

Acknowledgments

This study was supported by grant SFB F01808–B04 of the Austrian Science Funds, and in part by SFB F018–04 and SFB F018–05.

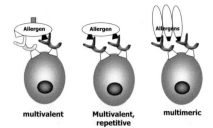

Figure 1. The triggering event of allergy effector cells is dependent on the crosslinking of FcεRI-bound IgE through allergens. Today mostly the concept of multivalent allergens is used to explain the crosslinking capability of these molecules. This is often illustrated by overdimensioned allergens exposing several IgE epitopes, which are then recognized by IgE antibodies harboring diverse epitope specificities (left panel). Some studies suggest that allergens may be multivalent, but expose similar epitopes in a repetitive manner (middle panel). There is increasing evidence that many allergens represent dimers or even higher oligomers (right drawing). This feature would facilitate crosslinking also in situations when the allergen is much smaller than IgE.

References

1. Ganglberger E, Grunberger K, Sponer B, Radauer C, Breiteneder H, Boltz-Nitulescu G, Scheiner O, Jensen-Jarolim E: Allergen mimotopes for 3-dimensional epitope search and induction of antibodies inhibiting human IgE. FASEB J 2000; 14:2177–2184.
2. Hantusch B, Krieger S, Untersmayr E, Schöll I, Knittelfelder R, Flicker S, Spitzauer S, Valenta R, Boluda L, Schweitzer-Stenner R, Jensen-Jarolim E: Mapping of conformational IgE-epitopes on Phl p 5 using mimotopes from a phage display library. J Allergy Clin Immunol 2004, in press.
3. Mirza O, Henriksen A, Ipsen H, Larsen JN, Wissenbach M, Spangfort MD, Gajhede M: Dominant epitopes and allergic cross-reactivity: complex formation between a Fab fragment of a monoclonal murine IgG antibody and the major allergen from birch pollen Bet v 1. J Immunol 2000; 165:331–338.
4. Spangfort MD, Mirza O, Ipsen H, Van Neerven RJ, Gajhede M, Larsen JN: Dominating IgE-binding epitope of Bet v 1, the major allergen of birch pollen, characterized by X-ray crystallography and site-directed mutagenesis. J Immunol 2003; 171:3084–3090.
5. Jarvinen KM, Chatchatee P, Bardina L, Beyer K, Sampson HA: IgE and IgG binding epitopes on

α-lactalbumin and β-lactoglobulin in cow's milk allergy. Int Arch Allergy Immunol 2001; 126: 111–118.

6. Cooke SK, Sampson HA: Allergenic properties of ovomucoid in man. J Immunol 1997; 159: 2026–2032.

7. Ball T, Sperr WR, Valent P, Lidholm J, Spitzauer S, Ebner C, Kraft D, Valenta R: Induction of antibody responses to new B-cell epitopes indicates vaccination character of allergen immunotherapy. Eur J Immunol 1999; 29:2026–2036.

8. Furmonaviciene R, Tighe PJ, Clark MR, Sewell HF, Shakib F: The use of phage-peptide libraries to define the epitope specificity of a mouse monoclonal anti-Der p 1 antibody representative of a major component of the human immunoglobulin E anti-Der p 1 response. Clin Exp Allergy 1999; 29:1563–1571.

9. Jensen-Jarolim E, Leitner A, Kalchhauser H, Zurcher A, Ganglberger E, Bohle B, Scheiner O, Boltz-Nitulescu G, Breiteneder H: Peptide mimotopes displayed by phage inhibit antibody binding to Bet v 1, the major birch pollen allergen, and induce specific IgG response in mice. FASEB J 1998; 12:1635–1642.

10. Jensen-Jarolim E, Wiedermann U, Ganglberger E, Zurcher A, Stadler BM, Boltz-Nitulescu G, Scheiner O, Breiteneder H: Allergen mimotopes in food enhance type I allergic reactions in mice. FASEB J 1999; 13:1586–1592.

11. Schöll I, Untersmayr E, Bakos N, Walter F, Boltz-Nitulescu G, Scheiner O, Jensen-Jarolim E: Anti-ulcer drugs promote oral sensitization and hypersensitivity to hazelnut allergens in BALB/c mice and humans. Am J Clin Nutr 2004, in press.

12. Untersmayr E, Scholl I, Swoboda I, Beil WJ, Forster-Waldl E, Walter F, Riemer A, Kraml G, Kinaciyan T, Spitzauer S, Boltz-Nitulescu G, Scheiner O, Jensen-Jarolim E: Antacid medication inhibits digestion of dietary proteins and causes food allergy: a fish allergy model in BALB/c mice. J Allergy Clin Immunol 2003; 112:616–623.

13. Ayuso R, Lehrer SB, Reese G: Identification of continuous, allergenic regions of the major shrimp allergen Pen a 1 (tropomyosin). Int Arch Allergy Immunol 2002; 127:27–37.

14. Beezhold DH, Hickey VL, Sutherland MF, O'Hehir RE: The latex allergen hev B 5 is an antigen with repetitive murine B-cell epitopes. Int Arch Allergy Immunol 2004; 134:334–340.

15. Pomes A, Vailes LD, Helm RM, Chapman MD: IgE reactivity of tandem repeats derived from cockroach allergen, Bla g 1. Eur J Biochem 2002; 269:3086–3092.

Erika Jensen-Jarolim

Center of Physiology and Pathophysiology, Medical University of Vienna, AKH, EBO 3Q, Waehringer Guertel 18–20, 1090 Vienna, Austria, Tel. +43 1 40400 5103, Fax +43 1 40400 5130, E-mail erika.jensen-jarolim@meduniwien.ac.at, www.allergology.at

Peroxisome Proliferator-Activated Receptor γ Ligands Have Antiviral and Anti-Inflammatory Activity

in the Course of Respiratory Syncytial Virus Infection

R. Arnold and W. König

Institute of Medical Microbiology, Otto von Guericke University, Magdeburg, Germany

Summary: *Background:* Respiratory syncytial virus (RSV) is worldwide the major causative agent of severe lower respiratory tract disease and death in infants. In the course of RSV-induced bronchiolitis and pneumonia overwhelming inflammatory host responses as well as direct viral cytopathic effects are responsible for the disease. Currently, there exists no effective vaccine or promising antiviral therapy. Therefore, to evolve new therapeutic strategies is a most important task. Evidence has been accumulated that activation of the peroxisome proliferator-activated receptor-γ (PPAR-γ) leads to anti-inflammatory cell responses. *Methods:* By means of FACS analysis and ELISA, in an *in vitro* infection model, we analyzed proinflammatory cell responses of RSV-infected human lung epithelial cells (A549) that were cultured in the presence of PPAR-γ agonists (ciglitazone, troglitazone, 15d-PGJ$_2$, FmocLeu) or medium alone. In addition, the replication of RSV was determined by FACS analysis. *Results:* Because A549 cells were pretreated with PPAR-γ agonists we observed a significantly reduced cell surface expression of ICAM-1 on RSV-infected A549 cells. Furthermore, the release of chemokines (IL-8, RANTES) as well as the replication of RSV was inhibited. *Conclusions:* Our data suggest that PPAR-γ agonists are able to inhibit the replication of RSV in human lung epithelial cells and to reduce significantly the detrimental inflammatory response induced by RSV-infection.

Keywords: ICAM-1, RANTES, IL-8, inflammation, RSV, PPAR-γ

The infection of the lung epithelial cell, the primary target for RSV, induces an overwhelming inflammatory response resulting in a prominent recruitment of inflammatory effector cells into the infected lung [1]. Especially, the increased cell surface expression of ICAM-1 as well as the prominent release of IL-8 from RSV-infected epithelial cells are early important proinflammatory cell responses of the innate immune response [2,3]. It was reported that following activation of the PPAR-γ epithelial cells show a reduced inflammatory response [4,5]. PPARs are ligand-activated transcription factors, which form a subfamily of the nuclear receptor gene family consisting of three isotypes: PPAR-α, PPAR-β, and PPAR-γ [6]. Moreover, HIV-1 replication in human macrophages was significantly impaired by PPAR-γ activators [7]. Therefore, we hypothesized that the inflammatory response induced

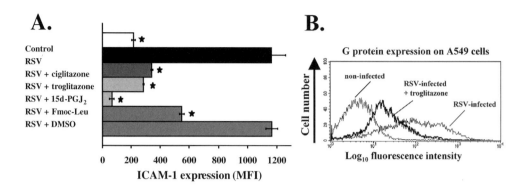

Figure 1. (A) Effect of PPAR-γ agonists on RSV-induced ICAM-1 cell surface expression of RSV-infected A549 cells. Results are means ± SEM (*n* = 3); *, *p* < 0.01 vs. RSV-infected cells. (B) Virus G protein expression on RSV-infected A549 cells cultured in medium alone or with troglitazone (20 μM) for 36 h. Results are representative of multiple experiments.

by RSV-infection and the replication of the virus might be influenced by the activation of PPAR-γ.

Material and Methods

Cell monolayers of the human pulmonary type II epithelial cell line A549 (ATCC) were pretreated for 30 min with ciglitazone (50 μM), troglitazone (50 μM), Fmoc-Leu (100 μM; Merck Biosciences), 15-deoxy-$\Delta^{12,14}$-prostaglandin J_2 (15d-PGJ$_2$; 20 μM; Biomol), and solvent (DMSO; 0.1%; Sigma), respectively. Thereafter, cells were infected with RSV (long strain, ATCC) at a multiplicity of infection (moi) of 3 for 2 h, washed, and then incubated with fresh medium (DMEM, 2% FCS; streptomycin, 100 μg/ml; penicillin, 100 IU/ml) in the presence of the substances until 36 h postinfection. No significant cell death (< 5%) occurred in any of the tested conditions. The cells were stained with PE-labeled mouse anti-human ICAM-1 mAb (clone: HA58, BD Biosciences) and mouse anti-RSV G protein mAb (clone: 131/G2) (Biotrend) plus Cy3-labeled AffiniPure goat anti-mouse IgG (H + L) (Dianova), respectively. Release of chemokines into the cell supernatant was determined by means of ELISAs specific for IL-8 and RANTES (R&D Systems, Wiesbaden, Germany), respectively.

Results and Discussion

As shown in Figure 1A, the RSV-infection of A549 cells increased the constitutive ICAM-1 expression in a significant manner. Cells infected and cultured in the presence of the PPAR-γ agonists ciglitazone, troglitazone, 15d-PGJ$_2$, and Fmoc-Leu, respectively, showed a significantly reduced expression of ICAM-1. For control, RSV-infected cells were incubated with DMSO alone, which was used as solvent for the PPAR-γ agonists (0.1%).

To further investigate the anti-inflammatory potential of PPAR-γ agonists in the course of primary RSV infection, we analyzed the release of the proinflammatory chemokine IL-8 and RANTES from RSV-infected cells cultured in the presence of PPAR-γ agonists. Our data show that the release of both chemokines was markedly diminished when cells were cultured in the presence of the above-mentioned agonists (data not shown).

Next, we asked whether PPAR-γ agonists might possess some inherent antiviral activity. For this purpose, the amount of virus G protein expressed on RSV-infected A549 was determined. We observed that the expression of virus G protein on RSV-infected cells was markedly reduced when cells were exposed to the thiazolidinediones ciglitazone and troglitazone. For example, Figure 1B shows a representative fluorescence histogram overlay of G protein expression on RSV-infected cells cultured in the presence of troglitazone or medium alone.

Our *in vitro* data presented herein supply evidence that PPAR-γ agonists are able to reduce detrimental inflammatory epithelial cell responses, i.e., the increased expression of ICAM-1 as well as the release of IL-8 and RANTES. The synthesis of high amounts of IL-8 seems to be responsible for the selective recruitment of neutrophils into the alveolar spaces of the RSV-infected lung [8]. Thereafter, recruited neutrophils contribute to the overwhelming inflammatory process by the release of their cytotoxic granular content [9]. Furthermore, the enhanced adherence of neutrophils to RSV-infected epithelial cells mediated by their increased ICAM-1 expression is responsible for the increased epithelial cell death observed in the RSV-infected lung [10].

Besides the reduction of these proinflammatory epithelial cell responses we also observed an antiviral activity of PPAR-γ agonists in our *in vitro* RSV infection model. The reduced expression of virus G protein in the plasma membrane of the infected lung epithelial cell suggests that PPAR-γ agonists, i.e., thiazolidinediones, interfere with the synthesis of virus proteins. Thus, PPAR-γ agonists may play an important role in controlling RSV-infection in human lung epithelial cells.

References

1. Aherne W, Bird T, Court S, Gardner P, McQuillin J: Pathological changes in virus infections of the lower respiratory tract in children. J Clin Pathol 1970; 23:7–18.
2. Arnold R, König W: ICAM-1 expression and low molecular weight G protein activation of human bronchial epithelial cells (A549) infected with RSV. J Leukoc Biol 1996; 60:766–771.
3. Arnold R, Humbert B, Werchau H, Gallati H, König W: Interleukin-8, interleukin-6, and soluble tumor necrosis factor receptor type I release from a human pulmonary epithelial cell line (A549) exposed to respiratory syncytial virus. Immunol 1994; 82:126–133.
4. Wang ACC, Dai X, Luu B, Conrad DJ: Peroxisome proliferator-activated receptor-γ regulates airway epithelial cell activation. Am J Respir Cell Mol Biol 2001; 24:688–693.
5. Su CG, Wen X, Bailey ST, Jiang W, Rangwala SM, Keilbaugh SA, Flanigan A, Murthy S, Lazar MA, Wu GD: A novel therapy for colitis utilizing PPAR-γ ligands to inhibit the epithelial inflammatory response. J Clin Invest 1999; 104:383–389.
6. Daynes RA, Jones DJ: Emerging roles of PPARs in inflammation and immunity. Nat Rev 2002; 2:748–759.
7. Hayes MM, Lane BR, King SR, Markowitz DM, Coffey MJ: Peroxisome proliferator-activated receptor γ agonists inhibit HIV-1 replication in macrophages by transcriptional and postranscriptional effects. J Biol Chem 2002; 277:16913–16919.
8. Everard ML, Awarbrick A, Wrightham M, McIntyre J, Dunkley C, James PD, Sewell HF, Milner AD: Analysis of cells obtained by bronchial lavage of infants with respiratory syncytial virus infection. Arch Dis Childhood 1994; 71:428–432.
9. Jaovisidha P, Peeples ME, Brees AA, Carpenter LR, Moy JN: Respiratory syncytial virus stimulates neutrophil degranulation and chemokine release. J Immunol 1999; 163:2816–2820.
10. Wang SZ, Xu H, Wraith A, Bowden JJ, Alpers JH, Forsyth KD: Neutrophils induce damage to respiratory epithelial cells infected with respiratory syncytial virus. Eur Respir J 1998; 12:612–618.

Wolfgang König

Otto von Guericke University, Institute of Medical Microbiology, Leipzigerstr. 44, D-39120 Magdeburg, Germany, Tel. +49 391 671-3393, Fax +49 391 671-3384, E-mail wolfgang.koenig@medizin.uni-magdeburg.de

Differences in *Bifido-bacterium* Species in Early Infancy and the Development of Allergy

S. Suzuki[1], N. Shimojo[1], Y. Tajiri[2], M. Kumemura[2], and Y. Kohno[1]

[1]*Division of Allergy and Clinical Immunology, Department of Pediatrics, Graduate School of Medicine, Chiba University, Japan,* [2]*Otsuka Pharmaceutical Co., Ltd. Otsu Nutraceuticals Research Institute, Japan*

Summary: *Background: Bifidobacterium*, which is the most common intestinal bacterium in infancy, may be related to the development of allergic diseases. Differences of *Bifidobacterium* species between allergic and nonallergic infants have not been studied in Japan. *Methods:* We prospectively followed infants born at a local hospital in Chiba prefecture until 2 years of age. Allergy was determined on the basis of skin status and SPT at 6 months and 2 years of age. Feces at 6 months and 2 years of age were cultured by Mitsuoka's method. Feces at 1, 3, 6 months and 2 years of age were analyzed for *Bifidobacterium* species by 16S rDNA targeted 10 species-specific PCR primers. *Results:* Eighteen infants were studied. *Bifidobacterium* were detected in all infants regardless of allergic status at 6 months and 2 years of age. No differences in counts of *Bifidobacterium* genus, and distributions of *Bifidobacterium* species were observed between allergics and nonallergics when they were grouped according to their allergic status by 2 years of age. In contrast, when they were grouped based on allergic status by 6 months of age, prevalence of *B. bifidum* was higher in allergics than nonallergics at 3 and 6 months and this tendency remained at 2 years of age, and that of *B. adolescentis* was lower at 3 months of age. *Conclusions:* Some intestinal *Bifidobacterium* species may be related to the allergic status in infancy, but not in later life.

Keywords: infant, allergy, intestinal flora, *Bifidobacterium*

Increasing prevalence of allergic diseases is a worldwide issue. Recent studies show a close link between decreased microbial exposure in early life and higher risk of development of allergic diseases in later life. Altered intestinal environment is related to the pathogenesis of atopic dermatitis (AD) and it is shown that administration of probiotics improve the symptoms or reduce the risk of the development of AD.

The *Bifidobacterium* genus, which consists of over 30 species, is the most common component of intestinal flora in infancy and considered to be an important immunomodula-tor. Studies performed in northern European countries have demonstrated decreased prevalence of *Bifidobacterium* or colonization of different species of *Bifidobacterium* in allergic infants [1–3]. However, the number of epidemiological studies on intestinal flora in relation to development of allergic diseases is still limited, and so far no prospective study has been performed on the difference in *Bifidobacterium* species. Here we report a prospective study of intestinal flora in Japan including the *Bifidobacterium* species and the development of allergic diseases.

Materials and Methods

Subjects

Newborns delivered from May 2001 to January 2002 at a local hospital in Chiba prefecture were followed at 1, 3, 6 months and 2 years of age for health checks. At 6 months and 2 years of age, SPTs with egg white, cow's milk, wheat, house dust, and mite were performed. Infants were determined as allergics if they had been diagnosed as AD based on criteria by the Japanese Dermatological Association [4] or they had more than one positive result of SPTs, and infants without any allergic diseases and a positive result of SPTs were determined as nonallergics.

Bacteriologic Analysis

Feces at 6 months and 2 years of age were cultured by the method of Mitsuoka [5] within 24 h after samples were obtained. Feces at 1, 3, 6 months and 2 years of age were preserved at –80 °C and analyzed for detection of *Bifidobacterium* species by 16S rDNA targeted 10 species-specific primers reported by Matsuki et al. [6].

Ethical Considerations

Written informed consents were obtained from the mothers of the infants. The study was conducted in accordance with the spirit of the Helsinki Declaration.

Statistical Methods

The Fisher exact test was used to compare allergic and nonallergic infants with respect to the prevalence of colonization. The counts and percentage of total counts of cultured bacteria were compared by Mann-Whitney rank sum test.

Results and Discussion

Eighteen infants (8 males and 10 females) were followed until 2 years of age. Twelve infants (5 males and 7 females) were determined

as allergics by 2 years of age. There were no differences between allergics and nonallergics in numbers of siblings, family size, body weight at birth, and feeding patterns until 6 months of age.

Bifidobacterium were detected in all infants regardless of allergic status at 6 months and 2 years of age. This is in accord with recent studies in Japan, which showed that *Bifidobacterium* were detected in almost all infants at 4 months of age [7], and young patients with AD [8]. These data in Japan are in contrast with northern European studies, which indicated lower prevalence of *Bifidobacterium* in both allergics and nonallergics in the first year of life [1]. Differences in methods including preservation of samples and media used for culture, genetic background, intestinal flora of mothers, and food customs may explain the differences described.

We could not find any significant differences in counts and percentage of *Bifidobacterium* between allergics and nonallergics. These results are similar to one of the studies in the northern European countries [1]. The previous study in Japan reported that lower counts or an absence of *Bifidobacterium* were observed in young patients with severe AD [7]. One reason why we obtained similar counts of *Bifidobacterium* between allergics and nonallergics is that none of the allergics had severe AD in our study.

Bacteroides of allergics at 2 years of age were significantly higher in counts (10.11 ± 0.38 vs. 9.54 ± 0.51, $p = 0.044$) and in percentage ($40\% \pm 14\%$ vs. $22\% \pm 7.4\%$, $p = 0.0017$). Since this difference was not observed at 6 months of age, the amounts of *Bacteroides* may not be related to pathogenesis of allergic diseases in young infants. Rather, these data suggest altered intestinal flora in allergics.

Distributions of *Bifidobacterium* species were similar between allergics and nonallergics when subjects were grouped by 2 years of age. Interestingly, when subjects were grouped on the basis of allergic status by 6 months of age (allergics 9, nonallergics 9), prevalence of *B. bifidum* in allergics at 3 and 6 months of age was higher (57% vs. 11%, 78% vs. 22%, respectively) and this tendency remained at 2 years of age, and that of *B. adolescentis* at 3 months of age was lower (14% vs. 67%). These results indicate that these two *Bifidobacterium* species can affect allergic status in infancy, but not in later life. Our results conflict with that of Ouwehand et al. [3], which reported *B. bifidum* were isolated mainly from healthy infants whereas *B. adolescentis* were isolated mainly from allergic infants. They identified *Bifidobacterium* species on the basis of morphological and metabolic characteristics of the *Bifidobacterium* cultured in the classical method. We used species-specific primers to identify *Bifidobacterium* species, which more directly reflects actual intestinal flora. Although the result is opposite, our data suggest that *B.bifidum* and *B. adolescentis* are involved in the pathogenesis of allergic diseases in infancy.

References

1. Bjorksten B, Sepp E, Julge K, Voor T, Mikelsaar M: Allergy development and the intestinal microflora during the first year of life. J Allergy Clin Immunol 2001; 108:516–520.
2. Bjorksten B, Naaber P, Sepp E, Mikelsaar M: The intestinal microflora in allergic Estonian and Swedish 2-year-old infants. Clin Exp Allergy 1999; 29:342–346.
3. Ouwehand AC, Isolauri E, He F, Hashimoto H, Benno Y, Salminen S: Differences in Bifidobacterium flora composition in allergic and healthy infants. J Allergy Clin Immunol 2001; 108:144–145.
4. The Japanese Dermatological Association: Japanese Dermatological Association criteria for the diagnosis of atopic dermatitis. Jap J Dermatol 1996; 106:64–65.
5. Mitsuoka T: A color atlas of anaerobic bacteria. Tokyo, Sobunsya, 1980, p. 341.
6. Matsuki T, Watanabe K, Tanaka R, Fukuda M, Oyaizu H: Distribution of bifidobacterial species in human intestinal microflora examined with 16S rRNA-gene-targeted species-specific primers. Appl Environ Microbiol 1999; 65:4506–4512.
7. Nambu M, Shintaku N, Ohta S: Intestinal microflora at 4 months of age and the development of allergy. Allergology Int 2004; 53:121–126.
8. Watanabe S, Narisawa Y, Arase S, Okamatsu H, Ikenaga T, Tajiri Y, Kumemura M: Differences in fecal microflora between patients with atopic dermatitis and healthy control subjects. J Allergy Clin Immunol 2003; 111:587–591.

Shuichi Suzuki

1-8-1 Inohana, Chuo-ku, Chiba, Japan 260-8670, Tel +81 43 226-2144, Fax +81 43 226-2145, E-mail seeyou@msj.biglobe.ne.jp

Comparison of Expression and Function of Toll-Like Receptors in Eosinophils and Neutrophils

H. Nagase[1], S. Okugawa[2], Y. Ota[2], M. Yamaguchi[3], K. Matsushima[4], K. Yamamoto[3], K. Ohta[1], and K. Hirai[5]

[1]Department of Internal Medicine, Teikyo University School of Medicine, Tokyo, Japan, [2]Departments of Infectious Diseases, [3]Allergy and Rheumatology, [4]Molecular Preventive Medicine and CREST, and [5]Bioregulatory Function, University of Tokyo Graduate School of Medicine, Tokyo, Japan

Summary: *Background:* The roles of eosinophils in innate immune responses have not been completely elucidated. Recently, Toll-like receptors (TLRs) were shown to play a critical role in innate immunity, but the expression profile of TLRs has not been precisely investigated in eosinophils. We compared the expression of a panel of TLRs and their functions in human eosinophils and neutrophils. *Methods:* The levels of TLR1 ~ 10 mRNA expression were quantitated by real-time PCR and functional activation by TLR ligands were also investigated. *Results:* Eosinophils constitutively expressed TLR1, TLR4, TLR7, TLR9, and TLR10 mRNAs (TLR4 > TLR1, TLR7, TLR9, TLR10 > TLR6). On the other hand, neutrophils expressed a larger variety of TLR mRNAs. Among various TLR ligands, only R-848, a ligand of TLR7/8, regulated adhesion molecule expression, prolonged survival, and induced superoxide generation in eosinophils. Stimulation of eosinophils by R-848 led to p38 MAP kinase activation. In contrast, neutrophils responded to a larger variety of TLR ligands (TLR2, TLR4, and TLR7/8). Although TLR8 mRNA expression was hardly detectable in freshly isolated eosinophils, mRNA expression of TLR8 as well as TLR7 was exclusively upregulated by IFN-γ but not by either IL-4 or IL-5. *Conclusions:* Recently, single-stranded RNA from RNA virus was identified as TLR7/8 ligands, and our results suggest that eosinophil TLR7/8 systems represent a potentially important mechanism linking viral infection with exacerbation of allergic inflammation and mechanisms of a host-defensive role against viral infection. A wide variety of functional expressions of TLR in neutrophils suggest its prominent role in host defense.

Keywords: eosinophils, neutrophils, toll-like receptor

Several lines of evidence have indicated that bacterial and/or viral infections modulate allergic inflammation. Viral or bacterial infections often precede asthma exacerbation in both children and adults. The link between infection and exacerbation of allergic diseases may consist of various pathways, but direct activation of eosinophils by microbe-derived molecules potentially represents one clear explanation of such mechanisms. As functionally important receptors for recognition of pathogens, the Toll-like receptors (TLRs) have been identified in mammals, and 10 different human TLR proteins have been identified and cloned to date. Expression of TLR4 in eosinophils has been reported by several groups, but the precise expression profiles and functions of other TLRs have remained largely unclear. We ex-

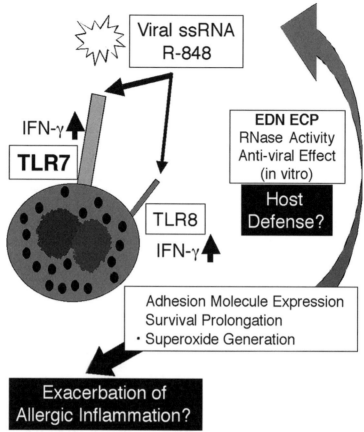

Figure 1. Hypothesis about the biological role of eosinophil TLR7 and 8.

plored and compared TLR expression and their functions in human eosinophils and neutrophils.

Material and Methods

Human eosinophils and neutrophils from normal volunteers were highly purified by density centrifugation followed by negative selection using CD16 or CD14-bound micromagnetic beads [1]. The levels of TLR1 ~ 10 mRNA expression were quantitated by real-time PCR. We also investigated the effect of various TLR ligands – Pam$_3$CSK$_4$ (TLR2), poly I:C (TLR3), LPS (TLR4), R-848 (TLR7/8), and CpG DNA 2006 (TLR9) – on several granulocyte functions, i.e., adhesion molecule expression, survival, IL-8 generation, and superoxide generation [1].

Results

Eosinophils constitutively expressed TLR1, 4, 7, 9, and TLR10 mRNAs (TLR4 > TLR1, 7, 9, 10 > TLR6) [1]. On the other hand, neutrophils expressed a larger variety of TLR mRNAs (TLR1, 2, 4, 6, 8 > TLR 5, 9, 10 > TLR7). Among various TLR ligands, only R-848, a ligand of TLR7/8, regulated adhesion molecule (CD11b and L-selectin) expression, prolonged survival, and induced superoxide generation in eosinophils [1]. In contrast, neutrophils responded to TLR2, TLR4, and TLR7/8 ligands, which induced survival prolongation, regulation of adhesion molecule expression, and IL-8 generation. Stimulation of eosinophils by R-848 led to p38 MAP kinase activation, and SB203580, a p38 MAP kinase inhibitor, almost completely attenuated R-848-induced superoxide generation. Although

TLR8 mRNA expression was hardly detectable in freshly isolated eosinophils, mRNA expression of TLR8 as well as TLR7 was exclusively upregulated by IFN-γ but not by either IL-4 or IL-5. The extent of R-848-induced modulation of adhesion molecule expression was significantly greater in eosinophils treated with IFN-γ compared with untreated eosinophils [1].

Discussion

Although we used R-848 for TLR7/8 ligand, single-stranded RNA from RNA virus was recently identified as TLR7/8 ligands [2,3]. In fact, expression of eosinophil TLR7 and 8 was exclusively upregulated by IFN-γ, lending support to the biological relevance of TLR7/8 systems under conditions associated with viral infections. Figure 1 shows our hypothesis about the biological role of eosinophil TLR7/8. When we assume viral compounds as TLR7/8 ligand, this activates eosinophils via TLR7. The fact that TLR8 mRNA expression became apparent during stimulation with IFN-γ suggests the possible involvement of TLR8 under certain conditions. TLR7/8 systems may represent potentially important mechanisms of eosinophil activation, linking viral infection with exacerbation of allergic inflammation.

On the other hand, TLR are assumed to have a host-defensive role by recognizing viral or bacterial products. Since EDN and ECP potentially exert antiviral effects because of their strong RNase activities, these receptors may also indicate a host-defensive role of eosinophils against viral infection. In contrast to limited response of eosinophils to TLR ligands, neutrophils responded to TLR2, TLR4, and TLR7/8 ligands. A wide variety of functional expressions of TLR in neutrophils suggests its prominent role in host defense.

Acknowledgments
We thank Ms. Chise Tamura and Ms. Masako Imanishi for their excellent technical assistance and Ms. Sachiko Takeyama for her valuable secretarial help.

References

1. Nagase H, Okugawa S, Ota Y, Yamaguchi M, Tomizawa H, Matsushima K, Ohta K, Yamamoto K, Hirai K: Expression and function of Toll-like receptors in eosinophils: activation by Toll-like receptor 7 ligand. J Immunol 2003; 171:3977–3982.
2. Heil F, Hemmi H, Hochrein H, Ampenberger F, Kirschning C, Akira S, Lipford G, Wagner H, Bauer S: Species-specific recognition of single-stranded RNA via Toll-like receptor 7 and 8. Science 2004; 303:1526–1529.
3. Diebold SS, Kaisho T, Hemmi H, Akira S, Reis E, Sousa C: Innate antiviral responses by means of TLR7-mediated recognition of single-stranded RNA. Science 2004; 303:1529–1531.

Hiroyuki Nagase

Department of Internal Medicine, Teikyo University School of Medicine, 2–11–1 Kaga, Itabashi-ku, Tokyo 173–8605, Japan, Tel. +81 3 3964-1211 (ext. 1591), Fax +81 3 3964-1291, E-mail nagaseh-tky@umin.ac.jp

Human T-Cells of Atopic and Nonatopic Donors Are Activated by Staphylococcal α-Toxin

K. Breuer[1,5], M. Wittmann[1], K. Kempe[1], A. Kapp[1], U. Mai[2],
O. Dittrich-Breiholz[3], M. Kracht[3], S. Mrabet-Dahbi[4], and T. Werfel[1]

[1]Department of Dermatology and Allergology, Hannover Medical University, Hannover, [2]Institute of Medical Microbiology and Hygiene, Hannover Medical Hospital, [3]Institute of Pharmacology, Hannover Medical University, [4]Department of Clinical Chemistry and Molecular Diagnostics, Central Laboratory, University of Marburg, [5]Nordseeklinik Norderney, Norderney, all Germany

Summary: *Background:* Staphylococcus aureus is a well known trigger factor of atopic inflammation and able to produce a variety of exotoxins. In this study we aimed to investigate the effect of sublytic α-toxin concentrations on human CD4[+] T-cells. *Methods:* Adult patients with atopic dermatitis (AD) were investigated for a colonization with α-toxin-producing *S. aureus* strains. Proliferation of CD4[+] T-lymphocytes incubated with sublytic concentrations of α-toxin was assessed. IFN-γ in the cell culture supernatants was measured by ELISA. Induction of IFN-γ on the mRNA level was determined by efficiency controlled real time RT-PCR. CD4[+] T-cells were assessed for the induction of t-bet translocation by α-toxin with the Electrophoretic Mobility-Shift Assay (EMSA). *Results:* A colonization with α-toxin producing *S. aureus* strains was found in 22/64 (34%) patients. α-toxin was detected in skin sections by immunohistochemistry. Sublytic concentrations of α-toxin induced marked proliferation of CD4[+] T-cells derived from atopic patients and healthy controls. Moreover IFN-γ was induced on the protein and the mRNA level. Stimulation of CD4[+] T-cells with α-toxin resulted in nuclear translocation and DNA binding of t-bet, known as a transcription factor involved into primary TH1 commitment. *Conclusion:* We show here for the first time that low concentrations of α-toxin are able to activate T-cells. Our results indicate that α-toxin may represent a factor relevant for the induction of a Th1-like cytokine response in inflammation. In AD this may facilitate the development of TH1 cell dominated chronic eczema.

Keywords: T-lymphocytes, α-toxin, α-hemolysin, IFN-γ, cytokines, atopic dermatitis

AD is a chronic inflammatory skin disease with a genetic background, which is influenced by various external factors [1]. Over the last decades, Staphylococcus aureus, a microorganism isolated from 80–100% of patients with AD has been identified as an important trigger factor of AD. An interrelation between *S. aureus* strains producing superantigens and the severity of AD has been demonstrated in a variety of studies [2, 3]. On the other hand, the severity of AD also decreased in patients colonized with nontoxigenic *S. aureus* strains upon antimicrobial treatment [4], which suggests the involvement of other pathogenic factors than superantigens derived from *S. aureus*. A distinct percentage of *S. aureus* strains are able to produce α-toxin, a potent 33000 Da cytotoxin that is particularly active against rabbit erythrocytes [5]. A wide range of human cells has been shown to be prone to lysis by α-toxin with greatly varying susceptibility, among them keratinocytes and lymphocytes [6, 7]. In the present study, we detected α-toxin in lesional skin of AD patients. Therefore, we investigated the effects of sublytic concentrations of α-toxin on human T-cells, since those represent the majority of inflammatory cells in lesional skin of AD [8–10].

Material and Methods

Isolation of Staphylococcus aureus and Identification of α-Toxin

Sixty-four adult patients with AD (mean age 36 years, mean SCORAD 40.1 points) were assessed for colonization with *S. aureus*. Isolates were screened for α-toxin production using the synergistic hemolysis (CAMP-like) test on Columbia 5% sheep blood agar plates (OXOID). 6 μm serial cryostat skin sections derived from patients colonized with α-toxin producing *S. aureus* were stained using the Vectastain ABC-AP kit (Vector Laboratories, Burlingame, CA). Polyclonal antistaphylococcal α-toxin antibodies (rabbit; Sigma, Munich, Germany) were used as primary antibody.

Cell Isolation, [please define]CFSE Labeling, Detection of IFN-γ

CD4+ T-cells were enriched from PBMC derived from healthy and atopic donors (i.e., patients with AD or allergic rhinitis) to > 95% purity by negative selection with the MACS CD4+ T-Cell Isolation Kit (Miltenyi Biotec). Proliferation of PBMC/CD4+ T-lymphocytes incubated with various α-toxin concentrations (Sigma-Aldrich, Munich, Germany) was assessed with the CFDA SE Cell Tracer Assay (Molecular Probes Inc., Eugene, OR, USA). Percentages of cells with a low CFSE fluorescence, which had undergone one or more cell divisions, were determined on a FACScan flow cytometer (Becton Dickenson, Heidelberg, Germany). Detection of IFN-γ in cell culture supernatants was performed using the

Human IFN-γ ELISA Ready-SET-Go kit (Biocarta, Hamburg, Germany).

DNA Microarray Experiments

Microarray experiments were performed using the Human Inflammation Array (MWG Biotech). This microarray contains validated oligonucleotide probes for 110 inflammatory genes as described previously [11].

mRNA Isolation and Reverse Transcription (RT)

mRNA was isolated from 1×10^5 cells (PBMC, CD4+ T-cells) stimulated with 10 ng/ml α-toxin for 24 h using the High Pure RNA Isolation kit (Roche Molecular Biochemicals, Mannheim, Germany) according to the supplier's instructions. Real-time fluorescence PCR for IFN-γ was performed using the Light Cycler (Roche) as described previously [12].

Electrophoretic Mobility-Shift Assay (EMSA)

DNA binding of t-bet was determined by EMSA. Isolated CD4+ T-cells were incubated for 2 h with 10 ng/ml α-toxin or with stimulating anti-CD3 (1 μg/ml) and anti-CD28 (0.2 μg/ml) antibodies (Peli Cluster, Amsterdam, Netherlands) as positive control. As a second signal, 100 ng/ml IL-12 was added and the cells were further incubated for 4 h. Nuclear extracts of 2×10^6 CD4+ T-cells per sample were prepared using the NE-PER™ Nuclear and Cytoplasmic Extraction Reagents kit (Pierce; Bonn, Germany). EMSA for T-bet were performed with equal amounts of protein. For detection of T-bet binding activity double-stranded, biotin-labeled oligonucleotides (5'- Biotin-AAT TTC ACA CCT AGG TGT GAA ATT-3') comprising the t-bet binding site of the IFN-γ gene were used . Mutant olignucleotides (5'-Biotin-AAT TTC AC*G T*CT AGG T*AC* GAA ATT-3') were used for specificity control.

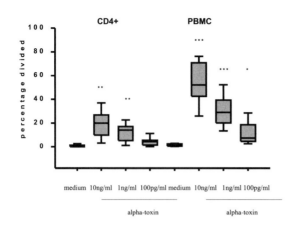

Figure 1. α-toxin induces concentration dependent proliferation of PBMC/CD4⁺ T lympho cytes. CD4⁺ cells/PBMC were incubated with different concentrations of α-toxin as indicated for four days. Percentages of cells that underwent one or more cell divisions are shown in comparison to the medium control. Rank Sum test, * $p < 0.05$, ** $p < 0.01$, *** $p < 0.001$ ($n = 25$ donors).

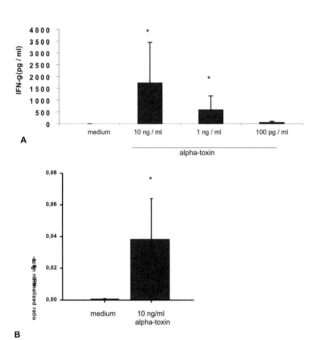

Figure 2. Upregulation of IFN-γ after incubation with α toxin. (A) CD4⁺ T cells were incubated with different concentrations of alpha-toxin for four days. Culture supernatants were harvested and IFN-γ was measured by ELISA. *t-test, $p < 0.05$ (13 healthy individuals, 8 atopic donors). (B) CD4⁺ T-cells were incubated with 10 ng/ml α-toxin for 24 h. An efficiency controlled real time RT-PCR was performed for IFN-γ. Target concentration relative to the reference gene (β-actin) of a calibrator normalized relative quantification are given as calculated by the relative quantification software. A significant upregulation of IFN-γ mRNA as compared with the medium control was observed. *t-test, $p = 0.025$. The results of 5 independent experiments are shown.

Results

α-toxin producing *S. aureus* strains were isolated from 22/64 (34%) adult patients with AD. α-toxin was detected by means of immunohistochemistry in sections of skin biopsy specimens obtained from lesional skin of patients with AD who were colonized with α-toxin-producing *S. aureus* strains. Specimens from healthy individuals did not stain with anti-α-toxin antibodies.

PBMC were incubated with 1 fg – 10 μg/ml of α-toxin. Concentrations of 1 μg/ml α-toxin and higher did not lead to proliferation due to cell death, similarly no proliferation was detected using concentrations of 1 pg/ml and lower (data not shown). Incubation of CD4⁺ T-cells isolated from the peripheral blood with α-toxin resulted in a concentration dependent proliferation. Proliferation induced in PBMC was even more pronounced than that induced in CD4⁺ cells (Figure 1). There was no difference between cells derived from atopic and nonatopic individuals (data not shown).

To investigate the effects of sublytic concentrations of α-toxin, we screened the expression of a selected set of genes with known relevance to inflammation in purified CD4+ T-cells and PBMC incubated with 10 ng/ml α-toxin for 24 h. Microarray analysis revealed that IFN-γ was the most strongly upregulated gene, in both CD4+ T-cells (22.3-fold induction) and PBMC (16.7-fold induction).

α-toxin induced a secretion of IFN-γ in CD4+ T-cells in a concentration dependent manner (Figure 2A) with no difference between atopic and nonatopic donors. Stimulation of PBMC with α-toxin resulted in even higher concentrations of IFN-γ in the cell culture supernatants (data not shown).

An efficiency controlled quantitative real time PCR for IFN-γ was performed. 24 h after stimulation of CD4+ T-cells with 10 ng/ml α-toxin, an upregulation of IFN-γ on the mRNA level as compared to unstimulated cells was detected (Figure 2B).

CD4+ T-cells were assessed for the induction of t-bet binding by α-toxin with the EMSA. We observed an induction of t-bet binding to the binding site of the IFN-γ gene in response to a treatment with α-toxin at a concentration of 10 ng/ml for 6 h. The specificity of the induced complexes was confirmed by using mutant oligonucleotides, which did not lead to t-bet binding.

Discussion

Staphylococcus aureus α-toxin is produced by a high percentage of human *S. aureus* isolates [5, 13]. By immunohistochemistry, we detected α-toxin in the epidermis and dermis of AD patients colonized with α-toxin producing *S. aureus* strains, where it may come into contact with various inflammatory cells. Since CD4+ T-cells comprise 80% of inflammatory cells in lesional skin of AD, we were interested in the effects of α-toxin on T-cells.

After incubation of CD4+ T-cells with low α-toxin concentrations a strong concentra-

tion and time dependent proliferation could be detected indicating activation of T-cells. We used microarray analysis to screen for potential proinflammatory effects of α-toxin and found that IFN-γ was induced in CD4+ T-cells and PBMC. Furthermore we could reproduce upregulation of IFN-γ on the mRNA and the protein level in CD4+ T-cells and PBMC. These effects were more pronounced in PBMC than in isolated CD4+ T-cells, which points to the fact that factors derived from monocytes, B-cells, NK cells, or CD8+ cytotoxic/helper cells may increase the response of CD4+ T-cells to α-toxin. In contrast, significant secretion of IL-4 was not induced by α-toxin. Since we were not able to detect effects on monocytes by a microarray focusing on genes with known relevance to inflammation and direct analysis of IL-12 and IL-18 (unpublished data), other lymphocyte populations besides T helper cells may be involved in the stronger induction of IFN-γ.

The mechanisms underlying the described effects in T-cells induced by subcytolytic concentrations of α-toxin are not clear. We found a strong t-bet binding activity upon incubation of human T-cells with α-toxin. T-bet, a member of the T box family of transcription factors, is expressed in developing and committed Th1 cells [14]. Incubation of CD4+ T-cells with α-toxin was followed by DNA binding of t-bet protein, comparable to TCR signaling through anti-CD3/anti-CD28 binding. The mechanisms underlying the induction of t-bet by α-toxin are not clear. Whether this activation is the result of membrane damage caused by formation of pores and subsequent ion flux or a direct effect of α-toxin on the transcriptional processes remains to be elucidated. However, our data suggest a new mechanism of T-cell activation.

Acknowledgment

We thank Viola Kohlrautz and Anja Neumann for excellent technical assistance. This study was supported by DFG grant WE 1289/6–1 and by a grant of the Dr.-Karl-Wilder-Stiftung, Germany.

References

1. Werfel T, Kapp A: Environmental and other major provocation factors in atopic dermatitis. Allergy 1998; 53:731–739.
2. Bunikowski R, Mielke M, Skarabis H, Worm M, Anagnostopoulos I, Kolde G et al.: Evidence for a disease-promoting effect of Staphylococcus aureus-derived exotoxins in atopic dermatitis. J Allergy Clin Immunol 2000; 105:814–819.
3. Skov L, Olsen JV, Giorno R, Schlievert PM, Baadsgaard O, Leung DYM: Application of staphylococcal enterotoxin B on normal and atopic skin induces up-regulation of T-cells by a superantigen-mediated mechanism. J Allergy Clin Immunol 2000; 105:820–826.
4. Breuer K, Häussler S, Kapp A, Werfel T: Staphylococcus aureus: colonizing features and influence of an antibacterial treatment in adults with atopic dermatitis. Br J Dermatol 2002; 147:55–61.
5. Dinges MM, Orwin PM, Schlievert PM: Exotoxins of Staphylococcus aureus. Clin Microbiol Rev 2000; 13:16–34.
6. Jonas D, Walev I, Berger T, Liebtrau M, Palmer M, Bhakdi S: Novel path to apoptosis: small transmembrane pores created by staphylococcal α-toxin in T-lymphocytes evoke internucleosomal DNA degradation. Infect Immun 1994; 62:1304–1312.
7. Walev I, Martin E, Jonas D, Mohamadzadeh M, Muller-Klieser W, Kunz L, Bhakdi S: Staphylococcal α-toxin kills human keratinocytes by permeabilizing the plasma membrane for monovalent ions. Infect Immun 1993; 61:4972–4979.
8. Reekers R, Schmidt P, Kapp A, Werfel T: Evidence of a lymphocyte response to birch pollen related food antigens in atopic dermatitis. J Allergy Clin Immunol 1999; 104:466–472.
9. Sager N, Feldmann A, Schilling G, Kreitsch P, Neumann C: House dust mite-specific T-cells in the skin of subjects with atopic dermatitis: Frequency and lymphokine profile in the allergen patch test. J Allergy Clin Immunol 1992; 89:801–810.
10. Werfel T, Morita A, Grewe M, Renz H, Wahn U, Krutmann J et al.: Allergen-specificity of skin-infiltrating T-cells is not restricted to a type 2 cytokine pattern in chronic skin lesions of atopic dermatitis. J Invest Dermatol 1996; 107:871–876.
11. Holzberg D, Knights CG, Dittrich-Breiholtz O, Schneider H, Dörrie A, Hoffmann E, Resch K, Kracht M: Disruption of the c-JUN-JNK complex by a cell-permeable peptide containing the c-Jun δ domain induces apoptosis and affects a distinct set of IL-1-induced inflammatory genes. J Biol Chem 2003; 278:40213–40223.
12. Wittmann M, Alter M, Stünkel T, Kapp A, Werfel T: Cell-to-cell contact between activated CD4+ T-lymphocytes and unprimed monocytes interferes with a Th1 response. J Allergy Clin Immunol 2004, in press.
13. Bhakdi S, Tranum-Jensen J: α-toxin of Staphylococcus aureus. Microbiol Rev 1991; 55:733–751.
14. Mullen AC, High FA, Hutchins AS, Lee HW, Villarino AV, Livingston DM, Kung AL, Cereb N, Yao TP, Yang SY, Reiner SL: Role of T-bet in commitment of TH1 cells before IL-12-dependent selection. Science 2001; 292:1907–1910.

Kristine Breuer

Nordseeklinik Norderney, Bülowallee 6, D-26548 Norderney, Germany, Tel. +49 4932 881500, Fax +49 4932 851702, E-mail breuer@nordsee-klinik-norderney.de

Increased Apoptosis of Circulating Memory/ Effector Th1 Cells in Atopic Diseases as Mechanism for Th2 Predominance

C.A. Akdis[1], T. Akkoc[1], E. Jensen-Jarolim[2], K. Blaser[1], and M. Akdis[1]

[1]Swiss Institute of Allergy and Asthma Research (SIAF), Davos, Switzerland, [2]Department of Pathophysiology, Medical University of Vienna, Austria

Summary: *Background:* Genetic predisposition and environmental instructions tune thresholds for the activation, effector functions and lifespan of T-cells, other inflammatory cells and resident tissue cells. Unequal apoptosis of Th1 and Th2 effector cells may lead to preferential deletion of one subset over another and cause a Th2-biased peripheral immune response in allergic diseases. *Methods:* Apoptosis and survival features of Th cell subsets were elucidated in several human and mouse models. *Results:* In atopic dermatitis (AD), circulating cutaneous lymphocyte-associated antigen-bearing (CLA$^+$) CD45RO$^+$ T-cells with skin-specific homing property represent an activated memory/effector T-cell subset. They express high levels of Fas and Fas-ligand and undergo activation-induced cell death (AICD). The freshly purified CLA$^+$ CD45RO$^+$ T-cells of atopic individuals display distinct features of *in vivo* triggered apoptosis such as procaspase degradation and active caspase-8 formation. Particularly, the Th1 compartment of activated memory/effector T-cells selectively undergoes AICD, skewing the immune response toward surviving Th2 cells in AD patients. The AICD of circulating memory/effector T-cells was confined to atopic individuals, whereas nonatopic patients such as psoriasis, intrinsic-type asthma, contact dermatitis, intrinsic type of AD, bee venom allergic patients, and healthy controls did not show any evidence for enhanced T-cell apoptosis. Studies with *in vitro* differentiated Th1 and Th2 cells and T-cells from allergic-inflammation susceptible and resistant mouse strains provided additional evidence for increased Th1 cell apoptosis in atopy. *Conclusion:* Unequal susceptibility to AICD between Th1 and Th2 cells causes an imbalance in T-cell subsets leading to Th2 response in atopic diseases.

Keywords: activation-induced cell death, atopy, cytokines, T-cells, asthma, atopic dermatitis, monoallergy, epithelial cells

There are three forms of allergic diseases with lung, nose, or skin involvement, which are overlapping in clinical features and sometimes not clearly distinguishable from each other. AD, allergic rhinitis, and asthma are typical atopic diseases that develop on a complex genetic background. Although they target differ-ent organs, in most patients they are characterized by the presence of elevated total serum IgE levels. The atopic form of allergic diseases is often initiated with the atopic march in infancy and the inflammation may involve one of the organs such as skin, lung, and nose, or appear in combination [1].

The second type of allergic disease is mono-allergy, so-called allergic breakthrough, characterized by development of allergen-specific IgE in the absence of high serum total IgE in nonatopic individuals [2]. It may develop at any time of life without any predisposing factor. It is manifested as an anaphylactoid type of allergy without any target organ inflammation in venom, some food and drug allergies, or with organ involvement as rhinitis, asthma, and dermatitis [3, 4]. One of the key questions in monoallergies has been to understand how an individual develops allergy to a single protein, while tolerating thousands of others exposed by ingestion or inhalation. Different subtypes of regulatory and suppressor cells and mechanisms that may play a role in peripheral tolerance have been demonstrated, and their biology has been the subject of intensive investigation during the last few years. There is increasing evidence that effector (allergen-specific Th2) and suppressor (allergen-specific Tr1) T-cells exist in both healthy and allergic individuals in certain amounts. Their ratio determines the development of a healthy or an allergic immune response and also plays a role in successful treatment [5–7].

A subgroup of patients with AD, asthma, and rhinitis show (a) clinical phenotype of asthma, AD or rhinitis; (b) negative type I skin hypersensitivity to aero- and food allergens; (c) normal serum IgE levels; (d) no detectable specific IgE antibodies to aero- and food allergens. These patients have been termed non-atopic form, nonallergic form, non-IgE-associated form, or intrinsic-types of asthma, dermatitis, and rhinitis [8, 9].

Increased Activation-Induced Cell Death in Th1 Cells as a Mechanism of Peripheral Th2 Dominance in Atopy

The balance between production and death is important in the control of cell numbers within physiological ranges. Cell accumulation in the tissues may be a consequence of either increased cell production or decreased cell death. The great majority of T-cells homing to skin are of the CD45RO+ memory/effector phenotype and express the skin-selective homing receptor, cutaneous lymphocyte-associated antigen (CLA). Peripheral blood CLA+ memory/effector cells demonstrate typical features of activated T-cells. Both CD4+ and CD8+ subsets of freshly isolated CLA+ T-cells express significantly higher levels of CD25, CD40-ligand, and HLA-DR. They show spontaneous proliferation, induce IgE production by B-cells, and enhance eosinophil survival [10–12].

It has been demonstrated that a fraction of circulating CLA+ CD45RO+ T-cells show direct evidence for in vivo initiated AICD [13]. Immediately after purification, these cells show active caspase-8 and increased caspase degradation, in contrast to their CLA− counterpart and CLA+ T-cells of healthy individuals and several nonatopic disorders, such as intrinsic types of asthma and AD, psoriasis, contact dermatitis, and bee venom allergy. In addition, AICD of CLA+ T-cells could be inhibited by caspase cascade inhibition and by blocking Fas/Fas-ligand interaction. Characterization of cytokine profile of T-cells, which resist or undergo AICD, revealed unequal death in Th1 and Th2 cells. In the absence of survival factors and Fas-pathway inhibitors, a Th2-skewed cytokine profile was observed in CD45RO+ T-cells as well as CLA+ CD45RO+ T-cell clones [13].

T-cells Induce Epithelial Cell Activation and Apoptosis

Transendothelial migration and influx into skin represent the first phase leading to dermal perivascular infiltration by T-cells in AD. Interestingly, a second step of chemotaxis takes place in the migration of T-cells closer to and into the epidermis, where they display effector functions [14]. Apoptosis of keratinocytes induced by T-cells and mediated by Fas is a crucial event in the formation of eczematous le-

Table 1. Immunological characterization of atopic, nonatopic, and monoallergic forms of allergic diseases.

	clinical outcome	total IgE	specific IgE	Th1 AICD	specific Th2	eosinophilia	epithelial apoptosis	Type 1 skin test reactivity
atopic diseases	AD asthma rhinitis	high	+ (multiple specificity)	+	+	+	+	+ (multiple specificity)
nonatopic diseases (non-IgE-associated, intrinsic)	dermatitis asthma rhinitis	normal	–	–	–	±	+	–
monoallergy (allergic-breakthrough)	without organ involvement (venom allergy)	normal	+ (single specificity)	–	+	–	–	+ (single specificity)
	with organ involvement dermatitis asthma rhinitis	normal	+ (single specificity)	–	+	–	+	+ (single specificity)

sions in AD and allergic contact dermatitis [15]. Similarly, the respiratory epithelium was demonstrated as an essential target of the inflammatory attack by T-cells and eosinophils in asthma [16]. In both asthmatic lung and eczematous skin, epithelial cells express functional Fas as an apoptosis receptor. IFN-γ upregulates Fas and renders keratinocytes susceptible to apoptosis. On the other hand, TNF-α upregulates both Fas and Fas-ligand as well as its own receptors, TNF-RI and II, on bronchial epithelial cells. Moderate to severe epithelial apoptosis was demonstrated to be relevant *in vivo* using bronchial biopsies in asthma and lesional skin biopsies in AD. It has to be noted here that receptor affinity and activation thresholds for IFN-γ and Th2 cytokines IL-4, IL-5, and IL-13 show a significant difference. For example, 1 ng/ml of IFN-γ can induce KC apoptosis, whereas 50 ng/ml of IL-4 and IL-13 are required to induce IgE production by B-cells and IL-5 to prolong eosinophil life span *in vitro* [6, 15]. This suggests that a Th2-like T-cell, which produces small quantities of IFN-γ, can also induce epithelial cell apoptosis. Apparently, bronchial epithelial apoptosis leads to epithelial shedding in asthma and keratinocyte apoptosis leads to spongiform morphology in AD [15–17].

Conclusion

Different immune response profiles and activation and apoptosis thresholds define at least three types of allergic diseases (Table 1). These three forms of diseases often overlap in terminology and mechanisms, however exact definitions related with the underlying pathomechanisms may become possible in the near future, because of rapid advancements in the field.

Acknowledgments
The authors' laboratories are supported by the Swiss National Science Foundation Grants No. 32–100266, 32–105865, 32–65436/2, United Bank of Switzerland, Zurich, and Niarchos Foundation, Monaco.

References

1. Spergel JM, Paller AS: Atopic dermatitis and the atopic march. J Allergy Clin Immunol 2003; 112:S118–127.
2. Katz DH, Bargatze RF, Bogowitz CA, Katz LR: Regulation of IgE antibody production by serum molecules. V. Evidence that coincidental sensitization and imbalance in the normal damping

mechanism results in "allergic breakthrough." J Immunol 1979; 122:2191–2197.

3. Müller UR: Recent developments and future strategies for immunotherapy of insect venom allergy. Curr Opin Allergy Clin Immunol 2003; 3: 299–303.

4. Pichler WJ: Lessons from drug allergy: against dogmata. Curr Allergy Asthma Rep 2003; 3:1–3.

5. Akdis M, Verhagen J, Taylor A, Karamloo F, Karagiannidis C, Crameri R, Thunberg S, Deniz G, Valenta R, Fiebig H, Kegel C, Disch R, Schmidt-Weber CB, Blaser K, Akdis CA: Immune responses in healthy and allergic individuals are characterized by a fine balance between allergen-specific T Regulatory 1 and Th2 Cells. J Exp Med 2004; 199:1567–1575.

6. Akdis CA, Blesken T, Akdis M, Wüthrich B, Blaser K: Role of IL-10 in specific immunotherapy. J Clin Invest 1998, 102:98–106.

7. Jutel M, Akdis M, Budak F, Aebischer-Casaulta C, Wrzyszcz M, Blaser K, Akdis AC: IL-10 and TGF-β cooperate in regulatory T-cell response to mucosal allergens in normal immunity and specific immunotherapy. Eur J Immunol 2003; 33: 1205–1214.

8. Schmid-Grendelmeier P, Simon D, Simon H-U, Akdis CA, Wüthrich B: Epidemiology, clinical features, and immunology of the "intrinsic" (non-IgE-mediated) type of atopic dermatitis (constitutional dermatitis). Allergy 2001; 56: 841–849.

9. Akdis CA, Akdis M: Immunological differences between intrinsic and extrinsic types of atopic dermatitis. Clin Exp Allergy 2003; 33:1618–1621.

10. Santamaria Babi LF, Picker LJ, Perez Soler MT, Drzimalla K, Flohr P, Blaser K, Hauser C: Circulating allergen-reactive T-cells from patients with atopic dermatitis and allergic contact dermatitis express the skin-selective homing receptor, the cutaneous lymphocyte-associated antigen. J Exp Med 1995; 181:1935–1940.

11. Akdis M, Akdis CA, Weigl L, Disch R, Blaser K: Skin-homing, CLA⁺ memory T-cells are activated in atopic dermatitis and regulate IgE by an IL-13-dominated cytokine pattern. IgG4 counter-regulation by CLA⁻ memory T-cells. J Immunol 1997; 159:4611–4619.

12. Akdis M, Simon H-U, Weigl L, Kreyden O, Blaser K, Akdis CA: Skin homing (cutaneous lymphocyte-associated antigen-positive) CD8⁺ T-cells respond to superantigen and contribute to eosinophilia and IgE production in atopic dermatitis. J Immunol 1999; 163:466–475.

13. Akdis M, Trautmann A, Klunker S, Daigle I, Küçüksezer UC, Deglmann W, Disch R, Blaser K, Akdis CA: Th2 predominance in atopic disease is due to preferential apoptosis of circulating memory/effector Th1 cells. FASEB J 2003; 17:1026–1035.

14. Klunker S, Trautmann A, Akdis M, Verhagen J, Schmid-Grendelmeier P, Blaser K, Akdis CA: A second step of chemotaxis after transendothelial migration: keratinocytes undergoing apoptosis release IFN-γ-inducible protein 10, monokine induced by IFN-γ, and IFN-γ-inducible α-chemoattractant for T-cell chemotaxis toward epidermis in atopic dermatitis. J Immunol 2003; 171: 1078–1084.

15. Trautmann A, Akdis M, Kleeman D, Altznauer F, Simon H-U, Graeve T, Noll M, Blaser K, Akdis CA: T-cell-mediated Fas-induced keratinocyte apoptosis plays a key pathogenetic role in eczematous dermatitis. J Clin Invest 2000; 106: 25–35.

16. Trautmann A, Schmid-Grendelmeier P, Krüger K, Crameri R, Akdis M, Akkaya A, Bröcker E-B, Blaser K, Akdis AC: T-cells and eosinophils cooperate in the induction of bronchial epithelial apoptosis in asthma. J Allergy Clin Immunol 2002; 109:329–337.

17. Trautmann A, Altznauer F, Akdis M, Simon H-U, Disch R, Bröcker E-B, Blaser K, Akdis CA: The differential fate of cadherins during T-cell-induced keratinocyte apoptosis leads to spongiosis in eczematous dermatitis. J Invest Derm 2001; 117:927–934.

Cezmi A. Akdis

Swiss Institute of Allergy and Asthma Research (SIAF), Obere Strasse 22, CH-7270 Davos, Switzerland, Tel. +41 81 4100848, Fax +41 81 4100840, E-mail akdisac@siaf.unizh.ch

Reduced Number of Cytokine-Expressing Inflammatory Cells in AD after Topical Tacrolimus Treatment

D. Simon[1], E. Vassina[2], S. Yousefi[2], E. Kozlowski[2], L.R. Braathen[1], and H.-U. Simon[2]

[1]Departments of Dermatology and [2]Pharmacology, University of Bern, Bern, Switzerland

Summary: In several clinical studies tacrolimus has been shown to be effective in the treatment of atopic dermatitis (AD). By inhibiting calcineurin it targets signaling pathways that control gene expression, in particular the expression of cytokines. We examined the cellular infiltrate and cytokine expression pattern in skin lesions of 10 AD patients before and after short-term topical therapy with tacrolimus 1% ointment. In parallel with a significant improvement of the skin lesions we observed a marked regression of spongiosis, acanthosis, and density of the cellular infiltrate in the dermis. The latter was due to reduced infiltration of T-cells, B-cells, and eosinophils. Moreover, the expression of the T helper (Th) 2 cytokines IL-5, IL-10, and IL-13 in CD4+ T-cells was reduced after therapy. Tacrolimus therapy was also associated with a reduction of CD8+ T-cells expressing the Th1 cytokine IFN-γ. Furthermore, the numbers of epidermal CD1a+ dendritic cells increased following treatment. In the peripheral blood, a decrease of granulocytes (eosinophils and neutrophils), but no changes in the distribution of lymphocyte subpopulations were noticed. Taken together, topical tacrolimus treatment exerts antiinflammatory effects on AD skin as indicated by reduced infiltration of cytokine expressing inflammatory cells. No evidence for drug-induced systemic immunosuppression was obtained.

Keywords: atopic dermatitis, cytokines, inflammation, tacrolimus, T-cells

AD is a chronic or relapsing eczematous skin disease. In the dermis of AD lesions, there is a marked perivascular infiltrate of both CD4+ and CD8+ T-cells [1,2] as well as of eosinophils [3]. The infiltration of cells is associated with increased expression of cytokines, in particular of IL-5 and IL-13 [4]. Despite a reduced capacity of PBMC to generate IFN-γ under *in vitro* conditions [5,6], IFN-γ-producing cells have been described in chronic skin lesions [7].

Tacrolimus decreases the phosphatase activity of calcineurin and, thus, inhibits intracellular signaling pathways leading to cytokine production in lymphocytes. Although several clinical trials have shown that topical tacrolimus is beneficial in the treatment of AD, little is known about its immunopharmacological effects in the skin.

The aim of our study was to investigate the effects of this drug on inflammatory cells and their cytokine gene expression in AD patients. For this purpose we obtained skin biopsies and peripheral blood from 10 patients (age 18–58 years) with moderate to severe AD before and after treatment with tacrolimus 0.1% ointment for 3 weeks.

To evaluate the clinical efficacy of the treatment with topical tacrolimus, the eczema area and severity index (EASI) was determined. Before treatment, the mean EASI was 25.7 ± 5.7. The patients experienced a rapid improvement of their AD lesions within the first week of treatment and further improvement within the next 2 weeks as indicated by mean EASI levels of 13.9 ± 3.4 and 10.8 ± 3.9, respectively.

Further, we semiquantitatively calculated the degree of hyperkeratosis, acanthosis, spongiosis, and inflammatory cell infiltration. Statistically different improvements were seen regarding spongiosis, dermal infiltrate, and acanthosis, although the after-treatment-scores were still higher compared to nonlesional AD skin. To identify the inflammatory cells infiltrating the dermis of lesional skin, we used a single immunofluorescence technique using antibodies against lineage-associated molecules. Tacrolimus treatment was associated with a significant reduction of CD4+ and CD8+ cells as well as B-cells and eosinophils. In contrast, the numbers of epidermal CD1a+ cells increased after treatment, perhaps because of a repopulation with high CD1a expressing LC and a reduction of low CD1a expressing inflammatory dendritic epidermal cells (IDEC) [8]. The numbers of mast cells remained unchanged following drug application.

Cytokine gene expression was analyzed by RNase protection assay in skin tissues taken from lesional skin of three patients before and after tacrolimus treatment. We observed in all three patients detectable levels of IL-2, IL-9, and IL-13 mRNA in acute skin lesions. IFN-γ mRNA was seen in two out of three patients. We noticed a clear reduction in the expression of these cytokine genes after treatment, suggesting that tacrolimus targets both Th1 and Th2 cytokines. To determine whether the difference in cytokine mRNA expressions is also seen at the protein level, we measured cytokine levels in crude tissue fluids obtained from skin biopsies before and after tacrolimus treatment. IL-5 and IL-13 were readily detectable.

IL-5 tissue levels (per g tissue protein) decreased from 3.8 ± 1.7 ng to 1.5 ± 0.5 ng, whereas levels of IL-13 in skin decreased from 24.4 ± 12.1 ng to 6.2 ± 1.7 ng. The levels of IL-2, IL-4, IL-10, TNF-α, and IFN-γ were usually below the detection limit even before therapy.

To analyze the Th1/Th2 cytokine expression pattern of CD4+ and CD8+ cells, we used a double immunofluorescence technique. We observed that at least a subpopulation of both cell types expressed IL-5, IL-10, IL-13, and IFN-γ. In general, the numbers of cytokine-expressing CD4+ cells were higher than cytokine-expressing CD8+ cells. The reduced expression of the Th2 cytokines IL-5, IL-10, and IL-13 during the tacrolimus treatment occurred mainly in CD4+ and less in CD8+ cells. Interestingly, tacrolimus appeared to reduce the expression of IFN-γ in CD8+ cells more effectively than in CD4+ cells.

The white blood cell count showed a decrease in the leukocyte numbers (from 8280 ± 530 to 6510 ± 500 per mm³; $p = 0.001$) because of decreased numbers of neutrophils and eosinophils after therapy. No significant differences before and after tacrolimus treatment were observed regarding lymphocyte subpopulations (CD4+ and CD8+ T-cells including activation markers, B-cells, NK cells). Despite the obvious suitability of HLA-DR as an indicator of T-cell activation, tacrolimus had no effect on the numbers of this T-cell subpopulation in blood.

We also analyzed the pattern of cytokine generation in PBMC induced by PHA-stimulation before and after tacrolimus treatment. PBMC had a slightly larger capacity in producing Th2 cytokines and generated less IFN-γ *in vitro* after tacrolimus treatment, although these differences did not reach statistical significance. PHA-induced lymphocyte proliferation was not affected by tacrolimus treatment.

Taken together, the results of this study provide evidence that many of the predicted mechanisms regarding the suppression of cytokine gene expression by tacrolimus indeed occur under *in vivo* conditions. Reduced cytokine expression was associated with reduced numbers of dermal infiltrating inflammatory cells in AD. The immunopharmacological effects correlated with dramatic improvements of the clinical condition. No systemic immunosuppressive effect after topical tacrolimus treatment has been observed.

Acknowledgments
This work was supported by grants from the Swiss National Science Foundation (grant no. 31–58916.99) and Fujisawa SA, Deutschland GmbH, Munich, Germany.

References

1. Braathen LR, Förre O, Natvig JB, Eeg-Larsen T: Predominance of T lymphocytes in the dermal infiltrate of atopic dermatitis. Brit J Dermatol 1979; 100:511–519.
2. Akdis CA, Akdis M, Simon D, Dibbert B, Weber M, Gratzl S, Kreyden O, Disch R, Wuethrich B, Blaser K, Simon H-U: T-cells and T-cell-derived cytokines as pathogenic factors in the nonallergic form of atopic dermatitis. J Invest Dermatol 1999; 113:628–634.
3. Simon D, Braathen LR, Simon HU: Eosinophils and atopic dermatitis. Allergy 2004; 59:561–570.
4. Hamid Q, Boguniewicz M, Leung DYM: Differential in situ cytokine expression in acute versus chronic atopic dermatitis. J Clin Invest 1994; 94:870–876.
5. Simon D, Borelli S, Braathen LR, Simon HU: Peripheral blood mononuclear cells from IgE and non-IgE associated allergic atopic eczema/dermatitis syndrome demonstrate increased capacity of generating IL-13 but differ in their potential of synthesizing INF-γ. Allergy 2002; 57:431–435.
6. Simon D, von Gunten S, Borelli S, Braathen LR, Simon H-U: IL-13 production by peripheral blood T-cells from extrinsic and intrinsic atopic dermatitis patients does not require CD2 costimulation. Int Arch Allergy Immunol 2003; 132: 148–155.
7. Grewe M, Gyufko K, Schopf E, Krutmann J: Lesional expression of INF-γ in atopic eczema. Lancet 1994; 343:25–26.
8. Wollenberg A, Sharma S, von Bubnoff D, Geiger E, Haberstock J, Bieber T: Topical tacrolimus leads to profound phenotypic and functional alterations of epidermal antigen-presenting dendritic cells in atopic dermatitis. J Allergy Clin Immunol 2001; 107:519–525.

Dagmar Simon

Department of Dermatology, Inselspital, University of Bern, CH-3010 Bern, Switzerland, Tel. +41 31 632-2278, Fax +41 31 381-5815, E-mail dagmar.simon@insel.ch

New Methods for Quantitative and Qualitative Assessment of Itch

U. Darsow[1,2], E. Ripphoff[2], S. Weissenbacher[1,2], H. Behrendt[2], and J. Ring[1]

[1]Department of Dermatology and Allergy Biederstein, Technical University Munich, Germany
[2]Division of Environmental Dermatology and Allergy GSF/TUM, Munich, Germany

Summary: We investigated instruments for qualitative and quantitative assessment of the itch sensation. Objective covariates of itch were shown using imaging techniques for the CNS: a complex pattern of cerebral activation after itch induction with histamine was observed in a $H_2{}^{15}O$ PET correlation study in healthy volunteers ($n = 6$). Subtraction analysis versus control revealed significant activation of the left primary sensory cortex and motor-associated areas, predominantly left-sided activations of frontal, orbitofrontal and superior temporal cortex and anterior cingulate. Quantity and quality of perceived itch show specific characteristics in different pruritic skin diseases: the multidimensional "Eppendorf Itch Questionnaire" (EIQ) was used in patients suffering from atopic eczema (AE, $n = 62$) and chronic urticaria (CU, $n = 58$). The total EIQ score was significantly higher in the AE group with 231.7 ± 11.6 vs. 175.2 ± 9.5. In 34 of 127 items, a significantly different rating was obtained, mostly with higher load for affective and some sensory items in AE. These findings can be interpreted as differences in CNS processing of a nociceptive sensation. The atopy patch test (APT) with aeroallergens can be used as a model for atopic eczema itch: a pilot study in 16 patients showed a significant correlation of APT itch intensity and qualitative total EIQ score. New models to measure itch may be useful for the development of new therapeutic strategies against pruritus.

Keywords: itch, CNS processing, Eppendorf itch questionnaire, imaging, positron emission tomography, atopy patch test

Itch is a major subjective symptom of allergic diseases; with its well-known psychophysiologic aspects it has substantial impact on the quality of life of patients [1]. We investigated new instruments for qualitative and quantitative assessment of the itch sensation.

Objective covariates of itch and differences to pain processing were shown using imaging techniques for the CNS: a complex pattern of cerebral activation after experimental itch induction with histamine dihydrochloride (0.03 to 8% [2]) at the right lower arm in healthy volunteers was observed in a $H_2{}^{15}O$ PET correlation study ($n = 6$) [3]. Subtraction analysis vs. control revealed significant activation of the left primary sensory cortex and motor-associated areas, predominantly left-sided activations of frontal, orbitofrontal, and superior temporal cortex and anterior cingulate. When compared to studies in a pain model, no thalamus activation, but significant activation in the insula region and differences in sensory, motor, and cingulate activation were seen. Activated areas significantly correlated with the subjective itch intensity (visual analog scale, VAS) are shown with their Brodmann area number (maximum) and known function in nociceptive processing in Figure 1.

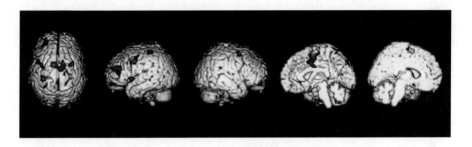

	BA	Region	Function
Left	9-10	Gyrus frontalis med.	Motivation, planning, cognition
Hemi-	6-9	Gyrus praecentralis/fr.med.	working memory, motor
sphere	-	Insula (posterior)	Sensory assessment
	3	Gyrus postcentralis	Sensory assessment
	6	SMA	Action planning
Right	6	SMA	Action planning
Hemi-	24-32	Anterior cingulate	Unpleasant sensation
sphere	24-32	Anterior cingulate	Coordination of aversive reactions

Figure 1. PET surface projections on MRI template: cerebral activation pattern after histamine stimuli at the right forearm. BA, Brodmann area.

These results give evidence for central nervous processing of itch, showing differences to pain processing. Planning of a scratch response is mirrored by extensive activation of motor areas in the cortex; other areas may be involved in the emotional evaluation of nociception.

Quantity and quality of perceived itch show specific characteristics in different pruritic skin diseases. The multidimensional "Eppendorf Itch Questionnaire" (EIQ) [4] was used for hospitalized patients suffering from atopic eczema (AE, $n = 62$) and chronic urticaria (CU, $n = 58$). Total scores (127 items), emotional and sensory ratings, reactive behavior, and VAS for itch intensity were evaluated. The mean VAS ratings of itch intensity showed no significant difference between the two diseases (Table 1). In contrast, the total EIQ score was significantly higher in the AE group with 231.6 ± 11.5 vs. 175.2 ± 9.4. In 34 of 127 items, a significantly different rating was obtained, mostly with higher load for affective and some sensory items in AE. Significant differences were also seen in the description of the scratch response.

Itch perception in AE and CU differs on a qualitative level, influencing items relevant

Table 1. Significantly higher total EIQ score in atopic eczema compared to chronic urticaria without differences in VAS itch intensities. $*p < 0.00001$.

Scales		N	Mean	SEM
VAS%	Atopic eczema	62	74.4	2.6
	Chronic urticaria	58	75.1	2.3
Total EIQ	Atopic eczema	62	231.6*	11.5
	Chronic urticaria	58	175.2*	9.4

for quality of life. Group-specific peculiarities not measurable with VAS were mirrored by the EIQ scores. These findings can be interpreted as differences in CNS processing of a nociceptive sensation.

Quality and intensity of itch induced by atopy patch test (APT) reactions in patients with AE were evaluated with the EIQ. In 16 patients with AE and a positive APT reaction to one of the four allergens – house dust mite (*D. pter.*), cat dander, grass pollen, or birch pollen – the corresponding aeroallergen was simultaneously retested on both forearms and the back. The test was read after 48 and 72 h (European Task Force on Atopic Dermatitis [ETFAD] key) [5]. Pruritus

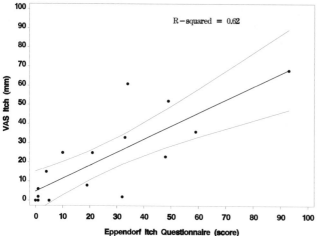

Figure 2. Correlation of itch intensity (mean VAS Itch Score) and qualitative Total Eppendorf Itch Questionnaire Score (48 h) in 16 patients with atopic eczema on the back. Regression line with 95% confidence limits.

was characterized by VAS mean itch score at baseline, 24, 48, 72 h and by EIQ at 48 and 72h. Results showed a high reproducibility (93.8%) of the APT model within an average of 16 months. There was no significant difference between arms and back in either quality or intensity of itch. In comparison, a positive APT reaction occurred more frequently on the back (93.8% on the back vs. 68.8% on the arms) and the intensity of reaction was significantly higher on the back compared to the arms ($p < 0.05$). There was no significant difference between both forearms with regard to the APT reaction. Itch (quality and intensity) and APT reaction both decreased at 72 h compared to 48 h. The most frequent items chosen in the EIQ were similar at all three application sites and at both time points: "itching, disturbing, annoying, unpleasant, tickling, crawling, and deterioration in warmth" with the positive control item "itching" being the first. A significant correlation of VAS itch intensity and EIQ total score was seen (Figure 2).

Apart from histamine, aeroallergens (APT) can be used as a model for atopic eczema itch, inducing medium VAS intensities. The APT reaction appears to be more reproducible if the back is used as the allergen application site.

New models to measure itch may be useful for the development of new therapeutic strategies against pruritus.

References

1. Darsow U, Ring J: Neural and psychophysiological aspects of itch. Jpn J Dermatoallergol 2002; 10:1–7.
2. Darsow U, Ring J, Scharein E, Bromm B: Correlations between histamine-induced wheal, flare, and itch. Arch Dermatol Res 1996; 288:436–441.
3. Darsow U, Drzezga A, Frisch M, Munz M, Weilke F, Bartenstein P, Schwaiger M, Ring J: Processing of histamine-induced itch in the human cerebral cortex: a correlation analysis with dermal reactions. J Invest Dermatol 2000; 115:1029–1033.
4. Darsow U, Scharein E, Simon D, Walter G, Bromm B, Ring J: New aspects of itch pathophysiology: component analysis of atopic itch using the "Eppendorf Itch Questionnaire." Int Arch Allergy Immunol 2001; 124:326–331.
5. Darsow U, Ring J: Airborne and dietary allergens in atopic eczema: a comprehensive review of diagnostic tests. Clin Exp Dermatol 2000; 25:544–551.

Ulf Darsow

Klinik und Poliklinik für Dermatologie und Allergologie am Biederstein, Technische Universität München, Biedersteiner Str. 29, D-80802 München, Germany, Fax +49 89 4140-3171, E-mail ulf.darsow@lrz.tum.de

Expression of Two Neuropeptide Receptors, Calcitonin-Gene-Related Peptide, and Somatostatin

in Peripheral Blood Mononuclear Cells from Patients with Atopic Dermatitis and Nonatopic Controls

M.J. Torres[1], C. Antúnez[1], C. Mayorga[1], L.F. Santamaría-Babi[2], J.A. Cornejo-García[1], and M. Blanca[1]

[1]*Research Unit for Allergic Diseases, Allergy Service, Carlos Haya Hospital, Málaga, Spain*
[2]*Almirall Prodesfarma, Barcelona, Spain*

Summary: There is increasing evidence that neuropeptides (NP) may be involved in the pathogenesis of atopic dermatitis (AD). Exacerbations of AD can be provoked by stress, and several studies have demonstrated changes in the skin levels NP in AD patients. The aim of the study was to evaluate the expression of the NP receptors (CGRPR and SSTR) in peripheral blood mononuclear cells from AD patients with both acute and chronic lesions, and from non-atopic controls. CGRPR and SSTR were amplified by semi-quantitative real-time PCR with SYBR-Green. We found a decrease in the expression of both CGRPR and SSTR in AD patients compared to controls, although this was only significant in the CGRPR. Comparisons between patients with acute and chronic lesions showed no differences for either receptor. We conclude that a down-regulation of CGRPR exists in peripheral blood mononuclear cells in AD patients compared to controls and that this down-regulation does not depend on the stage of the lesion, as there were no differences between patients with acute and chronic AD lesions.

Keywords: neuropeptide receptors, atopic dermatitis, real-time PCR

There is increasing evidence that the neuroendocrine and immune systems communicate with each other and this is probably mediated by the binding of different neuropeptides (NP) to their specific receptors. Somatostatin receptors (SSTR) have been found in T-cells [1] and are coded by five genes (SSTR1–5), which have been cloned and characterized [2]. At least three classes of calcitonin gene-related peptide receptors (CGRPR) have been identi-

fied, although only one has so far been identified; the calcitonin receptor-like receptor [3], which corresponds to the pharmacologically defined CGRPR1 subtype [4]. We have evaluated the expression of two NP receptors, CGRPR1 and SSTR3 in PBMC from patients with atopic dermatitis (AD) and nonatopic controls. We also compared the expression of both receptors in AD patients with acute and chronic lesions.

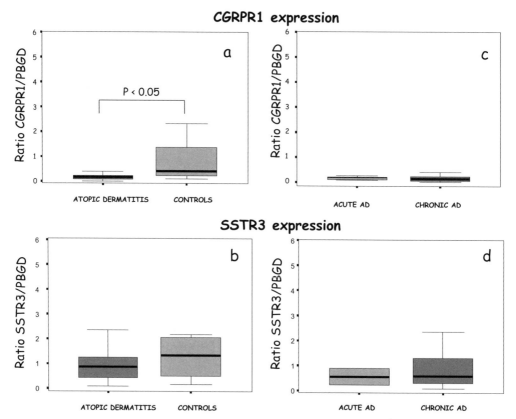

Figure 1. Box plot of the expression level of CGRPR1 (a) and SSTR3 (b) in PBMC from patients with atopic dermatitis and non-atopic controls and of CGRPR1 (c) and SSTR3 (d) in PBMC from patients with acute and chronic atopic dermatitis lesions.

Material and Methods

Patients

Thirteen patients with AD were studied and classified into two groups: Five with acute lesions (lesion onset less than 3 days before study) and eight with chronic lesions (lesion onset more than 2 weeks before study). Ten healthy nonatopic persons formed a control group. The study was approved by the institutional review board, and informed consent was obtained from patients and controls.

Quantification of Receptors

PBMC were obtained and total RNA was used for cDNA synthesis. CGRPR1 and SSTR3 were amplified by semi-quantitative real time-PCR with SYBR-Green, using PBGD (Por-

phobilinogen-Deaminase) transcript as a reference to normalize mRNA levels.

Primers

The primer used to amplify CGRPR1 mRNA sequence included 5'-TATTTGAAAGAT TGCTACCAC-3' and 5'-CCAACTGAATT GAGTCCT-3', for SSTR3 mRNA sequence included 5'-ACGGCCAGCCCTTCAGTC AC-3' and 5'-CGGCCAGGTAGCGGTCC AC-3', and for PBGD mRNA sequence included 5'-TCCAAGCGGAGCCATGTCTG-3' and 5'-AGAATCTTGTCCCCTGTGGTG GA-3'.

Statistical Study

Mean comparisons were done by nonparametric analysis (Mann-Whitney test). p-values represented two-tailed tests, with values < 0.05 considered statistically significant. The analysis was performed using the SPSS program version 11.5.

Results

The expression of both CGRPR1 and SSTR3 in AD patients and controls is shown in Figure 1A and 1B. There was a decreased expression of both CGRPR1 (median: 0.16, interquartile range [IR]: 0.23–0.072) and SSTR3 (median: 0.86, IR: 1.39–0.32) in AD patients compared with controls (CGRPR1, median: 0.41, IR: 2.31–0.17; SSTR3, median: 1.32, IR: 2.18–0.34), although the difference was only significant in CGRPR1 ($p < 0.05$). Comparison of the expression of CGRPR1 in AD patients with acute (median: 0.13, IR: 0.74–0.24) and chronic lesions (median: 0.14, IR: 0.23–0.057) showed no significant differences. Similar results were found when we analyzed the expression of SSTR3 in AD patients with acute (median: 0.54, IR: 0.87–0.22) and chronic lesions (median: 0.58, IR: 1.41– 0.24) (Figures 1C and 1D).

Discussion

Studies reporting the expression of NP receptors in different cells do not always agree. Some authors have described an increase in substance P expression in patients with AD compared to controls after *in vitro* stimulation with this NP [5]. Others, however, have found downregulation of VIP receptors in mast cells in AD lesions [6], and yet others have found no change in substance P receptor or SSRTR in skin biopsies of AD lesions [7].

In this study we evaluated the expression of SSTR3 and CGRPR1 in PBMC from AD patients and controls. We chose SSTR3 from the five types of receptors because it is the most widely expressed in T-cells [1] and CGRP1 because it is the best characterized [4]. We found no changes in the expression

of SSTR3 and a downregulation of CGRP1 in AD patients compared to controls and this downregulation does not depend on the time interval elapsed from the onset of AD. Possible explanations for this downregulation include: PBMC in AD may constitutively have fewer receptors, the chronic exposure to NP downregulates the PBMC receptors, or the PBMC that express more receptors have migrated and are, therefore, localized to the skin. However, the fact that there is no difference in the expression of NP receptors between AD patients with acute and chronic lesions makes the latter two possibilities less probable. In conclusion, our results suggest a role for CGRP1 in the pathophysiology of atopic dermatitis. Additional studies are under way to determine the presence of NP receptors in different memory T-cell populations in AD.

Acknowledgment

This study was partly supported by a grant from the Spanish Ministry of Health (01/0865).

References

1. Talme T, Ivanoff J, Hagglund M, et al.: Somatostatin receptor (SSTR) expression and function in normal and leukemic T-cells. Evidence for selective effects on adhesion to extracellular matrix components via SSTR2 and/or 3. Clin Exp Immunol 2001; 125:71–79.
2. Reisine T, Bell GI: Molecular biology of somatostatin receptors. Endocr Rev 1995; 16:427–442.
3. Chang CP, Pearse RV, O'Connell S, Rosenfeld MG: Identification of a seven trans-membrane helix receptor for corticotrophin-releasing factor and sauvagine in mammalian brain. Neuron 1993; 11:1187–1195.
4. Poyner D: Pharmacology of receptors for calcitonin gene-related peptide and amylin. Trends Pharmacol Sci 1995; 16:424–428.
5. Kim K, Park KC, Chung JH, Choi HR: The effect of substance P on peripheral blood mononuclear cells in patients with atopic dermatitis. J Dermatol Sci 2003; 32:115–124.
6. Groneberg DA, Welker P, Fisher TC, et al.: Downregulation of vasoactive intestinal polypeptide receptor expression in atopic dermatitis. J Allergy Clin Immunol 2003; 111:1099–1105.

7. Misery L, Bourchanny D, Kanitakis J, Schmitt D, Claudy A: Modulation of substance P and somatostatin receptors in cutaneous lymphocytic inflammatory an tumoral infiltrates. JEADV 2001; 15:238–241.

Maria José Torres

Allergy Service, Hospital Civil, Plaza del Hospital Civil s/n, 29009 Malaga, Spain, Tel. +34 951030346, Fax +34 951030302, E-mail mariaj.torres.sspa@juntadeandalucia.es

The Influence of Neuro-peptides on Cytokine Production in Peripheral T-Cells

in Atopic Dermatitis Patients with Acute and Chronic Lesions and in Controls

L.F. Santamaría-Babi[1], C. Antúnez[2], M.J. Torres[2], C. Mayorga[2], J.A. Cornejo-García[2], and M. Blanca[2]

[1]*Almirall Prodesfarma, Barcelona, Spain*
[2]*Research Unit for Allergic Diseases, Allergy Service, Carlos Haya Hospital, Málaga, Spain*

Summary: Atopic dermatitis (AD) is an inflammatory skin disease whose lesions can have two stages: acute and chronic, with two patterns of cytokine expression, Th2 in acute and Th1 in chronic lesions. Additionally, in AD pathogenic T lymphocytes express the cutaneous lymphocyte-associated antigen (CLA). Recently, it has been suggested that neuropeptides (NP) can modulate the cytokine production in memory T cells and this may influence the evolution of the disease. The aim of this study was to compare the effect on cytokine production of different NP (CGRP, somatostatin, and substance P) in patients with acute and chronic AD lesions and controls. We evaluated the cytokine production (IL-4, IL-5, IL-13 and IFN-g?) in CLA + and CLA- subsets, in peripheral T-lymphocytes with and without incubation with NP. We found that CGRP induced an increase in IL-13 production in AD patients with acute and chronic lesions and a decrease in IL-4 production in AD patients with chronic lesions and in controls, somatostatin induced an increase in IL-13 and IFN-g production in AD patients with acute lesions, and substance P induced no detectable changes. These changes were only observed in the CLA + but not in the CLA- subset. We conclude that the effect of the NP CGRP and somatostatin on cytokine production was limited to the CLA$^+$ subset, although with differing responses according to the type of lesion.

Keywords: neuropeptides, T-lymphocytes, CLA, atopic dermatitis

Atopic dermatitis (AD) is a chronic relapsing skin disease associated with abnormal activation and proliferation of different T-cell subpopulations. The disease is biphasic, with an initial stage predominated by T-cells producing Th2 cytokines but later switches to a Th1 pattern leading to chronic lesions [1]. Additionally, in AD the pathogenic T lymphocytes express the cutaneous lymphocyte-associated antigen (CLA).

There is increasing evidence that neuropeptides (NP) may be involved in the pathogenesis of AD [2]. NP change cytokine production in mouse T-cell lines [3]. Furthermore, it has been suggested that NP may modulate cytokine production in memory T-cells in AD patients and this may influence the course of the disease [4]. This effect, though, probably depends on the stage of the AD lesions, either acute or chronic. Accordingly, we compared the effect on cytokine production of different NP, calcitonin gene related peptide (CGRP), somatostatin (SOM), and substance P (SP), in patients with acute and chronic AD lesions and nonatopic controls.

Material and Methods

Patients

Ten patients with AD were studied and classified in two groups: five with acute lesions (lesion onset < 3 days before study) and five with chronic lesions (onset > 2 weeks). Ten healthy nonatopic persons formed a control group.

Cell Cultures with NP and Cytokine Production

PBMC from each patient were isolated by density gradient centrifugation and cultured at 2×10^{-6} cells/ml in complete RPMI with or without the different NP (CGRP, SOM and SP) at 10^{-8} M, and without any other stimulus, for 16 h at 37 °C at 5% CO_2. Cells were then cultured with ionomycin (Sigma,[where?]) at 1 µg/ml and monensin (Sigma,[where?]) at 10 µg/ml of cell suspension for 4 h. Cytokine production (IL-4, IL-5, IL-13 and IFN-γ) in both CLA$^+$ and CLA$^-$ subsets was performed as previously described [1]. Six parameters were analyzed on a Facscalibur flow cytometer using Cell Quest software.

Statistical Study

Mean comparisons were done by nonparametric analysis (Wilcoxon tests) with $p < 0.05$ considered statistically significant.

Results

To investigate whether the NP can directly change the T-cell cytokine production pattern

we tested the influence of the three NP on T-cell cultures. Figure 1 shows the cytokine production in the CLA$^+$ cells with and without NP stimuli.

CGRP induced an increase in IL-13 production in AD patients with acute lesions (with NP; median: 4.45; interquartile range (IR): 9.14–2.86), (without NP; median: 3.13; IR: 3.51–2.17), ($p < 0.05$), and in chronic lesions (with NP; median: 5.18; IR: 8.26–2.98), (without NP; median: 3.12; IR:3.95–1.92), ($p < 0.05$), and a decrease in IL-4 production in patients with chronic lesions (with NP; median: 1.97; IR:5.03–1.48), (without NP; median: 2.31; IR: 5.52–1.63), ($p > 0.05$), and controls (with NP; median: 1.90; IR:2.99–1.08), (without NP; median: 3.78; IR: 5.11–2.99), ($p < 0.05$). SOM induced an increase in IL-13 (with NP; median: 4.67; IR: 7.05–3.14), (without NP; median: 3.13; IR: 3.51–2.17), ($p < 0.05$) and IFN-γ (with NP; median: 5.07; IR: 7.09–3.27), (without NP; median: 4.19; IR: 5.98–1.57), ($p < 0.05$) in AD patients with acute lesions. SP induced no detectable changes in any cytokines. No changes were found in CLA$^-$ cells for any cytokine or NP (data not shown).

Discussion

Culture of mouse Th0, Th1, and Th2 T-cell lines with different NP induces changes in the cytokine patterns [3]. In humans similar studies have been performed using PBMC cultured with NP and anti-CD3 [5] or allergens [6]. To our knowledge, no studies using just NP stimulus have been performed on human PBMC. Accordingly, we decided to evaluate the cytokine production in patients with AD and controls after NP stimulus alone, separating patients into groups of those with chronic and acute lesions.

Our first conclusion is that NPs do directly induced changes in cytokine pattern in PBMC and limited to the CLA$^+$ subsets, with CGRP being the NP that induced the most change, with a significant increase in IL-13. Although IL-4 production runs in parallel with the production of IL-13, in our study we

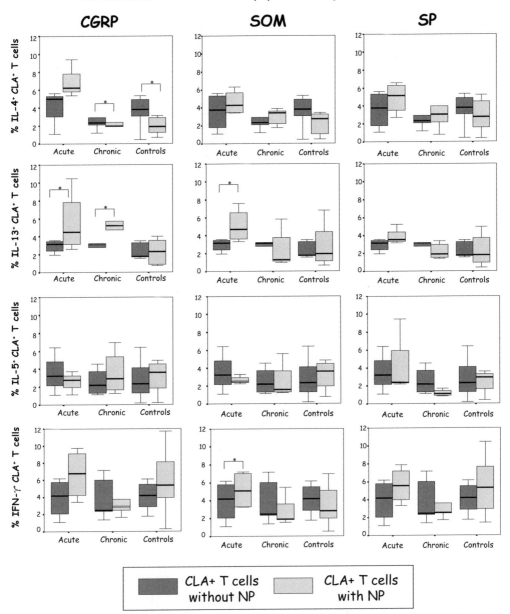

Figure 1. Box plot of the percentage of CD3⁺ CLA⁺ cells producing IL-4, IL-13, IL-5, and IFN-γ with or without stimulation with CGRP, SOM, or SP in AD patients with acute and chronic lesions and nonatopic controls.

only found a decrease in AD patients with chronic lesions and controls and we have no convincing explanation for these differences. Regarding SOM, we detected an increase in IFN-γ production in AD patients with acute lesions but no changes with SP for any of the cytokines evaluated.

Summarizing, the changes detected were lower than those described with the mouse T-cell line, with no clear switching of the cytokine pattern [3]. This may be because we analyzed PBMC instead of T-cell lines. Furthermore, since all the changes were only detected in the CLA⁺ cells, it may be of interest to evaluate the role of the different NP using purified CLA⁺ and CLA⁻ T-cells and this may constitute a relevant model to understand neuroimmunological mechanisms in AD.

Acknowledgments
This study was partly supported by a grant from the Spanish Ministry of Health (01/0865).

References

1. Antúnez C, Torres MJ, Mayorga C, et al.: Different cytokine production and activation marker profiles in circulating CLA$^+$ T-cells from patients with acute or chronic atopic dermatitis. Clin Exp Allergy 2004; 34:559–66.
2. Tobin D, Nabarro G, De Labarro G, et al.: Increased number of immunoreactive nerve fibers in atopic dermatitis. J Allergy Clin Immunol 1992; 90:613–622.
3. Levite M: Neuropeptides, by direct interaction with T-cells, induce cytokine secretion and break the commitment to a distinct T helper phenotype. Proc Natl Acad Sci USA 1998; 95:12544–12549.
4. Kang H, Byun DG, Kim JW: Effects of substance P and vasoactive intestinal peptide on INF-γ and IL-4 production in severe atopic dermatitis. Ann Allergy Asthma Immunol 2000; 85:227–232.
5. Goron DJ, Ostlere LS, Holden CA: Neuropeptide modulation of Th1 and Th2 cytokines in peripheral blood mononuclear leucocytes in atopic dermatitis and nonatopic controls. Br J Dermatol 1997; 137:921–927.
6. Yokote R, Yagi H, Furukawa F, Takigawa M: Regulation of peripheral blood mononuclear cell responses to *Dermatophagoides farinae* by substance P in patients with atopic dermatitis. Arch Dermatol Res 1998; 290:191–197.

Maria José Torres

Allergy Service, Hospital Civil, Plaza del Hospital Civil s/n, E-29009 Malaga, Spain, Tel. +34 951030346, Fax +34 951030302, E-mail mariaj.torres.sspa@juntadeandalucia.es

Eotaxin-1 SNP Associations in Allergic Conjunctivitis

H. Murakami, A. Nishimura, R.S. Campbell-Meltzer, and S.J. Ono

Department of Immunology, University College London, Institutes of Ophthalmology and Child Health, & Moorfields Eye Hospital, NHS Trust and Center for Genomics, UK

Summary: A role for genetic predisposition for allergic diseases can be assessed by analyzing associations between naturally occurring single nucleotide polymorphisms (SNPs) and disease phenotypes (e.g., serum IgE levels, allergen reactivities, and other clinical symptoms). For asthma, associations between genotype and pulmonary function are frequently assessed. In ocular allergy, associations are assessed with respect to well-established ophthalmic criteria such as lid edema and redness, tearing, photophobia, and conjunctival eosinophilia. In this study we have analyzed the eotaxin-1, -2, and -3 genes for SNPs associated with ocular allergy. Thirty-five SNPs in these genes were analyzed in 409 patients with moderate-severe seasonal allergic conjunctivitis, and a similar number of age/sex-matched normal controls. Logistic analyses were performed with codominant models with age and sex as covariables. While no associations were detected for eotaxin-2 and -3 SNPs, a significant association was observed between $-433C > A$ in the eotaxin-1 gene. This indicates that this gene product may contribute to genetic predisposition for severe-moderate SAC.

Keywords: genetics, ocular allergy, allergic conjunctivitis, eotaxin

Allergic reactions in the eye manifest as: seasonal allergic conjunctivitis (SAC), perennial allergic conjunctivitis (PAC), atopic keratoconjunctivitis (AKC), giant-papillary conjunctivitis (GPC), and vernal keratoconjunctivitis (VKC). These conditions range from transient phenomena that clear rapidly after allergen exposure (i.e., in mild SAC), to chronic diseases that both cause considerable discomfort and obscure vision [1]. While the conditions vary considerably in their severity and pathogenesis, each occurs most frequently in atopic individuals, suggesting a clear genetic component to each condition.

Several lines of evidence indicate that Th2 lymphocyte-driven, IgE-dependent type I hypersensitivity reactions underlie the pathogenesis of this group of conditions [2]. First, there is significant cosegregation of these diseases with other allergic diseases (e.g.,

rhinitis, asthma, dermatitis, and food allergy). This indicates that general atopy genes may predispose individuals to develop any of a number of allergic conditions. The linkage mapping of both shared and distinct regions of the human genome in different allergic diseases supports this concept, albeit also providing evidence for disease-specific susceptibility loci [3–5]. Second, there is a strong correlation between the number of mast cells detected in the epithelium and substantia propria of the conjunctiva and disease severity. Third, these diseases either follow allergen exposure, or are a consequence of prolonged allergen exposure. Fourth, analysis of tears from patients with conjunctivitis usually reveals high levels of mast cell mediators and proteases during ongoing disease. Finally, mast cell stabilizers (such as nedocromil) both decrease clinical symptoms and the number of inflammatory cells resident in the conjunctiva.

The severity of allergic responses in the eye correlates well with the degree of eosinophilia in the late phase reaction (when this does occur). Thus, strong acute responses in SAC usually include significant eosinophilia, while mild early responses often lack any evidence of a late phase reaction, and little or no eosinophilia. This is also true for AKC, GPC, and VKC [6]. For this reason, it is not surprising that the levels of eosinophil cationic protein found in the tears of VKC patients correlates well with other established ophthalmic criteria for disease severity. All of these data suggest that the eosinophil may play an important role in the pathogenesis of ocular allergy. Despite this, there is very little known about the pathways that recruit eosinophils into the conjunctiva, and no direct assessment of the importance of eosinophils in disease pathogenesis.

Vierucci and coworkers [7] carefully studied 110 Caucasian children with VKC and evaluated disease severity, evidence of allergen-sensitization, peripheral blood eosinophil counts, and serum eosinophil cationic protein levels in these and control patients. The striking finding in their work is that while eosinophilia does clearly correlate with disease severity, there is no strict requirement for atopy or allergen-specific sensitization for the eosinophilic response. Indeed, while tarsal and mixed forms of conjunctivitis showed a correlation with total and allergen-specific IgE titers and skin tests, bulbar forms of VKC showed no such correlation. These data suggest that there are likely both IgE-dependent and IgE-independent pathways driving eosinophilia in these two forms of VKC, and that eosinophils in the absence of a mast cell-driven response (in the bulbar forms) are sufficient to drive severe clinical symptoms in this mucosal tissue.

As part of a larger study to identify genes predisposing individuals to develop the different forms of ocular allergy, here we report an analysis of the eotaxin-1, -2, and -3 genes for associations with moderate-severe seasonal allergic conjunctivitis. A more compre-hensive study involving this patient cohort as well as 120 patients with VKC will be published separately.

Material and Methods

Thirty-five SNPs located throughout the eotaxin-1, -2, and -3 genes were detected and assessed in a patient cohort of 409 individuals. A similar number of age- and sex-matched controls was also assessed. Logistic analyses were performed with codominant models with age and sex as covariables, and p-values determined by the Stephens algorithm. SNP genotyping were performed using a high-throughput mass spectrometry approach. The impact of associated SNPs on the promoter activity of heterologous luciferase reporter constructs was determined by transient transfection into the airway epithelial cell line BEAS-2B. Eotaxin promoter-luciferase constructs were generated containing nucleotides −750 to +55 of the allelic promoters. Expression of the heterologous reporters was stimulated by addition of TNF-α and IL-4.

Results and Discussion

Although eosinophilia is often not observed in biopsies obtained from patients with mild seasonal allergic conjunctivitis (Ono and colleagues, unpublished data), a profound eosinophilia is almost always detected in the conjunctiva of patients with moderate/severe SAC and in patients with VKC. We, therefore, hy-

Table 1. Eotaxin-1 promoter SNP associations with moderate/severe SAC.

Locus	SAC	Ctl.	P
−521 C > T	0.43	0.40	ns
−433 C > A	0.28	0.17	0.003
−329 A > G	0.22	0.23	ns
+123G > A	0.15	0.16	ns
+361T > A	0.45	0.40	ns

pothesized that genetic polymorphisms within or near the eotaxin genes might be associated with ocular allergies, since these CC chemokines are potent eosinophil chemoattractants. Such SNPs might be in linkage disequilibrium with a disease-promoting gene allele, or might directly impact on disease by (1) altering the "potency" of the chemokine, or (2) by affecting the expression level of the chemokine.

Despite an exhaustive search of 30 SNPs within the eotaxin-2 and eotaxin-3 genes (and flanking regions), no associations with SAC in this patient population were detected relative to age- and sex-matched normal individuals. An analysis of five SNPs within the eotaxin-1 gene revealed a single significant association ($p = 0.003$) at $-433C > A$. No nonsynonymous replacements were detected in the coding region of the associated allele relative to at least one "normal" allele.

$-433C > A$ Impacts on Eotaxin-1 Promoter Activity in BEAS Stimulated with TNF-α and IL-4

Since the associated SNP is located within the proximal promoter of the eotaxin-1 gene, heterologous luciferase reporter constructs were generated containing nucleotides -750 to $+55$ of the allelic promoters cloned upstream of the reporter construct pTransLucent. The promoter fragments were inserted between the 5' BglII site and the 3' HindIII site of the 4.8 kilobase reporter. The -433 C and -433 A alleles were then transfected by lipofection using LipofectAMINE (Life Technologies, Inc.). Following transfection (at greater than 80% transfection efficiency), cells were stimulated with TNF-α and IL-4 to induce the expression of the endogenous and heterologous eotaxin-1 promoters. The reporter construct containing the -433 C allele was expressed at approximately 3.5 fold higher levels than the -433 A allele. Future studies will determine how the SNPs affect promoter occupancy *in vivo* following cytokine stimulation, and exactly what transcription factors are interacting with the altered TF binding site.

In conclusion, the thesis that conjunctival eosinophilia (a hallmark of moderate-severe SAC and VKC) might be controlled at least in part via SNPs within the eotaxin genes has been assessed in an SAC cohort. While no association has been detected within the eotaxin-2 and eotaxin-3 genes or their flanking regions (scanning 30 SNPs), a significant association has been detected at nucleotide -433 of the eotaxin-1 gene in SAC. This SNP impacts on the promoter "strength" of the associated allele in an *in vitro* system, where eotaxin gene expression is induced via TNF-α and IL-4 receptor engagement.

Future studies will extend these analyses to VKC, and will correlate genotype to eotaxin-expression detected in tears and via immunohistologic analyses. Taken together, the data do support the possibility that eosinophilia in the conjunctiva might be governed by both IgE-dependent and IgE-independent mechanisms (e.g., chemokine driven) and that antagonism of eotaxin-CCR3 interactions might be particularly effective in the treatment of ocular allergy. A comparison of these new data with similar studies performed in asthma and atopic dermatitis patients clearly illustrates divergence in specific associations between eotaxin genes and other allergic conditions [8,9].

References

1. Liu G, Keane-Myers A, Miyazaki D, Tai KF, Ono SJ: Hypersensitivity reactions in the conjunctiva. Chemical Immunology 1999; 73:39–58.
2. Toda M, Ono SJ: Genomics and proteomics of allergic disease. Immunology 2002; 106(1):1–10.
3. Casolaro V, Georas SN, Song Z, Ono SJ: Biology and genetics of atopic disease. Curr Opin Immunol 1996; 8:6.
4. Ono SJ: Genetics of atopic disease. Ann Rev Immunol 2000; 18:347–366.
5. Nishimura A, Campbell-Meltzer RS, Chute K, Orell J, Ono, SJ: Genetics of allergic disease: evidence for organ-specific susceptibility genes. Int Arch Allergy Immunol 2001; 124:197–200.
6. Leonardi A, Borghesan F, Faggian D, Secchi A, Plebani M: Eosinophil cationic protein in tears of normal subjects and patients affected by vernal keratoconjunctivitis. Allergy 1995; 50:610–613.
7. Pucci N, Novembre E, Lombardi E, Cianferoni A,

Bernardini R, Massai C, Caputo R, Campa L, Vierucci, A: Clin Exp Allergy 2003; 33(3):325–330.

8. Tsunemi Y, Saeki H, Nakamura K, Sekiya T, Hirai K, Fujita H, Asano N, Tanida Y, Kakinuma T, Wakugawa M, Torii H, Tamaki K: J Dermatol Sci 2002; 29(3):222–228.

9. Shin HD, Kim KH, Park BL, Jung JH, Kim JY, Chung I-Y, Kim JS, Lee JH, Chung SH, Kim YH, Park H-S, Choi JH, Lee YM, Park SW, Choi BW, Hong S-J, Park C-S: Association of eotaxing gene family with asthma and serum total IgE. Human Mol Genet 2003; 12(11): 1279–1285.

Santa Jeremy Ono

University College London, Institute of Ophthalmology, 11–43 Bath Street, London EC1V 9EL, UK, E-mail santa.ono@ucl.ac.uk

Neurotrophins in Allergic Bronchial Asthma

Modulators of Immunological and Neuronal Plasticity

H. Renz[1], C. Hahn[1], B. Schuhmann[1], S. Kerzel[1], C. Nassenstein[2], A. Braun[2], G. Päth[1], C. Virchow[3], and W.A. Nockher[1]

[1]Department of Clinical Chemistry and Molecular Diagnostics, Philipps University Marburg
[2]Frauenhofer Institute of Toxicology and Experimental Medicine, Hannover
[3]Department of Pneumology, University Hospital Rostock, all Germany

Summary: There is growing evidence that the immune and nervous systems are closely related not only in physiological but also in pathological reactions in the lung. Recent evidence from our group indicates that neurotrophin production, including nerve growth factor (NGF) and brain derived neurotrophic factor (BDNF), is upregulated in the lung. Both residential cells such as airway epithelium and inflammatory cells including macrophages, T-cells, and eosinophils serve as important sources. The effects of increased neurotrophin production are bidirectional. In addition they control sensory nerve fibers in terms of function, neuropeptide synthesis. and growth. On the other side, neurotrophins serve as important survival factors particularly for inflammatory cells such as eosinophils, T-cells, and macrophages. Utilizing the model of segmental allergen provocation of mild to moderate asthmatic patients, it has been shown that neurotrophins sufficiently prevent apoptotic cell death of lung, but not blood eosinophils. They augment the ongoing inflammatory reaction. The functional interaction between neurotrophins, immune, and nerve cells has been extensively studied in both human and mouse models of experimental allergic asthma. In the latter system, the crucial role of the pan-neurotrophin receptor p75 has been investigated in p75 Neurotrophinreceptor (NTR) –/– mice. Furthermore, NGF transgenic animals have been utilized to assess the contribution of NGF. The role of BDNF on differentiation and function of B-lymphocytes has been identified in BDNF –/– mice. In conclusion, our data support the concept that neurotrophins mediate immunological and neuronal plasticity within the neuro-immune network of bronchial asthma.

Keywords: asthma, allergy, neurotrophins, immunomodulation

Growing evidence indicates that the immune and the nervous system are closely related and that neurotrophins appear as mediators in the interaction between both immune and nerve cells. Our group has previously shown that the neurotrophin production including NGF and BDNF are upregulated in the inflamed lung [1]. Neurotrophins are produced by resident cells including airway epithelial cells [2] as well as a wide range of immune cells such as macrophages, T-cells, and eosinophils [3]. The effects of increased neurotrophin production are bidirectional. In addition, they are modulators of cell survival and differentiation throughout the nervous system. On the other hand, they act as survival factors for inflammatory cells such as eosinophils, T-cells, and macrophages [4, 5] and support the ongoing immune response. To illustrate the importance of neurotrophins as an immunological and neuronal modulator, the role of NGF as well as p75 NTR was studied in an animal model of allergic asthma. In addition, the functional relevance of neurotrophins for the activation and survival of eosinophils was analyzed after segmental allergen provocation of allergic patients.

Material and Methods

Patients

Segmental allergen provocation of allergic patients with mild asthma or healthy donors was performed [6].Patients were rebronchoscoped and lavaged with prewarmed PBS 18 h later. The study protocol was approved by the Ethics Committee of the University of Freiburg.

Animals

Mice were sensitized to OVA (Sigma Aldrich, Munich, Germany) by intraperitoneal injections on Days 1, 14, and 21. Before analysis animals received two consecutive allergen challenges via the airways delivered by nebulization of 1% OVA diluted in PBS on Days 27 and 28. A second group of mice were additionally challenged twice a week with OVA for a 12-week period. Nonimmunized mice received intraperitoneal injections with PBS and were challenged with OVA.

Assessment of Airway Hyperresponsiveness

Lung function was analyzed in nonanesthetized, spontaneously breathing mice in response to different stimuli by head-out bodyplethysmography as previously described [7]. For determination of bronchoconstriction, the midexpiratory airflow was measured after nebulization of methacholine or capsaicin (both Sigma Aldrich).

Analysis of Airway Inflammation

BAL was performed as previously described [8]. Cells were centrifuged onto slides and differentially stained with Diff-Quik (Baxter Dade, Marburg, Germany). Cells were classified by light microscopy according to classical morphologic criteria.

Immunohistochemistry

Lungs were preserved, filled with TissueTek (Sakura, Zouterwoude, The Netherlands), and cryo-fixed in liquid nitrogen. Cryostat sections were mounted, air-dried, and fixed in acetone. The sections were then subjected to standard immunohistochemical staining methods as previously described [9].

Determination of NT Levels in BAL Fluid

BAL fluid concentration of NGF and BDNF were measured by ELISA (Promega, Madison, WI, USA) according to the manufacturers' instructions.

Determination of Eosinophil Survival and Activation

Eosinophils were isolated from peripheral blood or from BAL fluid by centrifugation over a percoll gradient and subsequent immunomagnetic cell sorting (Miltenyi Biotech, Bergisch-Gladbach, Germany). The expression of NTR was assessed by RT-PCR or standard immunohistochemistry. The survival was measured with a standard flow cytometric dye exclusion assay (propidium iodide, BD, Mountain View, CA, USA).

Results and Discussion

To assess if allergic asthma is correlated with enhanced NT levels, mice were sensitized and challenged with OVA and NT levels were determined in the BAL fluid by ELISA. NGF and BDNF levels were elevated in the lavage fluid after OVA challenge (Figure 1A) [1] and increased further after a prolonged c7hallenge period.

To analyze the relationship between enhanced NT levels and allergic early-phase reactions, NGF transgenic mice overexpressing NGF in the airways (Clara-cell secretory protein promoter [CCSP-NGF-tg]) were sensitized using the same protocol. CCSP-NGF-tg mice showed mast cell degranulation and me-

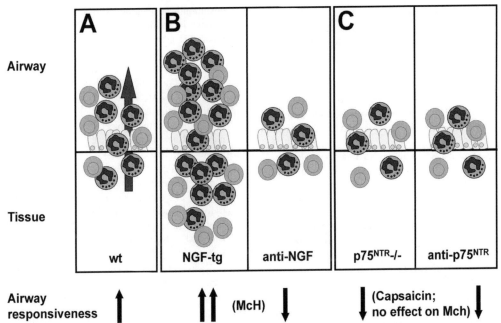

Figure 1. Neurotrophins mediate allergic airway inflammation and regulate airway hyperresponsiveness. (A) Allergic bronchial asthma is characterized by chronic airway inflammation and development of airway hyperresponsiveness. Levels of nerve growth factor (NGF) and brain derived neurotrophic factor (BDNF) levels were elevated in the lavage fluid of ovalbumin (OVA) sensitized and challenged mice [1]. (B) NGF transgenic mice overexpressing NGF showed an augmented airway inflammation and airway hyperresponsiveness, whereas anti-NGF treatment suppressed airway inflammation [10]. (C) In p75NTR -/- as well as anti-p75NTR treated mice airway inflammation and neuronal airway hyperreactivity to capsaicin was almost completely abolished [9].

diator release and the airway inflammation was strongly enhanced compared to wild-type mice. Furthermore, NGF transgenic mice developed an increased reactivity of sensory neurons in response to inhaled capsaicin [10] (Figure 1B). This observation provides evidence for a functional role of NGF in the development of the allergic early phase reaction in the airways of the lung.

Since NGF binds either to the specific tyrosine kinase receptor (trk) A or the pan-neurotrophin receptor p75NTR, the contribution of p75NTR to the pathology of allergic airway inflammation was assessed in p75NTR –/– mice. In wild-type mice p75NTR is expressed in noninflamed as well as asthmatic lungs and airways. Experiments performed in p75 NTR –/– mice revealed that airway inflammation depends to a large extent on this receptor and neuronal airway hyperresponsiveness to capsaicin depends entirely on this receptor (Figure 1C) [9]. These data

were confirmed in wild-type mice treated with an anti-p75NTR blocking antibody. Based on the data a molecular pathway in the neuroimmune pathogenesis of bronchial asthma could be defined.

To specify the role of NT on cells of the immune system we hypothesized that NT primarily act on eosinophils. Using the model of segmental allergen provocation of mild to moderate asthmatic patients, it has been shown that infiltrated and activated eosinophils have an elevated expression of the neurotrophin receptors p75NTR, trkA, trkB, and trkC [6]. Incubation with nerve growth factor, BDNF, neurotrophin-3, or neurotrophin 4 caused a significant increase in the viability and CD69 expression of isolated eosinophils from BAL fluid but not from peripheral blood from the same patients. This result indicates that NT-mediated activation of bronchial eosinophils plays a role in the regulation of eosinophilic inflammation in allergic asthma.

References

1. Virchow JC, Julius P, Lommatzsch M, Luttmann W, Renz H, Braun A: Neurotrophins are increased in bronchoalveolar lavage fluid after segmental allergen provocation. Am J Respir Crit Care Med 1998; 158(6):2002–2005.

2. Olgart HC, Frossard N: Nerve growth factor and asthma. Pulm Pharmacol Ther 2002; 15(1):51–60.

3. Barouch R, Appel E, Kazimirsky G, Braun A, Renz H, Brodie C: Differential regulation of neurotrophin expression by mitogens and neurotransmitters in mouse lymphocytes. J Neuroimmunol 2000; 103:112–121.

4. la Sala A, Corinti S, Federici M, Saragovi HU, Girolomoni G: Ligand activation of nerve growth factor receptor TrkA protects monocytes from apoptosis. J Leukoc Biol 2000; 68(1):104–110.

5. Garcia-Suarez O, Blanco-Gelaz MA, Lopez ML, Germana A, Cabo R, Diaz-Esnal B et al.: Massive lymphocyte apoptosis in the thymus of functionally deficient TrkB mice. J Neuroimmunol 2002; 129:25–14.

6. Nassenstein C, Braun A, Erpenbeck VJ, Lommatzsch M, Schmidt S, Krug N et al.: The neurotrophins nerve growth factor, brain-derived neurotrophic factor, neurotrophin-3, and neurotrophin-4 are survival and activation factors for eosinophils in patients with allergic bronchial asthma. J Exp Med 2003; 198:455–467.

7. Glaab T, Daser A, Braun A, Neuhaus-Steinmetz U, Fabel H, Alarie Y et al.: Tidal midexpiratory flow as a measure of airway hyperresponsiveness in allergic mice. Am J Physiol Lung Cell Mol Physiol 2001; 280(3):L565–L573.

8. Herz U, Braun A, Ruckert R, Renz H: Various immunological phenotypes are associated with increased airway responsiveness. Clin Exp Allergy 1998; 28(5):625–634.

9. Kerzel S, Path G, Nockher WA, Quarcoo D, Raap U, Groneberg DA et al.: Pan-neurotrophin receptor p75 contributes to neuronal hyperreactivity and airway inflammation in a murine model of experimental asthma. Am J Respir Cell Mol Biol 2003; 28(2):170–178.

10. Path G, Braun A, Meents N, Kerzel S, Quarcoo D, Raap U et al.: Augmentation of allergic early-phase reaction by nerve growth factor. Am J Respir Crit Care Med 2002; 166(6):818–826.

Harald Renz

Philipps-University Marburg, Department of Clinical Chemistry and Molecular Diagnostics; Central Laboratory, Baldinger Straße, D-35033 Marburg, Germany, Tel. +49 6421 28-66234, Fax +49 6421 28-65594, E-mail renzh@med.uni-marburg.de

Neuroimmunological Crosstalk in Atopic Dermatitis

Critical Role of Neurotrophins in Eosinophil Function

U. Raap, B. Wedi, and A. Kapp

Department of Dermatology and Allergology, Hannover Medical University, Germany

Summary: *Background:* Basic principles of immunology in atopic dermatitis (AD) have been well described, whereas neuroimmune interactions in AD still remain unknown. As AD is characterized by an increased density of sensory nerves, neurotrophins, produced by nerves, are suggested as possible mediators linking nervous and immunological interactions in AD. This study was designed to further reveal the role of neurotrophins on eosinophils as main effector cells of AD. *Methods:* Peripheral blood eosinophils of AD patients were purified by CD16 negative selection and stimulated with brain-derived neurotrophic factor (BDNF), neurotrophin (NT)-3, and nerve growth factor (NGF) for 24 to 120 h. Apoptotic eosinophils were investigated by determining their hypodiploid DNA peak. Chemotactic index was assessed in a modified Boyden chamber assay, respiratory burst by lucigenin-dependent chemiluminescence, BDNF production with BDNF-ELISA, and pan-neurotrophin receptor p75 (p75^{NTR}) and tyrosine kinase A-C (trkA-C) receptor expression with FACS analysis. *Results:* Stimulation with BDNF, NT-3, and NGF inhibited apoptosis of eosinophils from 24 up to 120 h ($p < 0.05$–0.01). P75^{NTR} and trkA-C were expressed on eosinophils. Chemotactic index was increased after stimulation with BDNF and NT-3 ($p < 0.05$–0.01). Respiratory burst of eosinophils was not modified after stimulation with BDNF, NT-3 or NGF. BDNF levels were higher in AD eosinophils compared to nonatopic controls ($p < 0.01$). *Conclusion:* To summarize, BDNF, NT-3 and NGF have a functional role on AD eosinophils, which express p75^{NTR} and trkA-C neurotrophin receptors. In addition, AD eosinophils are a source of neurotrophins such as BDNF itself. Therefore, neurotrophins are suggested as pivotal players of the neuroimmunological interaction in AD revealing new aspects of AD pathophysiology.

Keywords: atopic dermatitis, neuroimmunology, brain-derived neurotrophic factor, nerve growth factor, apoptosis, chemotaxis, eosinophils

Atopic dermatitis is a chronic inflammatory pruritic skin disease characterized by an influx of activated CD4$^+$ T-lymphocytes, eosinophils, and an increase of antigen presenting Langerhans-cells [1]. As AD is characterized by an increased density of sensory nerve fibers [2], the central hypothesis of our study was that nerve-mediators such as neurotrophins may have a role in the inflammatory response in AD. Recently, neurotrophins, which are increased in asthma, have been described as key players in allergic airway inflammation orchestrating inflammatory responses and neuronal hyperreactivity [3, 4]. Also in AD, NGF levels were found to be increased, correlating with disease activity [5]. Eosinophils, as target effector cells in AD, were suggested as possible NGF sources as they store NGF in the central core of granule proteins and contain higher levels compared to nonatopics [6]. Even though a functional role of NGF with inhibition of apoptosis and induction of reactive oxygen species has recently been described for peripheral blood eosinophils of healthy humans [7, 8], the direct effect on AD eosinophil function still remains unknown.

In our project we give the first evidence for a functional role of BDNF [9], NT-3, and NGF on AD eosinophils, i.e., inhibition of apoptosis (BDNF, NT-3, NGF) and induction of chemotaxis (BDNF, NT-3). In addition, we show for the first time that BDNF levels were increased in AD eosinophils, pointing to an autocrine source of neurotrophin in addition to NGF. Further, neurotrophin receptors such as p75^{NTR}, trkA-C were found to be expressed on AD eosinophils.

In conclusion, these data suggest that neurotrophins play a role in AD pathophysiology as they exert immunomodulatory functions on eosinophils, which are a source of neurotrophins such as BDNF itself. In this way, neurotrophins that act in concert with AD eosinophils might be closing the loop of neuroimmune interactions in this chronic inflammatory skin disease.

Acknowledgment

This project was funded by a young investigators grant of the Medical University of Hannover.

References

1. Leung DY, Boguniewicz M, Howell MD, Nomura I, Hamid QA: New insights into atopic dermatitis. J Clin Invest 2004; 113:651–657.
2. Tobin D, Nabarro G, Baart dlF, van Vloten WA, van der Putte SC, Schuurman HJ. Increased number of immunoreactive nerve fibers in atopic dermatitis. J Allergy Clin Immunol 1992; 90(4 Pt 1): 613–622.
3. Kerzel S, Path G, Nockher WA, Quarcoo D, Raap U, Groneberg DA et al.: Pan-neurotrophin receptor p75 contributes to neuronal hyperreactivity and airway inflammation in a murine model of experimental asthma. Am J Respir Cell Mol Biol 2003; 28:170–178.
4. Path G, Braun A, Meents N, Kerzel S, Quarcoo D, Raap U et al.: Augmentation of allergic early-phase reaction by nerve growth factor. Am J Respir Crit Care Med 2002; 166:818–826.
5. Toyoda M, Nakamura M, Makino T, Hino T, Kagoura M, Morohashi M: Nerve growth factor and substance P are useful plasma markers of disease activity in atopic dermatitis. Br J Dermatol 2002; 147:71–79.
6. Toyoda M, Nakamura M, Makino T, Morohashi M: Localization and content of nerve growth factor in peripheral blood eosinophils of atopic dermatitis patients. Clin Exp Allergy 2003; 33:950–955.
7. Solomon A, Aloe L, Pe'er J, Frucht-Pery J, Bonini S, Bonini S et al.: Nerve growth factor is preformed in and activates human peripheral blood eosinophils. J Allergy Clin Immunol 1998; 102: 454–460.
8. Kobayashi H, Gleich GJ, Butterfield JH, Kita H: Human eosinophils produce neurotrophins and secrete nerve growth factor on immunologic stimuli. Blood 2002; 99:2214–2220.
9. Raap U, Goltz C, Deneka N, Bruder M, Renz H, Kapp A, Wedi B: Brain-derived neurotrophic factor is increased in atopic dermatitis and modulates eosinophil functions compared with that seen in nonatopic subjects. J Allergy Clin Immunol 2005; 115:1268–1275.

Ulrike Raap

Department of Dermatology and Allergology, Hannover Medical University, Ricklingerstr. 5, D-30449 Hannover, Germany, Tel. +49 511 9246-232, Fax. +49 511 9246-234, E-mail mail@ulrike-raap.de

Kinetics of Cytokine Production by Human Lung Tissue

T.-L. Hackett and J.A. Warner

University of Southampton, Biomedical Sciences Building

Summary: *Background:* We have examined the effect of 100 ng/ml lipopolysaccharide (LPS) on the production of seven different mediators from human lung tissue over 48 h. Tissue came from 25 patients (9F/16M, average age 60.3 ± 2.6 yrs, average FEV1/FVC = 0.7 ± 0.02) undergoing resection for cancer. *Methods:* Tissue was maintained in culture and supernatant collected at 1, 2, 4, 6, 24, and 48 h time points. Supernatant was analyzed for TNF-α, IL-6, IL-8, and IL-10 using commercial ELISAs, and results confirmed using Western blot. *Results:* Release of the proinflammatory cytokine TNF-α, was statistically elevated in the LPS-stimulated lung at 1, 2, and 4 h, peaking at 6 h (median = 9.9 ng/mg of tissue vs. 0.1 ng/mg of tissue in the control, $p < .05$) and remained elevated until 48 h. A second proinflammatory cytokine, IL-6, was statistically increased in the LPS-stimulated supernatant at 6 h, with a maximum response at 24 h (median = 510.0 ng/mg of tissue compared to 48.5 ng/mg of tissue in the control, $p < .05$) and remained elevated at 48 h. The release of the chemokine IL-8 followed a similar pattern with a maximum response at 24 h (median = 1060.0 ng/mg of tissue vs. median = 1925.0 ng/mg of tissue in the control, $p < .05$) and remained elevated. Intriguingly, the antiinflammatory cytokine IL-10 was elevated at 24 h (median = 12.5 ng/mg of tissue compared to undetectable levels in the control, $p < .05$) and remained elevated at 48 h. *Conclusions:* In summary, LPS stimulated production of TNF-α early on in the response of human lung tissue. This was followed by IL-6, IL-8, and IL-10 production at 24 h.

Keywords: human lung tissue, TNF-α, IL-6, IL-8, IL-10, LPS

Cytokines have many roles to play within the human lung, including proinflammatory, antiinflammatory, and modulation of long term responses. Many cytokines are pleotrophic, with multiple functions including regulation of other cytokines. Identifying the sequence in which cytokines are released may, therefore, help to focus on key inflammatory cytokines, which regulate downstream events. We have looked in detail at the kinetics of cytokine production in human lung tissue stimulated with LPS. We have concentrated on proinflammatory cytokines TNF-α, IL-6, the chemokine IL-8, and the antiinflammatory cytokine IL-10.

Materials and Methods

Characterization of Human Lung Tissue

Human lung tissue was collected from patients undergoing resection for carcinoma; tissue used was the normal margin from around the tumour. The patient groups consisted of 25 patients (9F/16M, average age 60.3 ± 2.6 years, average FEV1/FVC = 0.7 ± 0.02). There were 10 ex-smokers, who had given up smoking for more than 3 years, 13 current smokers and 2 nonsmokers.

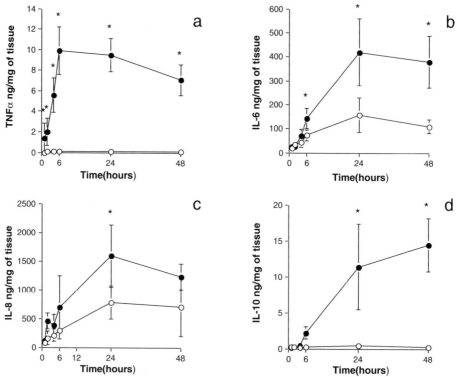

Figure 1. A. TNF-α release from human lung tissue. Human lung tissue (*n* = 25) was stimulated with 100 ng/ml LPS (purple circles) or buffer control (yellow circles). The release of TNF-α into the supernatant was measured by ELISA. Values shown are the mean ± SEM and * indicates a *p* < .05. B. IL-6 release from human lung tissue. Supernatants from figure 1A were analyzed for IL-6 using ELISA. Values given are the mean ± SEM and * indicates a *p* < .05. C. IL-8 release from human lung tissue. Supernatants from Figure 1A were analyzed for IL-8 using ELISA. Values given are the mean ± SEM and * indicates a *p* < .05. D. IL-10 release from human lung tissue. Supernatants from Figure 1A were analyzed for IL-10 using ELISA. Values given are the mean ± SEM and * indicates a *p* < .05.

Preparation of Human Lung Tissue for Primary Cell Culture

Human lung tissue was finely chopped using dissection scissors into fragments and given several washes with Tyrode's buffer. Fragments were stimulated with 100 ng/ml LPS (Sigma Chemical Company, Poole, UK) using a modified method of Bochner [1]. Supernatants were harvested at 1, 2, 4, 6, 24, and 48 h time points and the lung fragments weighed; both were stored at –80°C.

TNF-α ELISA

TNF-α levels were measured in lung supernatant using commercially available ELISAs from RnD Systems (Minneapolis, MN, USA). The assay was carried out as per manufactur-

er's instructions, the limit of detection being 0.31 pg/ml.

IL-6, IL-8, and IL-10 ELISAs

IL-6, IL-8, and IL-10 were all measured in lung supernatant using commercially available ELISA Duosets from Biosource (Europe, SA) as per manufacturers instructions. The limits of detection for IL-6, IL-8, and IL-10 were 0.28 ng/ml, 0.26 pg/ml, and 0.25 pg/ml, respectively.

Statistical Analysis

Nonparametric analysis was used throughout and results were considered statistically significant if *p* < .05.

Results

As shown in Figure 1A, release of the proinflammatory cytokine TNF-α was statistically elevated in the LPS-stimulated tissue at 1, 2, and 4 h, peaking at 6 h (median = 9.9 ng/mg of tissue vs. 0.1 ng/mg of tissue in the control, $p < .05$) and remained elevated until 48 h. A second proinflammatory cytokine, IL-6, was statistically increased in the LPS-stimulated supernatant at 6 h, with a maximum response at 24 h (median = 510.0 ng/mg of tissue compared to 48.5 ng/mg of tissue in the control, $p < .05$) and remained elevated at 48 h (see Figure 1B). The release of the chemokine IL-8 followed a similar pattern with a maximum response at 24 h (median = 1925 ng/mg of tissue vs. median = 1060 ng/mg of tissue in the control, $p < .05$) and remained elevated as shown in Figure 1C. Intriguingly, Figure 1D shows that the antiinflammatory cytokine IL-10 was elevated at 24 h (median = 12.5 ng/mg of tissue compared to undetectable levels in the control, $p < .05$) and remained elevated at 48 h.

Discussion

TNF-α is one of the most important proinflammatory cytokines, with roles in acute inflammation and also host defense. We found that LPS stimulated production of the proinflammatory cytokine TNF-α from human lung tissue. TNF-α release was rapid and statistically elevated from 1 h post-challenge, reaching a maximum by 6 h and was maintained at 48 h. TNF-α is released earlier than the other cytokines measured, indicating TNF-α may play a key role in the response to LPS. Studies in rodents have also shown early release of TNF-α in pulmonary inflammation [2]. The acute release of TNF-α is followed by elevated levels of IL-6 and IL-8, both peaking at 24 h. Elevat-

ed levels of IL-10 were detected at 24 h and were still increasing at 48 h.

While TNF-α was the first cytokine to be released, levels of TNF-α recorded were much lower than the other cytokines. Concentrations of IL-6 were up to 60 fold greater than TNF-α. The temporal relationship between cytokines may, therefore, be more important than the concentrations of cytokines released.

Our data also suggests the lung tissue may have two phases of response to LPS. The acute inflammatory phase driven by TNF-α, followed by the release of IL-6 and IL-8. Secondly, later release of the antiinflammatory cytokine IL-10 may indicate a repair or remodeling phase.

In conclusion, our findings show TNF-α is a key cytokine in the kinetics of an inflammatory response. TNF-α would, therefore, be a therapeutic target in pulmonary inflammation.

Acknowledgment

This study was funded by Arakis Ltd, Chesterford, UK.

References

1. Bochner BS, Rutledge BK, Schleimer RP: IL-1 production by human lung tissue. II. Inhibition by antiinflammatory steroids. J Immunol Oct 1987; 139:2303–2307.
2. Bergeron Y, Ouellet N, Deslauries A-M, Simard M, Oliver M, Bergeron MG: Cytokine kinetics and other host factors in response to pneumococcal pulmonary infection in mice. Infection and Immunity, Mar 1998; 912–922.

J.A. Warner

University of Southampton, Biomedical Sciences Building, Bassett Crescent East, Southampton, SO16 7PX, UK, Tel. +44 23 8059-4363, Fax +44 23 8059-4459, E-mail jawarner@soton.ac.uk

21-Year Longitudinal Study of Healthy Infants

Correlates with Atopy, Allergic Disease, and Asthma (The RIFYL Study)

K. Lemmert[1,2], R. Clancy[1,2], M. Gleeson[1,2]

[1]*Immunology Unit, Hunter Area Pathology Service, John Hunter Hospital, New Lambton, Australia,* [2]*School of Biomedical Sciences, Faculty of Health, University of Newcastle, Callaghan, Australia*

Summary: The RIFYL study was a 21 year prospective study of 263 healthy term children born into an Australian coastal suburban population, with a focus on parameters that influence the evolution of atopy, allergic disease and asthma. The initial study (1979–1984) obtained comprehensive records of feeding, demography, immunisation and health events as well as determining the pattern of normal development of mucosal immunity using saliva markers. Subsequent studies in 1985, 1991, 1993 and 2001 correlate atopic status, bronchial hyperreactivity, induced sputum cell count and cytokine patterns with clinical events. The 1985 study concluded that there was no relationship in pre-school children between atopy and asthma (23% asthmatics atopic). In 1991 transient early absence of IgA predict increased bronchial hyperreactivity – with a lower incidence of atopy but no relationship with asthma. In 1993 36% had asthma, 63% of whom were atopic. Sputum eosinophil counts correlated with bronchial hyperreactivity and asthma. The current study (2001) evaluated events over 21 years with risk factors. Environmental exposure in infancy had a time dependant effect on clinical outcome – an issue not considered in previous studies. Example (1), pets had no influence on atopic disease at any age, but exposure to birds was linked to less atopic disease in early adulthood. (2) Early introduction of cows milk linked to an early acquisition of atopy, but with no effect on later prevalence of atopy or atopic disease. (3) Early introduction of solids was associated with a higher prevalence of allergic disease but only in school aged children. (4) Age of immunisation was linked to a higher or lower rate of asthma, depending on age study. It is concluded that correlations between mechanisms, risk factors and clinical events vary over time, which needs to be recognised in epidemiological studies.

Keywords: atopy, allergic disease, asthma, skin prick test, bronchial hyperreactivity, birth cohort, breast feeding, respiratory infections

The prevalence of atopy and associated allergic diseases has increased since 1960 in affluent countries, especially in higher socioeconomic groups, in comparison to poorer countries or rural areas [1]. The factors contributing to this increase remain unclear but appear to be a complex interaction between socioeconomic, environmental, genetic, and immunologic factors. The evolution of atopy, allergic disease, and asthma was examined prospectively over a 21-year period in a birth cohort of 263 healthy infants born into an Australian coastal suburban population. The focus of the longitudinal study was to evaluate the influence of risk factors identified in the first year of life on the evolutionary patterns of these disease outcomes at critical developmental ages throughout childhood.

It has been recommended that studies assessing changes in prevalence rates should use the same population and the same objective methods on more than one occasion [2]. The

Respiratory Illness in the First Year of Life (RIFYL) Study [3] has provided an opportunity to investigate the changes in rates of asthma, atopy, and allergic disease in a birth cohort followed over a 21-year period. The RIFYL subjects were recruited prior to birth between 1979–1984 and studied prospectively for between 2 to 5 years, depending on the year of enrollment, for risk factors known to be associated with the development of asthma and allergic disease. Comprehensive demographic, socioeconomic, and medical records were kept on each subject during this initial study period, including the feeding history for each child, immunization dates, and health events relating to respiratory illness, allergy, and asthma.

Follow-up studies on the RIFYL cohort were conducted at critical developmental ages in 1985, 1991, 1993, and 2001. Objective measures of atopy, allergic disease, and asthma were recorded in all follow-up studies [4, 5, 6] using the same validated questionnaires and test protocols.

Methods

The atopic status of each subject was defined in each study year by standard SPT to common aeroallergens [4, 5, 6]. Specialist physicians using a validated questionnaire and clinical examinations determined the presence of allergic diseases and asthma in each subject during each study. Bronchial hyperreactivity responses to histamine [5] and saline challenges [6] and induced sputum eosinophil counts [6] were also used to assess current asthma status in the 1991 and 1993 studies. Allergic disease was defined as the presence of either allergic rhinoconjunctivitis and/or eczema.

Results

Longitudinal Prevalence

The prevalence of SPT atopy to the aeroallergens increased significantly with age from 12% in 1985 to 47% in 1991–93 ($p = < 0.01$) and 80% in 2001 ($p = < 0.01$). The prevalence

of allergic diseases increased significantly with age from 18% in 1985 to 38% in 1991–93 ($p = 0.01$) and remained steady at 41% in 2001. The prevalence of asthma increased significantly from 26% in 1985 to 38% in 1991–93 ($p = 0.03$) but decreased significantly in 2001 to 22% ($p = 0.05$) of the study population.

1985 (Age Range 2–6 Years)

In the 1985 study there were significant relationships between increased SPT atopy to common aeroallergens and a parental history of food allergy; and being introduced to cow's milk early in the first year of life. Conversely, having an infection (especially early) in the first year of life was associated with a decreased risk of atopy. A maternal history of eczema was associated with increased eczema in the child [4]. Asthma was found to be more prevalent in boys and was also associated with an older age at first immunization, but the difference was only 7 days.

1991 (Age Range 7–12 Years)

In the 1991 study a transient salivary IgA deficiency in the first year of life was associated with a decreased risk of atopy but an increased risk of bronchial hyperresponsiveness (BHR) but not asthma [5]. An increased risk of allergic disease was found in subjects introduced to solid foods early in the first year of life and a lower risk of allergic disease in those who were breast fed longer, or who had older siblings. A familial history of allergic disease in either the parents or the siblings increased the likelihood that the subject would have asthma in 1991.

1993 (Age Range 9–14 Years)

The 1993 study confirmed the findings of the 1991 study. The presence of older siblings protected against the development of allergic disease but increased the risk if those siblings had allergic disease. The duration of exclusive breast-feeding was inversely correlated with the risk of allergic disease. The results for the BHR and induced sputum eosinophil tests [6] showed a positive correlation with asthma in 1993, and a parental history of allergic disease was also associated with an increased risk of asthma.

2001 (Age Range 16–22 Years)

The most recent follow-up study in 2001 identified the early life risk factors for allergy and asthma in the cohort as young adults. A higher socioeconomic-level household, early introduction to cow's milk, and exposure to cigarette smoke during the first year of life were all associated with increased atopic sensitization, but not necessarily clinical disease as adults. Exposure to pets (cats, dogs, horses) showed no positive associations with atopy or allergic diseases, however, exposure to birds during the first year of life was associated with a decreased risk of allergic disease as adults. The presence of older siblings in the household continued to show the same decreased risk of allergic disease found at younger ages, but if the siblings had allergic disease then the subjects were also more likely to have asthma as young adults. The young adults with asthma had a parental history of allergic disease and received solid foods at an earlier age. The finding of an increased risk of asthma with delayed immunization in 1985 was not confirmed in the young adults. The data indicted the converse and asthma was more likely if the subjects were immunized earlier.

Conclusions

It is apparent from the 21-year longitudinal study of the RIFYL cohort that risk factors in the first year of life influence the clinical expression of allergic disease and asthma at different ages. Epidemiological studies focusing on a single time point (age group) may not predict the long-term development of these disease outcomes and may account for some of the discrepancies observed between studies. The RIFYL cohort studies have demonstrated that while some of the early risk factors were common to allergic disease and asthma at all ages, different early life factors can influence

clinical outcomes in childhood and as young adults.

A familial history of allergic disease was the most consistent risk factor for developing atopy, allergic disease, and asthma. High socioeconomic status, exposure to cigarette smoke, and infant feeding practices all influenced the development and persistence of these diseases over time. The early introduction of solid foods increased the risk of developing SPT atopy and asthma. A longer duration of exclusive breast-feeding reduced the risk of SPT atopy and allergic disease. The only consistent protective factors identified with a decreased risk of developing atopy and allergic diseases were: having nonallergic siblings; having an infection early in the first year of life; and exposure to birds in the first year.

Acknowledgments
Funding for the 2001 follow-up study was provided by grants from the Hunter Medical Research Institute and the John Hunter Children's Hospital, Newcastle, Australia. The study was conducted in the Hunter Area Pathology Service research laboratories at John Hunter Hospital.

References

1. Ring J, Kramer U, Schafer T, Behrendt H: Why are allergies increasing? Curr Opin Immunol 2001; 13:701–708.
2. Devereux G: The increase in allergic disease: environment and susceptibility. Proceedings of a symposium held at the Royal Society of Edinburgh, 4th June 2002. Clin Exp Allergy 2003; 33:394–406.
3. Cripps AW, Gleeson M, Clancy RL: Ontogeny of the mucosal immune response in children. In: Immunology of milk and the neonate (pp. 87–92). New York: J Mestecky, 1991.
4. Hensley MJ, Henry RL, Wlodarczyk JH, Clover K, Gleeson M, Firman DW, Dobson AJ, Clancy RL, Cripps AW: Determinants of atopy, eczema, and asthma in a community-based cohort study of preschool children. Am Rev Respir Dis 1986; 133(4):A41.
5. Gleeson M, Clancy RL, Hensley MJ, Cripps AW, Henry RL, Wlodarczyk JH, Gibson PG: Development of bronchial hyperreactivity following

transient absence of salivary IgA. Am J Respir Crit Care Med 1996; 153:1785–1789.

6. Gibson PG, Wlodarczyk JH, Hensley MJ, Gleeson M, Henry RL, Cripps AW, Clancy RL: Epidemiological association of airway inflammation with asthma symptoms and airway responsiveness in childhood. Am J Respir Crit Care Med 1998; 158:36–41.

Karla Lemmert

Immunology Unit, Hunter Area Pathology Service, Locked Bag 1, Hunter Region Mail Centre, NSW, 2310, Australia, Tel. +61 2 4921-4018, Fax +61 2 4921-4440, E-mail klemmert@ hunter.health.nsw.gov.au

Angiogenesis and Remodeling of Airway Vasculature in Asthma

M. Hoshino and T. Nakagawa

Division of Respiratory and Infectious Diseases, Department of Internal Medicine,
St. Marianna University School of Medicine, Kawasaki, Japan

Summary: *Background:* Histological examination of biopsies from asthma obtained during broncho-scopy has highlighted the presence of increased vessel numbers and vascularity in the submucosa. We hypothesized that cytokines and chemokines may play an important role in angiogenesis associated with asthma. *Methods:* We examined the expression of vascular endothelial growth factor (VEGF), basic fibroblast growth factor (bFGF), angiogenin, and stromal cell-derived factor-1 (SDF-1) immu-noreactivity in endobronchial biopsy specimens obtained from asthma and control subjects. The num-ber of vessels and the vascular area per unit area on a histologic section were estimated by computerized image analysis after staining for type IV collagen in vessel walls. *Results:* The airways of asthmatic subjects had significantly more vessels and greater vascular area than controls. Asthmatic subjects exhibited higher VEGF and bFGF, and angiogenin immunoreactivity in the submucosa than controls. Furthermore using *in situ* hybridization methods, VEGF and its receptor mRNA[+] cells were overex-pressed in asthma. Finally, we have demonstrated that the number of SDF-1[+] cells, one of the CXC chemokine, is higher in asthma than that of controls. *Conclusion:* These findings provide evidence that angiogenic factors may play an important role in angiogenesis of asthma.

Keywords: airway inflammation, airway remodeling, angiogenesis, angiogenin, asthma, basic fibro-blast growth factor, vascular endothelial growth factor, stromal cell-derived factor-1

Increased vessel numbers resulting from an-giogenesis in the airway wall contribute to air-way remodeling in asthma. Immunohisto-chemical methods using antibodies to vascular markers have made it much easier to visualize these vessels in bronchial biopsies and autopsy specimens, and changes in the airway micro-vasculature in human inflammatory respirato-ry disease are now better documented. Some of the cytokines associated with airway inflam-mation may also play roles in airway remodel-ing, and may be responsible for the increased vascularity in asthmatic airways. Several an-giogenic factors, such as vascular endothelial growth factor (VEGF), which is involved in vascular permeability, basic fibroblast growth factor (bFGF), hepatocyte growth factor, plate-let-derived growth factor have been identified.

Material and Methods

Endobronchial biopsy specimens were exam-ined by staining for VEGF, bFGF, and angio-genin and stromal cell-derived factor-1 (SDF-1) from asthmatic and control subjects. Spec-imens were also analyzed for the presence of the mRNA of VEGF and its receptors with *in situ* hybridization. The number of vessels and the vascular area were estimated by using computer-assisted image analysis.

Results

The airways of asthmatic subjects had signif-icantly more vessels and greater vascular area than that observed in controls. Asthmatic subjects exhibited higher VEGF and bFGF and angiogenin immunoreactivity in the submucosa than did control subjects. Significant correlations were detected between vascular area and the number of each angiogenic factor-positive cells within the asthmatic airways. Furthermore, asthmatic subjects exhibited a greater expression of VEGF and receptors mRNA[+] cells in the airway mucosa compared with control subjects. Finally, we have demonstrated that asthmatic subjects exhibited a greater number of SDF-1[+] cells in the airway mucosa than controls.

Concluding Remarks

Angiogenesis may lead to produce enlarged congested mucosal blood vessels which contribute to the increased airway wall thickness. These findings provide evidence that angiogenesis can be proposed to contribute to the airway remodeling process in patients with asthma.

References

1. Hoshino M et al.: Expression of vascular endothelial growth factor, basic fibroblast growth factor, and angiogenin immunoreactivity in asthmatic airways and its relationship to angiogenesis. J Allergy Clin Immunol 2001; 107:295–301.

2. Hoshino M et al.: Gene expression of vascular endothelial growth factor and its receptors and angiogenesis in bronchial asthma. J Allergy Clin Immunol 2001; 107:1034–1038.

3. Hoshino M et al.: Increased immunoreactivity of stromal cell-derived factor-1 and angiogenesis in asthma. Eur Respir J 2003; 21:804–809.

Makoto Hoshino

Division of Respiratory and Infectious Diseases, Department of Internal Medicine, St. Marianna University School of Medicine, 2-16-1 Sugao, Miyamae-ku, Kawasaki, 216-8511, Japan, Tel. +81 44 977-8111, Fax +81 44 977-8361, E-mail mhoshino@marianna-u.ac.jp

Protease-Activated Receptor-2 Enhances Allergen-Induced Airway Inflammation and Airway Hyperresponsiveness

H. Vliagoftis[1], C. Ebeling[1], and M. Hollenberg[2]

[1]*Pulmonary Research Group, University of Alberta, Edmonton, AB, Canada*
[2]*Department of Pharmacology and Therapeutics, University of Calgary, Calgary, AB, Canada*

Summary: *Background:* Certain allergens with serine protease activity can activate the Proteinase-Activated Receptor-2 (PAR-2), which has been shown to be upregulated in asthmatic airways. We investigated the effects of PAR-2 activation in the airways during allergen challenge on the two principle features of asthma: airway inflammation and airway hyperresponsiveness (AHR). *Methods:* PAR-2 activating peptide (PAR-2 AP) or control peptide (PAR-2 CP) were administered alone or in conjunction with ovalbumin (OVA) intranasally to mice sensitized to ovalbumin and AHR and airway inflammation were evaluated. *Results:* PAR-2 AP did not induce AHR or airway inflammation in OVA-sensitized mice that had not been challenged with OVA. When administered with OVA, PAR-2 AP enhanced AHR and airway inflammation compared to OVA administered alone or with PAR-2 CP. Mice administered PAR-2 AP alone during the 5 days following the final antigen challenge demonstrated an additional enhancement to airway inflammation when compared to the control animals. PAR-2 AP administered with allergen increased IL-13 and TNF in BAL fluid. *Conclusions:* Exogenous PAR-2 activation enhances allergen-mediated AHR and airway inflammation. PAR-2 activation can also enhance established airway inflammation even when dissociated from exposure to allergen. Therefore, PAR-2 activation may play a pathogenic role in the development of AHR and airway inflammation.

Keywords: airway inflammation, airway hyperresponsiveness, animal models, asthma, protease-activated receptor-2

PAR-2 is of particular interest in asthma because it has been implicated in inflammatory reactions and can be activated by a number of clinical important aeroallergens [1]. PAR-2 knockout mice exhibit delayed and decreased OVA-mediated eosinophilic airway inflammation and AHR compared to wild-type mice [2]. PAR-2 is upregulated on the airway epithelium of asthmatics [3]. PAR-2-mediated activation of airway epithelial cells induces the release of mediators involved in eosinophil recruitment [4]. However, other studies have shown a protective effect of PAR-2 against bronchoconstriction *in vivo* [5]. It is therefore, not clear whether PAR-2 activated in the airway is protective, i.e., induces bronchodilation, or detrimental by inducing inflammation and/or hyperresponsiveness.

We hypothesized that *in vivo* activation of PAR-2 in the airways has proinflammatory effects. Our recent studies show that PAR-2 activation in the respiratory tract increases allergen-mediated recruitment of eosinophils and mononuclear cells in the airways and AHR. These effects may be mediated through the release of IL-13 and TNF following PAR-2 activation.

Materials and Methods

Immunohistochemistry

Frozen sections or cytospins were stained for the presence of PAR-2 using the anti-PAR-2 B5 rabbit polyclonal antibody.

Sensitization and Challenge with OVA

Male Balb/c mice were sensitized via intraperitoneal injection of OVA. They were later challenged intranasally with OVA (50 µg) together with saline, PAR-2 activating peptide (PAR-2 AP, 100 µM), or PAR-2 control peptide (PAR-2 CP, 100 µM) twice on alternate days. Mice were assessed for AHR and airway inflammation the day after the last challenge or 5 days later by plethysmography and bronchoalveolar lavage (BAL) respectively.

Inflammatory Cytokine Analysis

Total lung RNA was extracted and analyzed for TNF, IL-4, IL-5, IL-10, IL-13, MIP-1α, MIP-2, MCP-1, IL-6, IFN-γ, L32, and GAPDH by RNase protection assay. IL-4, IL-5, IL-9, IL-10, IL-13, TNF, and IFN-γ were measured in BAL fluid by ELISA.

Results

PAR-2 was localized to the airway epithelium, endothelium, and airway smooth muscle of Balb/c mice. PAR-2 was also abundantly expressed on the nasal cavity epithelium and on alveolar macrophages (AM). In OVA-challenged mice BAL eosinophils and mononuc-

lear cells were positive for PAR-2, although at low levels.

Intranasal administration of PAR-2 AP to naïve or OVA-sensitized mice had no effects on airway inflammation and AHR. Coadministration of PAR-2 AP with OVA increased AHR and total inflammatory cell numbers in the BAL the day after the last challenge, while PAR-2 CP administered with OVA did not induce any changes compared to OVA alone. Mice treated with PAR-2 AP with OVA had increased numbers of eosinophils and mononuclear cells in the BAL when compared to mice given the PAR-2 CP with OVA.

We also evaluated other animals 5 days after the last challenge. AHR was still enhanced in the PAR-2 AP treated mice while there were no differences in total BAL numbers between the treatment groups. Therefore, the enhanced airway inflammation seen following PAR-2 AP administration dissipated 5 days after the last PAR-2 AP administration.

Finally, other mice were treated with PAR-2 peptides alone twice more during the 5 days after the last OVA challenge. In this case again PAR-2 AP administration with OVA increased total inflammatory cell numbers in the BAL compared to PAR-2 CP with OVA.

To define the mechanism of enhanced AHR and airway inflammation we studied cytokine expression in the lung following PAR-2 AP administration. Intranasally administered PAR-2 AP alone upregulated TNF and MIP-2 and to a smaller extent IL-13 mRNA levels in the lungs of naïve mice 4 h after administration. In all protocols in which the mice were given the PAR-2 AP the cytokine levels of IL-13 and TNF were elevated in BAL fluid compared to mice receiving PAR-2 CP. IL-4, IL-9, IL-10, and IFN-γ were not significantly altered although IL-5 showed an upward trend.

Discussion

A role for PAR-2 in airway inflammation has already been demonstrated [2]. However, our studies have shown for the first time that although PAR-2 may be involved in both AHR and airway inflammation, it regulates these

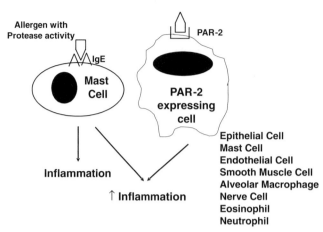

Figure 1. PAR-2-mediated enhancement of allergic inflammation.

two principle features of asthma through different pathways. We have demonstrated that AHR remains elevated for over 5 days following exogenous PAR-2 activation while the enhancement to airway inflammation was short lived. We have also shown, for the first time, that PAR-2 activation in inflamed airways increases airway inflammation even in the absence of continued allergen exposure. This observation indicates that in cases of established allergic airway inflammation nonspecific signals that can activate PAR-2, such as exogenous or endogenous serine proteinases, are sufficient to perpetuate airway inflammation. This observation may explain why allergen avoidance may not be a very effective therapeutic measure as long as airway inflammation persists.

The changes in AHR shown were consistent with the increase in IL-13 seen in the BAL fluid of mice that were administered PAR-2 AP. IL-13 has been shown to be critical for the development of allergen-induced AHR in mice [6]. The increased TNF seen following PAR-2 activation may be responsible for the increased airway inflammation by a number of mechanisms including increased adhesion molecule expression on the endothelium [7].

The current literature indicates that PAR-2 activation in the airways may have both protective and pathogenic roles in inflammatory airway diseases depending on the model used and the route of PAR-2 activation. Our results indicate that PAR-2 activation in the airways may have detrimental effects in asthma. Cross-linking of IgE on the surface of mast cells by the relevant allergen, initiates a cascade of inflammatory mediator production that leads to the recruitment of eosinophils and a number of other immune cells and the development of allergic inflammation. We propose that allergens with serine protease activity are also able to activate PAR-2 expressing cells. These PAR-2 expressing cells release a number of inflammatory mediators, which act together with the mediators released from mast cells to increase the inflammatory reaction (Figure 1).

References

1. Dery O, Corvera CU, Steinhoff M, Bunnett NW: Proteinase-activated receptors: novel mechanisms of signaling by serine proteases. Am J Physiol 1998; 274:C1429–C1452.
2. Schmidlin F, Amadesi S, Dabbagh K, Lewis DE, Knott P, Bunnett NW, Gater PR, Geppetti P, Bertrand C, Stevens ME: Protease-activated receptor 2 mediates eosinophil infiltration and hyperreactivity in allergic inflammation of the airway. J Immunol 2002; 169:5315–5321.
3. Knight DA, Lim S, Scaffidi AK, Roche N, Chung KF, Stewart GA, Thompson PJ: Protease-activated receptors in human airways: upregulation of PAR-2 in respiratory epithelium from patients with asthma. J Allergy Clin Immunol 2001; 108:797–803.
4. Vliagoftis H, Befus AD, Hollenberg MD, Moqbel R: Airway epithelial cells release eosinophil survival-promoting factors (GM-CSF) after stimulation of proteinase-activated receptor 2. J Allergy Clin Immunol 2001; 107:679–685.

5. Cocks TM, Fong B, Chow JM, Anderson GP, Frauman AG, Goldie RG, Henry PJ, Carr MJ, Hamilton JR, Moffatt JD: A protective role for protease-activated receptors in the airways. Nature 1999; 398:156–160.
6. Walter DM, McIntire JJ, Berry G, McKenzie AN, Donaldson DD, DeKruyff RH, Umetsu DT: Critical role for IL-13 in the development of allergen-induced airway hyperreactivity. J Immunol 2001; 167:4668–4675.
7. Haraldsen G, Kvale D, Lien B, Farstad IN, Brandtzaeg P: Cytokine-regulated expression of E-selectin, intercellular adhesion molecule-1 (ICAM-1), and vascular cell adhesion molecule-1 (VCAM-1) in human microvascular endothelial cells. J Immunol 1996; 156:2558–2565.

Harissios Vliagoftis

Pulmonary Research Group, Department of Medicine, 550 HMRC, University of Alberta, Edmonton, AB, Canada T6G 2S2, Tel. +1 780 492-9295, Fax +1 780 492-5329, E-mail harissios.vliagoftis@ualberta.ca

Glucocorticoids Promote T Regulatory Cells in Asthma by Increasing FOXP3 Expression

C. Karagiannidis[1], G. Menz[2], M. Akdis[1], P. Holopainen[1], G. Hense[2], B. Rückert[1], P.-Y. Mantel[1], C.A. Akdis[1], K. Blaser[1], and C.B. Schmidt-Weber[1]

[1]*Swiss Institute of Allergy and Asthma Research (SIAF), Davos, Switzerland*
[2]*Hochgebirgsklinik Davos Wolfgang, Davos-Wolfgang, Switzerland*

Summary: T regulatory (T_{reg}) cells are balancing immune responses and play a key role in maintenance of peripheral tolerance against antigens, including autoantigens and allergens. Glucocorticoids (GC) are used to control inflammatory diseases and are assumed to target particularly lymphocytes, but their impact on T_{reg} cells is currently unknown. We, therefore, investigated local and systemic GC treatment and its impact on asthmatic patients' T_{reg} cells *in vivo*. $CD4^+$ T-cells from healthy donors and 50 asthmatic, GC-treated patients were isolated and mRNA expression of FOXP3, a crucial T_{reg} marker, along with IL-10 and TFG-β_1 was determined. FOXP3 and IL-10 mRNA expression correlated with each other and FOXP3 was significantly increased in asthmatic patients receiving inhalative or/and systemic GC treatment. However asthma patients who suffered from moderate asthma and who were not GC-treated showed neither increased FOXP3 nor IL-10 expression. In contrast, TFG-β_1 expression was even significantly decreased in GC-naïve patients and not different to healthy donors regarding the GC-treated groups. No correlation of FOXP3 mRNA expression was observed in relation to a known microsatellite polymorphism. This study shows that GCs are promoting the Tr1 phenotype of T_{reg} cells by a FOXP3-dependent mechanism.

Keywords: lymphocytes, glucocorticoids, asthma

T_{reg} cells balance the immune responses to maintain peripheral tolerance against antigens, including autoantigens and allergens. This new paradigm in immunology suggests that T_{reg} cells are characterized by their ability to suppress effector T-cells of either Th1 or Th2 phenotype involved in mediating inflammation [1–3]. T_{reg} cells have been described expressing $CD4^+$ $CD25^+$ surface molecules and suppressive cytokines such as IL-10 (Tr1 cells) and TFG-β_1 (Th3 cells) [4–8]. T_{reg} cells mediate their suppressive capacity in a cell contact and antigen-specific manner [9–11].

This new paradigm of peripheral tolerance was shown to control allergen reactivity in healthy individuals and in mono-allergic disease, however more complex diseases such as asthma have not, so far, been investigated. Asthma is therapeutically controlled by immunosuppressive drugs, which may be more efficiently employed if their ability to alter the regulatory function of T_{reg} cells is known. The effectivity of GCs has been at least partially attributed to reduced T-cell activation and cytokine expression. However, it is currently unknown how GCs affects the activity of T_{reg} cells. To investigate the role of T_{reg} cells we investigated the expression of IL-10, TFG-β, and the currently most specific marker for T_{reg} cell, FOXP3 [12–15].

Materials and Methods

PBMC were isolated from blood of healthy donors and asthmatic patients by Ficoll (Biochrom KG, Berlin, Germany) density gradient centrifugation. CD4+ T-cells were purified as previously described [16]. RNA was isolated using the RNeasy Mini Kit (Qiagen, Hamburg, Germany) according to the manufacturer's protocol. The PCR primers detecting EF-1a, FOXP3, IL-10, and TFG-β were described previously [17]. The cDNAs were prepared from T-cell RNA and amplified using SYBR-PCR mastermix (Applied Biosystems) according to the recommendations of the manufacturer (Applied Biosystems). Relative quantification and calculation of the range of confidence was performed using the comparative $\Delta\Delta CT$ method as described [18]. All amplifications were carried out at least in triplicate.

Results

A significant increase in FOXP3 mRNA expression was observed in freshly isolated, unstimulated CD4+ T-cells of patients with moderate steroid treated asthma (2.25-fold, $n = 24$, $p \leq 0.05$, Figure 1A) compared to healthy non-allergic subjects or untreated patients. The group of severe asthmatics treated with systemic steroids showed a significant increase in FOXP3 mRNA expression in freshly isolated CD4+ T-cells (2.92-fold, $n = 18$, $p \leq 0.05$, Figure 1A) in comparison to untreated patients with moderate asthma or healthy control subjects. No difference was observed between the two groups of GC-treated asthmatic patients ($p > 0.05$, Figure 1A). Untreated patients with moderate asthma showed a remarkable lower expression of FOXP3 mRNA compared to both groups of treated asthmatic patients ($p < 0.01$, Figure 1A).

A significant increase in IL-10 expression was observed in the groups of GC-treated mod-erate (2.43-fold, $n = 24$, $p \leq 0.05$) and severe asthmatics (2.70-fold, $p \leq 0.05$, Figure 1C) compared to healthy controls and untreated asthmatics. A significant decrease of TFG-β_1 mRNA expression was observed in untreated asthmatic patients in relation to the group of healthy individuals and also in comparison to GCtreated asthmatic patients ($p > 0.05$, Figure 1C). Since patients with genetic FOXP3 defects (IPEX syndrome) show high total serum IgE levels, FOXP3 mRNA expression and serum IgE levels were also analyzed. Although a tendency toward lower IgE levels with higher FOXP3 mRNA expression in CD4+ T-cells was detected, there was no statistically significant correlation between FOXP3 expression and total serum IgE level ($n = 43$, Spearman $r_s = -0.205$, $p > 0.05$, Figure 1B).

FOXP3 and IL-10 mRNA expression showed a significant correlation in freshly isolated CD4+ T-cells of asthmatic patients ($n = 57$, Spearman $r_s = 0.588$, $p \leq 0.0001$, Figure 1D). A moderate correlation was observed between FOXP3 and TFG-β_1 mRNA expression ($n = 47$, Spearman $r_s = 0.327$, $p \leq 0.03$, Figure 1F). However, the correlation is only half as tight as was observed for IL-10.

Discussion

Current results demonstrate increased T_{reg} cell activity in asthmatic patients treated with GCs. Significantly increased FOXP3 mRNA expression was found in unstimulated peripheral blood CD4+ T-cells of both severe asthmatic patients, treated with systemic GCs, and patients with moderate asthma treated with inhaled GCs, but not in patients with untreated moderate asthma. The higher T_{reg} cell activity in GC treated asthmatic patients is demonstrated by increased IL-10 mRNA expression, which tightly correlated with the FOXP3 expression. In contrast, TFG-β_1 showed only a moderate correlation. This underlines the distinct role of TFG-β_1 in T_{reg} cells and the different regulatory pathways of this suppressive cytokine [10]. The role of TFG-β_1 in context of T_{reg} cells has been recently described to be in the induction phase of regulatory processes

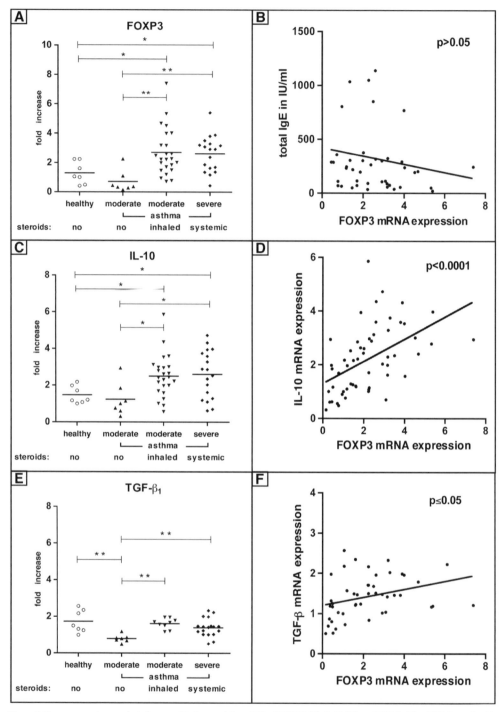

Figure 1. Gene expression analysis by quantitative real time PCR of FOXP3 (A), IL-10 (C) and TFG-β₁ (E) mRNA from freshly isolated, unstimulated CD4⁺ T-cells of healthy nonallergic donors and asthmatic patients. The correlation of the individual values of FOXP3 mRNA versus total IgE serum levels (B), IL-10 (D) or TFG-β (F) mRNA are analyzed on the basis of spearman rank correlation. Data were normalized to one randomly chosen healthy donor and set as one. Statistical significance was tested using Student's t-Test and is indicated by asterisks (* = $p \le 0.05$).

and not necessarily in the suppression itself. The present study shows that patients suffering from moderate asthma, which is not treated with GCs, show significantly lower TFG-β$_1$ mRNA expression, which may indicate a lowered ability to induce T$_{reg}$ cells. Interestingly, there was no difference in FOXP3 mRNA expression between moderate and severe, intrinsic or extrinsic asthmatic patients. Serum IgE levels of the investigated asthmatic patients only show a tendency to correlate with FOXP3 expression, possibly caused by the concomitant IgE-enhancing effect of GCs. It is interesting to note that all patients with high IgE serum levels of more than 1000 IU/ml expressed low amounts of FOXP3.

The presented data demonstrate that GC treatment is not only immunosuppressive and antiinflammatory, it also promotes or initiates the differentiation of effector cells into Tr1 cells in a FOXP3 dependent manner. However analysis of GC treatment in a time course suggests that GC induced T$_{reg}$ cells only transiently occur in the periphery (data not shown). These findings are important for an advanced understanding of GC therapy and the development of new therapeutic approaches aiming at the generation of T$_{reg}$ cells.

Acknowledgments

This work was supported by the Swiss National Foundation Grants Nr: 31–65436.01 and 3100A0–100164, the Ehmann Foundation Chur, the Ernst Goehner Foundation Zug, the Saurer Foundation Zurich, and the Swiss Life Zurich.

References

1. Schmidt-Weber CB, Blaser K: Immunological mechanisms in specific immunotherapy. Springer Semin Immunopathol 2004; 25(3–4):377–390.

2. Schmidt-Weber CB, Blaser K: Immunological mechanisms of specific allergen immunotherapy. Curr Drug Targets Inflamm Allergy 2004, in press.

3. Schmidt-Weber CB, Blaser K: Regulation and role of transforming growth factor β in immune tolerance induction and development of inflammatory disease. Curr Opin Immunol, in press.

4. Sakaguchi S: Regulatory T-cells: key controllers of immunologic self-tolerance. Cell 2000; 101:455–458.

5. Shimizu J, Yamazaki S, Takahashi T, Ishida Y, Sakaguchi S: Stimulation of CD25$^+$ CD4$^+$ regulatory T-cells through GITR breaks immunological self-tolerance. Nat Immunol 2002; 3:135–142.

6. Takahashi T, Tagami T, Yamazaki S, Uede T, Shimizu J, Sakaguchi N, et al.: Immunologic self-tolerance maintained by CD25$^+$ CD4$^+$ regulatory T-cells constitutively expressing cytotoxic T lymphocyte-associated antigen 4. J Exp Med 2000; 192:303–310.

7. Wakkach A, Fournier N, Brun V, Breittmayer JP, Cottrez F, Groux H: Characterization of dendritic cells that induce tolerance and T regulatory 1 cell differentiation *in vivo*. Immunity 2003; 18:605–617.

8. Weiner HL: Induction and mechanism of action of transforming growth factor-β-secreting Th3 regulatory cells. Immunol Rev 2001; 182(1):207–214.

9. Dieckmann D, Bruett CH, Ploettner H, Lutz MB, Schuler G: Human CD4$^+$CD25$^+$ regulatory, contact-dependent T-cells induce IL- 10-producing, contact-independent type 1-like regulatory T-cells [corrected]. J Exp Med 2002; 196:247–153.

10. Piccirillo CA, Letterio JJ, Thornton AM, McHugh RS, Mamura M, Mizuhara H, et al.: CD4$^+$CD25$^+$ regulatory T-cells can mediate suppressor function in the absence of transforming growth factor β1 production and responsiveness. J Exp Med 2002; 196:237–246.

11. Nakamura K, Kitani A, Strober W: Cell contact-dependent immunosuppression by CD4$^+$CD25$^+$ regulatory T-cells is mediated by cell surface-bound transforming growth factor β. J Exp Med 2001; 194:629–644.

12. Khattri R, Cox T, Yasayko SA, Ramsdell F: An essential role for Scurfin in CD4$^+$ CD25$^+$ T regulatory cells. Nat Immunol 2003; 4:337–342.

13. Fontenot JD, Gavin MA, Rudensky AY: Foxp3 programs the development and function of CD4$^+$CD25$^+$ regulatory T-cells. Nat Immunol 2003; 4:330–336.

14. O'Garra A, Vieira P: Twenty-first century Foxp3. Nat Immunol 2003; 4:304–306.

15. Hori S, Nomura T, Sakaguchi S: Control of regulatory T-cell development by the transcription factor Foxp3. Science 2003; 299:1057–1061.

16. Wohlfahrt JG, Karagiannidis C, Kunzmann S, Epstein MM, Kempf W, Blaser K, et al.: Ephrin-

A1 suppresses Th2 cell activation and provides a regulatory link to lung epithelial cells. J Immunol 2004; 172(2):843–850.

17. Karagiannidis C, Akdis M, Holopainen P, Woolley NJ, Hense G, Rueckert B, et al.: Glucocorticoids upregulate FoxP3 expression and regulatory T cells in asthma. J Allergy Clin Immunol, 2004; 114:1425–1433.

18. Kunzmann S, Wohlfahrt JG, Itoh S, Asao H, Komada M, Akdis CA, et al.: SARA and Hgs attenuate susceptibility to TFG-β_1-mediated T-cell suppression. FASEB J 2003; 17:194–202.

Carsten B. Schmidt-Weber

SIAF, Obere Str. 22, CH-7270 Davos, Switzerland, E-mail csweber@siaf.unizh.ch

The Phenotype of Steroid-Dependent Severe Asthma Is Not Associated with Increased Lung Levels of Th-2 Cytokines

S.E. Wenzel, S. Balzar, H.W. Chu, and M. Cundall

National Jewish Medical and Research Center, Denver, CO, USA

Summary: Severe, steroid-dependent asthma represents a poorly understood portion of the asthma population. We hypothesized increased IL-4 or IL-13 would be found in severe asthma, as compared to mild-moderate asthma and normal control lungs. *Methods:* BAL cell and tissue biopsy specimens were collected from 17 normal controls, 11 mild-moderate asthmatics, and 23 severe steroid-dependent asthmatics. The BAL cell pellet (macrophages, lymphocytes, and granulocytes) was analyzed at baseline and after 24 h in culture for IL-4 and IL-13 mRNA by quantitative real-time (RT)-PCR. The supernatant was collected for analysis of IL-4 and IL-13 protein by immunoassay. IL-4 and-13 mRNA were also measured in endobronchial tissue by RT-PCR. BAL and biopsy cell differentials were obtained. *Results:* IL-4 mRNA or protein were not reliably detected in any compartment. IL-13 mRNA and protein levels in all compartments and subjects were low. Severe asthma subjects had the lowest levels of BAL cell IL-13 mRNA after 24 h in culture ($p = 0.008$), despite the highest BAL lymphocyte numbers ($p = 0.05$). The IL-13 BAL cell supernatant protein and mRNA levels from biopsies of mild-moderate subjects also tended to be the highest ($p = 0.10$ and 0.13, respectively), with severe asthmatics having the lowest levels. The 24 h BAL cell IL-13 mRNA correlated with tissue eosinophils ($r^2 = 0.23$, $p = 0.02$) and with FEV1 ($r^2 = 0.29$, $p = 0.005$). *Conclusions:* These results suggest that although Th-2 cytokines may have a role in mild-moderate asthma, they are not contributing factors in most severe asthma patients. Other mechanisms for severe asthma should be investigated.

Keywords: asthma, interleukin-13, inflammation

The phenotype of severe asthma is often assumed to be accompanied by an active Th2 inflammatory process, believed to drive associated symptoms and lung function abnormalities. Most of these assumptions are based on animal models and evaluation of patients with milder disease. In severe asthma, this process has been suggested to be "un- or poorly" responsive to steroids, thereby contributing to the refractory nature of these patients [1,2].

Classic Th2 cytokines, such as IL-4, IL-5, and IL-13 have been described in the lung tissue and BAL fluid of patients with asthma [2–4]. Interestingly, as the primary sources for both IL-4 and IL-13 are believed to be Th2 lymphocytes, which do not store the protein, most studies have evaluated mRNA, most commonly by *in situ* hybridization. However, some studies have described the protein, as well, where the likely source is the mast cell.

We hypothesized that increases in IL-4/-13 play a significant role in severe asthma. To evaluate this, BAL cells, their supernatant, and biopsy tissue were evaluated for IL-4/-13 mRNA and protein from severe steroid-dependent or mild-moderate asthmatics, as well as normal subjects. The results suggest these Th2 cytokines are not major contributors to severe asthma.

Methods

Subjects

Asthmatic subjects were divided into severity category as previously described [5]. Mild-moderate asthmatics had a prebronchodilator FEV1 of 60% predicted and were treated with β-agonists and/or low dose inhaled corticosteroids (ICS) (<400 µg/day). None had required oral steroids in the last year. Severe asthmatics required treatment with oral steroids for 50% of the previous year, as well as high dose ICS with at least one other long-term controller. They continued to have symptoms and utilize urgent health care. Normal controls had normal pulmonary function and no history of any respiratory illness. The National Jewish Institutional Review Board approved the study and all subjects gave informed consent.

Procedures

Endobronchial biopsies were taken from the subcarinae of the 3rd to 4th generation bronchi of the left or right lower lobes. BAL was performed in subsegments of the right middle lobe. Biopsies were placed in acetone for immunohistochemistry (IHC) or TriZol for mRNA. BAL fluid was pooled and centrifuged to separate fluid from cells. Cell counts on tissue were performed as previously described [5].

Isolation and Culture of BAL cells

10^6 BAL cells were placed into Teflon-coated wells and cultured in Dulbecco's modified eagle medium (DMEM)/0.1% bovine serum albumin (BSA) for 24 h (37 °C, 5% CO_2). RNA was extracted from the *ex vivo* cultured BAL cells placed in TriZol, while the supernatant was collected for IL-4/-13 protein levels.

Real-time PCR for Measurement of IL-4/-13 mRNA

IL-4 and IL-13 mRNA expression in BAL cells and biopsy tissue was determined by reverse transcription, followed by real-time quantitative PCR. The IL-4/-13 and 18sRNA primers and probes were purchased from Applied Biosystems (Forster City, CA) and labeled with fluorescein (FAM) or VIC. RT-PCR was performed on the ABI Prism 7700 system (Applied Biosystems). IL-4/-13 mRNA was indexed to 18s rRNA (multiplication factor 1×10^6).

IL-4/-13 Protein

Il-4/-13 protein was measured by commercial high or ultrasensitivity enzyme-linked immunosorbant assay kits from R&D systems (Minneapolis, MN, USA).

Statistics

Log-transformed data were analyzed by ANOVA, with Tukey-Kramer intergroup comparisons. Data are presented as mean ± standard error of the means (SEM). Correlation analysis was done using Pearson's correlation coefficient of the log-transformed data.

Results

Seventeen normal, 11 mild-moderate, and 22 severe asthmatic subjects were evaluated. They were well matched for age, gender, and atopy, with eosinophils highest in mild-moderate, and mast cells lowest in severe asthma (Table 1). There were no differences in BAL cell eosinophils, but there was a trend to higher lymphocytes in severe asthma BAL (overall $p = 0.06$).

IL-4 and IL-13 mRNA and Protein Levels

IL-4 mRNA or protein were not reliably detectable in any sample. IL-13 mRNA was present in both tissue and BAL cell pellets from subjects in all groups. IL-13 mRNA was significantly increased in the BAL cell pellet from mild-moderate asthma, as compared to severe asthma subjects (overall $p = 0.008$, intergroup comparison $p < 0.05$; Figure 1). Similarly, there was a trend for increased BAL cell supernatant IL-13 protein levels in mild-moderate asthmatics, as compared to the other groups ($p = 0.07$). mRNA levels of IL-13 in biopsy tissue were also not different among the groups, but were numerically highest in mild-moderate asthma, with little difference between normals and severe asthma (overall $p = 0.06$). The presence/absence of atopy did not influence the results. IL-13 mRNA and protein levels correlated across compartments, supporting the validity of the measures (r-values of 0.3 to 0.55) .

Correlations with Inflammation and FEV1

There were no correlations of IL-13 mRNA or protein with BAL or tissue lymphocytes. However, there was a modest correlation of IL-13 BAL cell mRNA with tryptase (+) mast cells ($r = 0.3$, $p = 0.09$), and a correlation of BAL cell IL-13 mRNA levels with tissue eosinophils ($r = 0.36$, $p = 0.03$). There was a

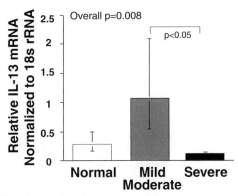

Figure 1. Legend missing, please supply!

strong positive correlation of BAL cell IL-13 mRNA levels with FEV. ($r = 0.55$, $p = 0.005$).

Discussion

The results suggest that although Th2 cytokines, in particular IL-13, are measured in mild-moderate asthma, significantly lower levels of mRNA and a trend toward lower protein levels are measured in severe asthma than in control groups. These findings suggest that persistent Th2 inflammation is not a major contributor to the pathophysiology of severe asthma.

Th2 cytokines have been the focus of intensive investigation in asthma with animal and human data suggesting that Th2 cytokines contribute to many if not all the immunopathologic and physiologic changes. Yet, in this study, in most severe asthmatics, with the

Table 1. Baseline characteristics.

	Atopy (%)	FEV1 (%)*	Eos†/mm²	Lymphs†/mm²	Mast cells†/mm²
Normal	76	NL	3.4 (2.2–5.2)	47 (33–66)	71 (64–80)
Mild-Moderate	83	86±11	21.5 (16.1–28.8)	41 (26–73)	55 (34–77)
Severe	78	52±15	5.5 (3.3–8.0)	23 (17–32)	14 (10–20)
$p =$	NS	0.001	0.03	0.31	0.005

*mean ± standard deviation; †log transformed means and standard errors of the mean, reformatted to original scale

worst disease, they could not be found. IL-4 mRNA or protein could not be reliably detected in any subject. While it is certainly conceivable that they "were" present in severe asthma and that the high doses of corticosteroids suppressed them, the implication remains the same. In their absence, severe asthma exists unabated. Interestingly, in two previous studies of "steroid resistant" severe asthma, Th2 cytokines remained elevated despite high doses of systemic steroids [1, 2]. The current results contradict those, perhaps caused by differing methodology (*in situ* hybridization vs. RT-PCR) and the much more severe nature of the patients studied here. Additionally, the levels of IL-13 did not correlate with lung lymphocytes, but marginally correlated with mast cells, bringing into question the source of the IL-13 in asthma. Although not reported here, IL-13(+) mast cells can be identified by IHC, although the numbers are not particularly higher in one group or another.

Another surprising finding was the correlation of IL-13 with lung function in asthma. Even in mild-moderate patients, higher levels correlated with better lung function. The adaptive immune response associated with IL-13, although initiating allergic/IgE related responses, may also have protective effects on lung function. Further study is indicated.

In conclusion, these data question the importance of Th2 cytokines to the evolution of severe asthma. Future studies will need to address interactions with other inflammatory mediators and structural changes, which may be more important to this phenotype.

References

1. Leung DY, Martin RJ, Szefler SJ, Sher ER, Ying S, Kay AB, et al.: Dysregulation of interleukin 4, interleukin 5, and interferon γ gene expression in steroid-resistant asthma. J Exp Med 1995; 181: 33–40.
2. Naseer T, Minshall EM, Leung DY, Laberge S, Ernst P, Martin RJ, et al.: Expression of IL-12 and IL-13 mRNA in asthma and their modulation in response to steroid therapy. Am J Respir Crit Care Med 1997; 155:845–851.
3. Humbert M, Durham SR, Kimmitt P, Powell N, Assoufi B, Pfister R, et al.: Elevated expression of messenger ribonucleic acid encoding IL-13 in the bronchial mucosa of atopic and nonatopic subjects with asthma. J. Allergy Clin Immunol 1997; 99:657–665.
4. Virchow JC Jr, Kroegel C, Walker C, Matthys H: Inflammatory determinants of asthma severity: mediator and cellular changes in bronchoalveolar lavage fluid of patients with severe asthma. J Allergy Clin Immunol 1996; 98(5 Pt 2):27–33; discussion S. 33–40.
5. Wenzel SE, Schwartz LB, Langmack EL, Halliday JL, Trudeau JB, Gibbs RL, et al.: Evidence that severe asthma can be divided pathologically into two inflammatory subtypes with distinct physiologic and clinical characteristics. Am J Respir Crit Care Med 1999; 160(3):1001–1008.

Sally E. Wenzel

National Jewish Medical and Research Center, 1400 Jackson St., Denver, CO 80206, USA, Tel. +1 303 398-1521, Fax +1 303 398-1476, E-mail wenzels@njc.org

Bronchial Smooth Muscle Cells Apoptosis in Airway Remodeling

K. Solarewicz[1], M. Jutel[1], T. Basinski[1], J. Verhagen[2], R. Crameri[2], M. Akdis[2], K. Blaser[2], and C.A. Akdis[2]

[1] *Wroclaw Medical University, Department of Internal Medicine and Allergology, Wroclaw, Poland,* [2]*Swiss Institute of Allergy and Asthma Research (SIAF), Davos, Switzerland*

Summary: *Background:* Chronic inflammatory diseases of the lung like asthma and chronic obstructive pulmonary disease (COPD) are associated with pathological remodeling of airway tissues, disrupting their proper structure and function. Bronchial smooth muscle cells (SMC) are an active cellular component able to proliferate, express adhesion molecules, and secrete cytokines. The structural changes in bronchial SMC refer to the size, mass, and number of the cells with a remarkably increased death index. *Aim:* Investigation of the mechanisms and factors responsible for the bronchial SMC death process in asthma and COPD. *Methods:* Cultured primary bronchial SMC were stimulated with *in vitro* differentiated Th1 and Th2 cell supernatants, activated eosinophil and neutrophil lysates, IFN-γ, TNF-α, and soluble Fas-ligand (sFasL). Viability, expression of apoptosis receptors, apoptosis-indicating enzymes and other molecules, and morphologic features of SMC were investigated by flow cytometry and immunocytology. *Results:* Bronchial SMC death showed characteristic morphological features of apoptosis. The viability of SMC, assessed by ethidium bromide uptake, was markedly decreased in comparison to the control cells after 3–6 days of incubation with the death-inducing cytokines (IFN-γ, TNF-α, sFasL) and activated Th1 and Th2 cell supernatants. Whereas IL-5-stimulated eosinophils induced apoptosis, SMC were resistant to GM-CSF- and IFN-γ-activated eosinophil lysates as well as to IFN-γ-activated neutrophil lysates. Death receptor expression on SMC was regulated. Unstimulated SMC expressed the death receptors: TNFR 1&2, Fas, TRAIL 1&2, and membrane Fas-Ligand. IFN-γ and TNF-α appeared to be the effector molecules rendering the bronchial SMC susceptible to apoptosis. They upregulated TNFR1, TNFR2, and Fas as well as the membrane FasL expression on SMC after 48 h of coincubation. TNF-α upregulated both TRAIL 1&2 receptors and soluble FasL upregulated TNFR2. Supporting these findings, intracellular caspase-3 activation in SMC was significantly increased by IFN-γ, sFasL, TRAIL, Th1, and Th2 supernatants. *Conclusion:* Bronchial SMC appear as the essential target of the inflammatory attack by T-cells and eosinophils. These data demonstrate an important pathogenetic event leading to morphological changes and functional contraction/relaxation disorder in the bronchial wall in asthma and COPD.

Keywords: smooth muscle, T-cells, eosinophils, apoptosis

Bronchial hyperresponsiveness and variable airway obstruction are cardinal features of asthma. Persistent airway inflammation and irreversible structural changes of the bronchial wall (defined as airway remodeling) are crucial processes in asthma development [1, 2]. These alterations involve changed expression and/or function for a variety of proinflammatory cytokines, growth factors and their receptors, as well as a dysregulation in the differentiation, proliferation, and apoptosis of multiple cell types [3, 4]. In particular, the increase in SMC content can explain the mechanical consequences of airway remodeling, such as airway luminal narrowing and the permanent reduction of the airway caliber [3, 5, 6]. Bidirectional stimulatory cross-talk was recently found to exist between activated T-cells and airway smooth muscle (ASM) cells, a process that results in the induction of asthmatic changes in ASM responsiveness [7]. Also the eosinophils can be the source of proinflammatory cytokines including GM-CSF, IL-4, IL-5, IL-6, IL-8, and TNF-α [8]. This study demonstrates a mechanism by which T-cells and eosinophils can cause injury to airway SMC.

Material and Methods

Cell Cultures

Primary normal bronchial smooth muscle cells (BSMC) were purchased (Clonetics, BioWhittaker, Cambrex Company, San Diego, CA, USA). Cells were grown in smooth muscle cell growth medium (SMCGM, supplemented accordingly to the manufacturer's protocol), in humidified atmosphere containing 5% CO_2 at 37 °C. The cytokines were added to the cell-cultures and incubated for 2, 4, 24, 48, or 72 h.

Human *in vitro* Th1 and Th2 Cell Differentiation

Th1 and Th2 cells were obtained by differentiation of purified cord blood CD45RA$^+$ T-cells as previously described in detail [11]. Cytokine production by Th1 and Th2 revealed distinct profiles.

Isolation of Eosinophils

Granulocyte-enriched cell pellets were isolated by Ficoll (Biochrom KG) density gradient centrifugation of venous blood and depleted of erythrocytes by use of hypotonic saline lysis. Eosinophils were negatively selected by using the MACS system (Miltenyi Biotec) as described [12].

Demonstration of BSMC Viability and Apoptosis in Cultures

For the analysis of apoptosis in SMC cultures, cells were examined under phase-contrast microscopy to evaluate the morphologic characteristics. SMC viability was evaluated by ethidium bromide (1 μmol/L) uptake and flow cytometry. Annexin V is a phosphatidylserine binding protein that was also used to detect apoptotic cells [13]. Hoechst staining was performed as described [13]. SMC cultures were evaluated with an inverted microscope equipped with interference contrast and UV light (Axiovert 405M; Carl Zeiss AG, Feldbach, Switzerland).

Results

The viability of SMC was assessed by ethidium bromide uptake. Stimulation with IFN-γ or TNF-α induced cell death after 3–6 days of culture. However, an additive effect was observed when the cells were stimulated with both cytokines. Similar results were obtained when supernatants from *in vitro* differentiated activated Th1 cells were added to the SMC cultures. Supernatants from Th2 cells induced less cell death. Resting T-cell supernatants did not induce SMC death.

Unstimulated SMC expressed the death receptors: TNFR1, TNFR2, Fas, TRAIL 1, TRAIL2, and membrane Fas-Ligand. IFN-γ and TNF-α appear to be the effector molecules rendering the bronchial SMC susceptible to apoptosis. They upregulated TNFR1, TNFR2, and Fas as well as the membrane FasL expression on SMC 48 h after stimulation. Soluble FasL upregulated TNFR2. The apoptosis receptors DR4 (TRAIL-1) and DR5 (TRAIL 2) were present on the surface of unstimulated SMC. TNF-α significantly upregulated both TRAIL 1 and 2 receptors. Stimulation of the cells with IFN-γ, sFasL, TRAIL, Th1 cell supernatants, or Th2 cell supernatants resulted in increased caspase-3 activity in SMC.

SMC were stimulated with IFN-γ, TNF-α, or recombinant ECP. The type of keratinocyte (KC) death was investigated by demonstration of apoptotic features such as chromatin condensation and fragmented nuclei shown in Hoechst staining. There was substantial staining with annexin V in SMC, which were exposed to activated T-cells, IFN-γ, and TNF-α.

SMC death appeared in 6-day cultures after treatment with lysates of IL-5-primed eosinophils. SMCs were resistant to GM-CSF- and IFN-γ- activated eosinophil lysates as well as to IFN-γ-activated neutrophil lysates. ECP is a potent eosinophil-derived cytotoxic substance released into the microenvironment. Human recombinant ECP was used to induce SMC death. ECP induced cell death as assessed by ethidium bromide exclusion and propidium iodide staining and subsequent flow cytometry assessment.

Discussion

The study shows that the apoptosis of bronchial SMC is a key pathogenic event of the tissue injury that leads to airway remodeling. BSMC appear as an essential target of the inflammatory attack by T-cells and eosinophils. The inflammatory cells induce apoptosis in the SMC through secreted cytokines and contact, thus triggering the important mechanisms leading to morphological changes and functional contraction/relaxation disorder in the bronchial wall in asthma.

The crucial role of infiltrating T-cells and eosinophils is suggested in pathogenic mechanisms responsible for disintegration of airway tissue and damage of structural cells such as mesenchymal cells and bronchial epithelial and smooth muscle cells [7, 13–17].

It has previously been demonstrated that Fas protein is expressed by SMC tissue *in vivo* and on the surface of cultured human airway myocytes *in vitro* [14]. It has also been reported that Fas cross-linking induces apoptosis in TNF-α-treated vascular smooth muscle cells [18, 19].

We showed that IFN-γ and TNF-α are the effector molecules rendering the bronchial SMC susceptible to apoptosis. They upregulate TNFR1, TNFR2, and Fas as well as the membrane FasL on SMC. The large numbers of activated eosinophils are present in the mucosa of asthmatic patients and they are believed to be the central effector cells in asthma [20, 21].

Human ECP induced cell death only 3 h after SMC stimulation and no elevation of acti-

vated intracellular caspase-3 was found, which accounts for necrosis as the mechanism of cell death.

T-cells are well documented to contact ASM cells [7, 14]. The concept that the asthmatic inflammation is fully mediated by type 2 T-cells should be reconsidered [21]. In humans there is not a straight bias for type 1 and type 2 differentiated T-cell subsets in disease [22, 23]. The amount of IFN-γ and TNF-α is elevated in supernatants from cultures of unstimulated and stimulated BAL cells from asthma patients [24]. During exacerbations of asthma, viral infections may also contribute to the IFN-γ level in the airway mucosa [3]. In this study Th1 cells induced stronger apoptotic cell death of SMC than Th2 cells by the mechanism dependent on the effects of IFN-γ. The demonstration of bronchial SMC apoptosis accounts for the essential role of T-cells and eosinophils in induction of bronchial hyperresponsiveness in the altered pro-asthmatic constrictor and relaxant phenotype. This process is mediated by IFN-γ and TNF-α and characterized by apoptosis and subsequent proliferation and hypertrophy of bronchial SMC resulting in remodeling of the SM layer.

Acknowledgments

This study has been supported by Polish Committee of Scientific Research grant No 1387/PO5/2000/19.

References

1. Elias JA, Zhu Z, Chupp G, Homer RJ: Airway remodeling in asthma. J Clin Invest 1999; 104:1001–1006.

2. Busse W, Elias J, Sheppard D, Banks-Schlegel S: Airway remodeling and repair. Am J Respir Crit Care Med 1999; 160:1035–1042.

3. Bousquet J, Jeffery P, Busse WW, Johnson M, Vignola AM: Asthma. From bronchoconstriction to airways inflammation and remodeling. Am J Respir Crit Care Med 2000; 161:1720–1745.

4. Holgate ST, Davies DE, Lackie PM, Wilson SJ, Puddicombe SM, Lordan JL: Epithelial-mesenchymal interactions in the pathogenesis of asthma. Eur Respir J 2000; 105:193–204.

5. Hirst SJ, Lee TH: Airway smooth muscle as a target of glucocorticoid action in the treatment of asthma. Am J Respir Crit Care Med 1998; 158:201–206.

6. Seow CY, Schellenberg R, Pare PD: Structural and functional changes in the airway smooth muscle of asthmatic subjects. Am J Respir Crit Care Med 1998; 158:179–186.

7. Hakonarson H, Grunstein MM: Autocrine regulation of airway smooth muscle responsiveness. Respir Physiol Neurobiol 2003, 137:263–276.

8. Weller PF: Human eosinophils. J Allergy Clin Immunol 1997; 100:283–287.

9. Trautmann A, Akdis M, Kleemann D, Altznauer F, Simon HU, Graeve T, et al.: T-cell-mediated Fas-induced keratinocyte apoptosis plays a key pathogenetic role in eczematous dermatitis. J Clin Invest 2000; 106:25–35.

10. Trautmann A, Altznauer F, Akdis M, Simon HU, Disch R, Bröcker EB, et al.: The differential fate of cadherins during T-cell-induced keratinocyte apoptosis leads to spongiosis in eczematous dermatitis. J Invest Dermatol 2001; 117:927–934.

11. Sallusto F, Mackay CR, Lanzavecchia A: Selective expression of the eotaxin receptor CCR3 by human T helper 2 cells. Science 1997; 277: 2005–2007.

12. Hansel TT, de Vries IJM, Carballido JM, Braun RK, Carballido-Perrig N, Rihs S, et al.: Induction and function of eosinophil intercellular adhesion molecule-1 and HLA-DR. J Immunol 1992; 149: 2130–2136.

13. Trautmann A, Schmid-Grendelmeier P, Kruger K, Crameri R, Akdis M, Akkaya A, Brocker EB, Blaser K, Akdis CA: T-cells and eosinophils cooperate in the induction of bronchial epithelial cell apoptosis in asthma. J Allergy Clin Immunol 2002; 109:329–337.

14. Hamann KJ, Vieira JE, Halayko AJ, Dorscheid D, White SR, Forsythe SM, Camoretti-Mercado B, Rabe KF, Solway J: Fas cross-linking induces apoptosis in human airway smooth muscle cells. Am J Physiol Lung Cell Mol Physiol 2000; 278:618–624.

15. Shenberger JS, Dixon PS: Oxygen induces S-phase growth arrest and increases p53 and p21(WAF1/CIP1) expression in human bronchial smooth-muscle cells. Am J Respir Cell Mol Biol 1999; 21:395–402.

16. Montefort S, Herbert CA, Robinson C, Holgate ST: The bronchial epithelium as a target for the inflammatory attack in asthma. Clin Exp Allergy 1992; 22:511–520.

17. Ohashi Y, Motojima S, Fukuda T, Makino S: Airway hyperresponsiveness, increased intracellular spaces of bronchial epithelium, and increased infiltration of eosinophils and lymphocytes in bronchial mucosa in asthma. Am Rev Respir Dis 1992; 145:1469–1476.

18. Geng Y-J, Henderson LE, Levesque EB, Muszynski M, Libby P: Fas is expressed in human atherosclerotic intima and promotes apoptosis of cytokine-primed human vascular smooth muscle cells. Arterioscler Thromb Vasc Biol 1997; 17:2200–2208.

19. Geng Y-J, Wu Q, Muszynski M, Hansson GK, Libby P: Apoptosis of vascular smooth muscle cells induced by in vitro stimulation with interferon-γ, tumor necrosis factor-α, and interleukin-1β. Arterioscler Thromb Vasc Biol 1996; 6:19–27.

20. Lee NA, Gelfand EW, Lee JJ: Pulmonary T-cells and eosinophils: coconspirators or independent triggers of allergic respiratory pathology. J Allergy Clin Immunol 2001; 107:945–957.

21. Boushey HA, Fahy JV: Targeting cytokines in asthma therapy: round one. Lancet 2000; 356: 2114–2116.

22. Krug N, Madden J, Redington AE, Lackie P, Djukanovic R, Schauer U, et al.: T-cell cytokine profile evaluated at the single cell level in BAL and blood in allergic asthma. Am J Respir Cell Mol Biol 1996; 14:319–326.

23. Parronchi P, Macchia D, Piccini MP, Biswas P, Simonelli C, Maggi E, et al.: Allergen- and bacterial antigen-specific T-cell clones established from atopic donors show a different profile of cytokine production. Proc Natl Acad Sci USA 1991; 88:4538–4542.

24. Cembrzynska-Nowak M, Szklarz E, Inglot AD, Teodorczyk-Injeyan JA: Elevated release of tumor necrosis factor-α and interferon-γ by bronchoalveolar leukocytes from patients with asthma. Am Rev Respir Dis 1993; 147:291–295.

Marek Jutel

Department of Internal Medicine and Allergology, Wroclaw Medical University, Traugutta 57, 50–417 Wroclaw, Poland, Tel./Fax +48 71 3700129, E-mail mjutel@dilnet.wroc.pl

In vitro Methods for Monitoring the Development of Clinical Tolerance to Foods

L.P.C. Shek[1], L. Soderstrom[2], S. Ahlstedt[2,3], K. Beyer[1], and H.A. Sampson[1]

[1]*Mount Sinai School of Medicine, New York, NY, USA,* [2]*Pharmacia Diagnostics AB, Uppsala, Sweden,* [3]*Institute of Environmental Medicine and Center for Allergy Research, Karolinska Institute, Stockholm, Sweden*

Summary: About 3–4% of young children in the US are allergic to cow's milk, hen's egg and/or peanut. While the vast majority of children outgrow cow's milk and hen's egg allergy, there are no good indices to predict when and in whom this occurs. This study aimed to determine whether monitoring food-specific IgE levels over time could be used as a predictor for if and when patients develop clinical tolerance. 88 patients with egg and 49 patients with milk allergy were included in the study and underwent repeated double-blind placebo-controlled food challenges (DBPCFC). Using the Pharmacia CAP-System FEIA®, specific IgE levels to milk and egg were determined retrospectively from stored serum samples obtained at the time of the food challenges. Logistic regression was used to evaluate the relationship between tolerance development and the decrease in sIgE levels over a specific time period between the two challenges. For egg, the decrease in sIgE levels ($p = 0.0014$) was significantly related to the probability of outgrowing the allergy, with the duration between challenges having an influence ($p = 0.06$). For milk there was also a significant relation of decrease in sIgE levels ($p = 0.0175$) to the probability of outgrowing milk allergy, but without any significant contribution with regard to time. Using these results, we developed a model for predicting the likelihood of outgrowing milk and egg allergy based on the decrease in food-specific IgE over time. Using the likelihood estimates from this study physicians could be helped in predicting development of tolerance and in timing of need of subsequent food challenges, thereby decreasing the number of premature and unnecessary DBPCFCs.

Keywords: specific IgE, tolerance, food

Food allergy affects up to 8% of children under the age of 5, and the incidence appears to be rising [1]. Levels of food-specific IgE that could predict clinical reactivity to egg and milk with greater than 95% certainty have been previously established and confirmed prospectively [2,3].

Fortunately, the majority of children develop tolerance within the first 3 to 5 years of life. The two foods responsible for most of these reactions are cow's milk and hen's eggs. About 85% and 50% of children with cow's milk and hen's egg allergy, respectively, become clinically tolerant by the third year of life [2,3]. To date, there are no good indices to predict when and in whom this occurs. The objective of this study was to evaluate whether the decrease in IgE antibody level could predict development of tolerance for milk and egg and if the magnitude and time for the change would influence the outcome.

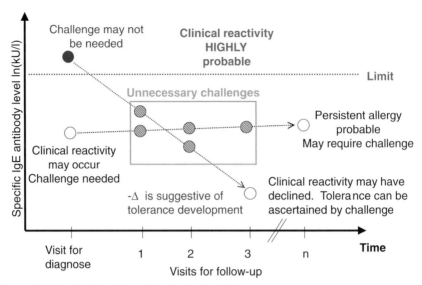

Figure 1. Proposed strategy for diagnosing and monitoring food allergy.

Materials and Methods

Eighty-eight patients with hen's egg and 49 patients with cow's milk allergy who had undergone two or more DBPCFCs to cow's milk or hen's egg were included in the study. Patients were divided into 2 groups; (a) patients with at least two positive DBPCFCs representing those who remained allergic, and (b) patients with an initial positive DBPCFC followed by a negative one representing those who became tolerant. The primary outcome was a "tolerant" group or "persistent allergy" group, determined by DBPCFC to egg or milk. Specific IgE to milk and egg were measured retrospectively from stored serum samples using the Pharmacia CAP-System FEIA®, with a range of detection from ≥ 0.35 to ≤ 100 kU/L. Serum was obtained at the time of the food challenge and stored at $-80\,^\circ$C until analysis. Logistic regression was used to evaluate the relationship with the decrease in sIgE levels between the first and last challenge and also the time period between these two challenges.

Results

Twenty-eight of the 66 egg- and 16 of the 33 milk-allergic patients lost their allergy over time. For egg, the decrease in sIgE levels ($p = 0.0014$) was significantly related to the probability of outgrowing the allergy, with the duration between challenges having an influence ($p = 0.06$). For milk there was also a significant relation of decrease in sIgE levels ($p = 0.0175$) to the probability of outgrowing milk allergy, but no significant contribution with regard to time. Using these results, we developed a model for predicting the likelihood of outgrowing milk and egg allergy based on the decrease in food-specific IgE over time, Figure 1.

Discussion

In this study, we included only patients whose initial diagnosis and final evaluation of tolerance development was by DBPCFC, eliminating the problem of uncertain diagnoses. There was a relationship between the degree of decrease in food-specific IgE antibody concentrations over time and the likelihood of developing tolerance. A greater decrease in sIgE levels over a shorter period of time was indicative of a greater likelihood of developing tolerance. If a repeated measurement a year later fell by 90%, our estimates demonstrated that the clinician could be confident that the patient had at least a 78% chance of passing the food challenge at that point.

Levels of food-specific IgE that could predict clinical reactivity to egg and milk with greater than 95% certainty have been previously established and confirmed prospectively [2,3]. Our estimates used in conjunction with these decision points could reduce the number of DBPCFCs performed for the benefit of the patients and the health care system. The clinician could then recommend a repeat food challenge at the time point the egg-specific IgE levels have fallen, thereby eliminating the discomfort, expense, risks, and time wasted should the second challenge fail (Figure 1).

Conclusion

In summary, we have used a simple, standardized, reproducible, and objective test, the measurement of food-specific IgE by Pharmacia CAP System FEIA®, to develop a model for predicting the likelihood of developing tolerance in milk and egg allergy. This adds to the previously published levels of IgE antibody levels to detect clinical reactivity with 95% probability. The confirmation of this model, and subsequent application in clinical practice, would aid clinicians in the timing of food challenges, and in providing prognostic information for patients and their families, thereby reducing the discomfort, expense, risks, and time wasted should the second challenge fail.

References

1. Sampson HA: Food allergy. Part 1: immunopathogenesis and clinical disorders. J Allergy Clin Immunol 1999; 103:717–728.
2. Sampson HA, Ho DG: Relationship between food-specific IgE concentrations and the risk of positive food challenges in children and adolescents. J Allergy Clin Immunol 1997; 100:444–451.
3. Sampson HA: Utility of food-specific IgE concentrations in predicting symptomatic food allergy. J Allergy Clin Immunol 2001; 107:891–896.

Staffan Ahlstedt

Institute of Environmental Medicine, Center for Allergy Research, Karolinska Institute, BOX 210, 17177 Stockholm, Sweden, Tel. +46 70 396-9213, Fax +46 18 166390, E-mail staffan.ahlstedt@pharmacia.com

In vitro Methods for Assessing the Potential Severity of Food Allergic Reactions

H.A. Sampson[1], W.G. Shreffler[1], K. Beyer[2], T.H.T. Chu[1], A.W. Burks[3], and S. Ahlstedt[4]

[1]*Mount Sinai School of Medicine, New York, USA*, [2]*Charité Hospital, Berlin, Germany*, [3]*Duke University School of Medicine, Durham, NC, USA*, [4]*Pharmacia Diagnostics, Uppsala, Sweden*

Summary: Food allergies affect about 4% of the U. S. population and are the single leading cause of anaphylaxis treated in American emergency departments. While the double-blind oral food challenge remains the "gold standard" for diagnosing food allergy, quantitative assays of food-specific IgE have improved the diagnostic specificity of *in vitro* testing. However, several studies have shown that there is no correlation between the level of food-specific IgE antibodies and the severity of allergic reactions experienced when a patient ingests the food. In evaluating IgE binding to sequential epitopes of allergenic proteins utilizing peptide microarray technology, we found a correlation between the number of allergenic peanut epitopes recognized by patient IgE antibodies [epitope diversity] and the severity of reactions experienced by the patient. *In vitro* sensitization of basophils with IgE of "high" diversity revealed increased releasability compared to IgE of "low" diversity. Further studies are underway to explore the validity of this assay in predicting the severity of IgE-mediated reactions to foods.

Keywords: food allergy, diagnostics, anaphylaxis, peanut allergy, sequential epitope, peptide microarray

In the United States, food allergies affect up to 8% of the pediatric population less than 3 years of age, with IgE-mediated reactions accounting for about 60% of these reactions [1]. Recent epidemiological surveys indicate that about 4% of the overall U. S. population is afflicted with food allergies [2]. Several studies suggest that the prevalence of food allergy, like most atopic disorders, is increasing in "westernized" countries, with a doubling of peanut allergy recently noted in American children less than 5 years of age [3].

Patient history, SPTs and/or RASTs, and elimination diets have provided the mainstay of diagnosis in most clinical settings. However,

a number of studies have demonstrated the relatively low predictive value of these diagnostic tools with respect to predicting clinical reactivity. The "gold standard" for diagnosing food allergy is the blinded food challenge. SPTs and blood tests measuring food-specific IgE antibodies (RASTs) can identify foods that may be responsible for a patient's food allergic symptoms, but their ability to accurately predict who will experience an allergic reaction to a food remains unsatisfactory. However, new advances in our understanding of how the immune system interacts with food proteins and in our ability to examine how an allergic patient's IgE antibodies "see" these allergenic proteins are leading to more useful *in vitro* diagnostic tests.

In the last several years, studies have shown that there is an association between the quantity of food-specific IgE antibody a patient has and the likelihood that they will experience an allergic reaction to the food. As depicted in Figure 1, the greater the amount of egg-specific IgE, the more likely the individual will experience an allergic reaction to egg. There are now commercial tests available that can accurately quantitate the amount of food-specific IgE antibodies in the blood, i.e., CAP-System FEIA® and Uni-Cap® (Pharmacia Diagnostics, Uppsala, Sweden).

As indicated in Figure 1, any individual who has 7 kU/L or more of peanut-specific IgE is more than 95% likely to react to an ingested egg [4]. This level is considered "diagnostic" for egg allergy. As the level of egg-specific IgE decreases, the probability that the patient will react to egg also decreases. Depending on the clinical history and level of food-specific IgE, the clinician can decide whether a food challenge is warranted [4, 5]. Similar diagnostic levels have been established for other common food allergens, but these diagnostic levels differ for different foods and are influenced by age; the younger the patient, the lower the diagnostic level of food-specific IgE [6].

Recent advances in technology have enabled investigators to evaluate the food-allergic response at the molecular level. Allergenic proteins within foods have been identified, isolated and sequenced, and in many cases, full-length cDNAs coding for these proteins have been isolated. Using SPOTS peptide technology or more recently peptide microarrays, investigators have been able to identify IgE-binding (allergenic) epitopes and determine which amino acids within these epitopes are critical for IgE binding. Utilizing peptides of different lengths, 10-, 15- and 20-mers, it appears that IgE antibodies recognize epitopes of 10–12 amino acids in length.

As depicted in Figure 2a, epitopes may be comprised of a sequence of amino acids along the peptide chain, i.e., *"sequential epitope,"* or a sequence of amino acids from adjacent parts of the chain as it folds back upon itself, i.e., *"conformational epitope."* The conformational epitope is dependent upon the protein maintaining its native shape, because if the chain is stretched out, the amino acids making

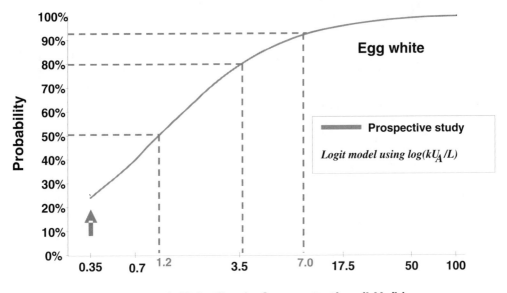

Figure 1. Probability of reacting to egg.

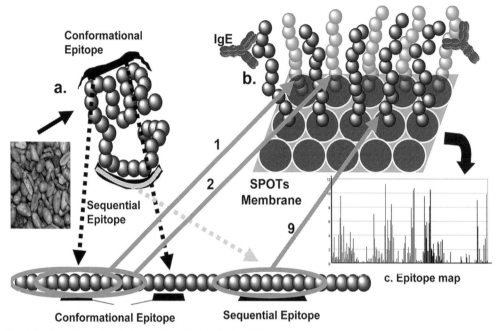

Figure 2. Determining where IgE antibodies attach to food proteins.

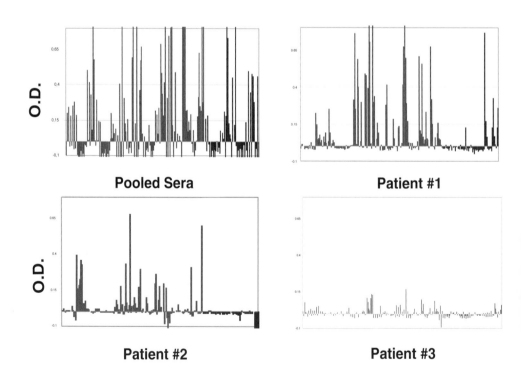

From Shreffler et al. *JACI* 2004; 113:776-782

Figure 3. Epitope map of Ara h1–3.

up the sequence are no longer together and the epitope disappears (bottom of Figure 2). When serum from a food allergic patient is incubated with a series of overlapping 20-mer peptides spanning the full length of the protein, IgE antibodies will attach to those segments that replicate the amino acid sequence of the *sequential epitope*. In this way, a map can be generated (Figure 2c representing 3 major peanut proteins) showing which epitopes each patient recognizes. Recent studies indicate that patients who have life-long egg, milk, or peanut allergy recognize certain epitopes that are not recognized by patients who "outgrow" their allergy [7–9].

In a recent report, we utilized a microarray-based immunoassay that allowed parallel analysis of IgE binding to a complete set of overlapping peptides from the sequences of the peanut allergens Ara h1, Ara h2 and Ara h3, as well as the recombinant proteins, using microliter amounts of patient serum per assay [10]. Using this assay, we analyzed serum samples from more than 75 individual peanut-sensitized patients. The antigenic/allergenic regions identified correlated well with previously reported results of epitope mapping. However, use of this microarray immunoassay revealed a marked degree of heterogeneity among sensitized individuals with respect to their epitope binding patterns, which had not been appreciated previously (Figure 3). Interestingly, the degree of diversification of epitope recognition correlated poorly with peanut-specific IgE levels, i.e., patients with high levels of peanut-specific IgE did not uniformly recognize greater numbers of IgE-binding epitopes.

Patients who had antibodies to many epitopes were found to have more severe allergic reactions than those who had IgE antibodies reacting to relatively few epitopes. When all peanut-sensitized patients were segregated by median number of allergenic epitopes recognized, those recognizing more epitopes (high diversity) had a history of significantly more severe reactions. For those recognizing relatively few epitopes (low diversity), the 95% confidence interval for the reaction severity score [11] was 0.67 to 1.5, while for the high diversity group the 95% confidence interval was 1.3 to 2.2 ($p < 0.05$). Similar findings were not seen when patients were segregated by peanut-specific IgE levels. The number of documented reactions experienced by patients in each group, a related trend, failed to reach statistical significance. The high diversity group had a median of 1.5 reactions (range 0 to 6) compared to the low diversity group with a median of 0 reactions (range 0 to 3, $p = 0.08$).

The differences found among the patients' histories of reactions suggested that epitope diversity could be related to IgE function. This was tested by adapting two bioassays of IgE function. In the first set of experiments, basophils from nonpeanut allergic donors were passively sensitized with pooled sera from individuals with high or low diversity peanut-specific IgE ($n = 4$; median IgE > 100 kU/L for each group). These pooled sera were matched for ratio of peanut-specific to total IgE and used at equal concentrations. Following sensitization, cells were stimulated with peanut extract and degranulation was measured as increased surface expression of CD63. The high diversity IgE sera conferred significantly greater sensitivity to peanut extract. The greater response was specific to peanut allergen, with no difference in the response to anti-IgE seen for either donor group. To further test the functional capacity of these two pooled sera, the rat basophilic leukemia cell line expressing human FcεRI (RBL-SX38, kindly provided by JP Kinet) was passively sensitized. Consistent with the results in passively sensitized human basophils, the more diverse IgE-containing sera conferred greater effector response as measured by basophil degranulation ($p < 0.001$).

New miniaturized technology under development (*peptide microarray*) may enable physicians to screen patients to a variety of foods with a "finger-stick" blood draw and tell whether they will experience an allergic reaction to a food, how severe their reaction may be, and whether they are likely to "outgrow" their allergy. The latter will be important since treatments for food allergy should be available in the next 5–10 years.

References

1. Sampson HA: Update of food allergy. J Allergy Clin Immun 2004; 113:805–819.
2. Sicherer SH, Munoz-Furlong A, Sampson HA: Prevalence of seafood allergy in the United States determined by a random telephone survey. J Allergy Clin Immun 2004; 114:159–165.
3. Sicherer SH, Munoz-Furlong A, Sampson HA: Prevalence of peanut and tree nut allergy in the United States determined by means of a random digit dial telephone survey: a 5-year follow-up study. J Allergy Clin Immun 2003; 112:1203–1207.
4. Sampson HA: Utility of food-specific IgE concentrations in predicting symptomatic food allergy. J Allergy Clin Immun 2001; 107:891–896.
5. Perry TT, Matsui EC, Connover-Walker MK, Wood RA: The relationship of allergen-specific IgE levels and oral food challenge outcome. Journal of Allergy Clin Immunology 2004; 114: 144–149.
6. Garcia-Ara C, Boyano-Martinez T, Diaz-Pena JM, Martin-Munoz F, Reche-Frutos M, Martin-Esteban M: Specific IgE levels in the diagnosis of immediate hypersensitivity to cows' milk protein in the infant. J Allergy Clin Immunol 2001; 107:185–190.
7. Vila L, Beyer K, Jarvinen KM, Chatchatee P, Bardina L, Sampson HA: Role of conformational and linear epitopes in the achievement of tolerance in cow's milk allergy. Clin Exp Allergy 2001; 31:1599–1606.
8. Jarvinen KM, Beyer K, Vila L, Chatchatee P, Busse PJ, Sampson HA: B-cell epitopes as a screening instrument for persistent cow's milk allergy. J Allergy Clin Immunol 2002; 110:293–297.
9. Beyer K, Ellman-Grunther L, Jarvinen KM, Wood RA, Hourihane JO'B, Sampson HA: Measurement of peptide-specific IgE as an additional tool in identifying patients with clinical reactivity to peanuts. J Allergy Clin Immunol 2003; 112: 202–208.
10. Shreffler WG, Beyer K, Burks AW, Sampson HA: Microarray immunoassay: association of clinical history, in vitro IgE function, and heterogeneity of allergenic peanut epitopes. J Allergy Clin Immun 2004, 113:776–782.
11. Sampson HA: Anaphylaxis and emergency treatment. Pediatr 2004; 111:1601–1608.

Hugh A. Sampson

Mount Sinai School of Medicine, 1 Gustave L. Levy Place, Box 1192, New York, NY 10029, USA, Tel. +1 212 241-5548, E-mail hugh.sampson@mssm.edu

Eosinophilic Esophagitis

New Clinical and Pathophysiological Insights

A. Straumann[1] and H.-U. Simon[2]

[1]Department of Gastroenterology, Kantonsspital Olten, Switzerland
[2]Department of Pharmacology, University of Bern, Switzerland

Summary: Eosinophilic esophagitis (EE), is a leading cause of dysphagia. Today, neither the natural course of EE nor the mechanisms leading to the eosinophilic tissue infiltration are clearly understood. The intention of our analyses was to characterize the natural course of EE and to determine the activation patterns of the eosinophils in inflamed and noninflamed tissue. Thirty patients with previously confirmed EE underwent a follow-up examination including endoscopy and histometric analyses. Additionally, the expressions of CD25 and of several Th2 cytokines were determined in esophageal, intestinal, and blood eosinophils. Dysphagia and eosinophil infiltration persisted in almost all patients, although the cell number decreased significantly. No extension of the infiltration to other sections of the digestive tract appeared but the inflammation led to esophageal fibrosis. In healthy individuals, a subgroup of intestinal, but not blood, eosinophils expressed CD25 and IL-13, suggesting a physiologic activation. In EE, eosinophils infiltrating the inflamed esophageal mucosa also demonstrated heterogeneity, but the majority expressed CD25, IL-4, and IL-13. Moreover, IL-13 positive intestinal eosinophils were increased in patients compared to the normal intestinal mucosa. EE is a primary-chronic, esophageal-restricted inflammation, which leads to persistent dysphagia and structural alterations of the esophagus. Three activation patterns of mucosal eosinophils are suggested in EE: *Primary Activation* observed at the inflammation site, reflecting eosinophils' involvement in the inflammatory process; *Remote Activation* noted far from the inflammatory process, consistent with a systemic activation; and *Baseline Activation* seen in the intestinal mucosa of healthy subjects, indicating eosinophils' involvement in barrier function.

Keywords: eosinophilic esophagitis, natural history, tissue-dwelling eosinophils, eosinophil activation patterns, CD25, interleukin-13

EE is an increasingly recognized, inflammatory disorder of the esophagus, characterized by a dense eosinophilic infiltration of the esophageal epithelium [1, 2, 3]. Adult EE patients complain almost exclusively of acute and recurrent dysphagia with impaction of solid foods [4]. The natural history of EE is still poorly defined and information describing the potential long-term risks, such as disabling dysphagia or the development of malignancies, has simply not been available. Furthermore, neither the function of resident intestinal eosinophils nor the mechanisms driving resting mucosal eosinophils to become activated cells with tissue-damaging effects, are clearly defined. We hypothesized

that, in EE patients, different populations of tissue-dwelling eosinophils may coexist in the digestive tract: an activated population with tissue-damaging effects infiltrating the esophagus and a resident, nonactivated population in the intestine. Using this unique model, it was hoped to characterize resting and activated eosinophils based on their cytokine expression patterns under *in vivo* conditions.

In a prospective case series we examined 30 adult patients with EE (22 males, 8 females; mean age 40.6 years) whose diagnosis had been previously made based on: (1) typical history, (2) consistent endoscopic abnormalities, and (3) infiltration of the esophageal ep-

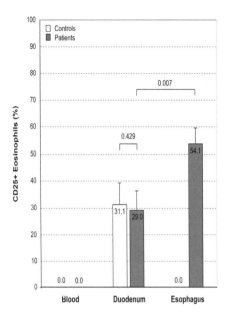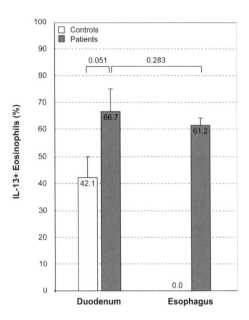

Figure 1. CD25 and IL-13 expression by blood, duodenal, and esophageal eosinophils in control individuals and in EE patients. Blood eosinophils did not express CD25 in either group as assessed by flow cytometry. A subgroup of duodenal eosinophils expressed CD25 in both groups as assessed by immunofluorescence and confocal microscopy. Expression of IL-13 was significantly enhanced in esophageal and duodenal eosinophils of EE patients compared to control individuals. No esophageal eosinophil infiltration was seen in control individuals. Data are means ± SEM. The results of the statistical analysis (*p* values) are indicated.

ithelium with > 24 eosinophils/hpf. After a mean 7.2 years, patients underwent a comprehensive follow-up examination consisting of a detailed history, physical examination, blood analyses, upper endoscopy, and histomorphometric examinations. Furthermore, immunofluorescence and immunoassays charted the expression of CD25 and of the Th2 cytokines IL-4, IL-5, IL-10, and IL-13 in esophageal, intestinal, and blood eosinophils in eight representative EE patients and in four healthy controls.

All patients survived the study period in a stable nutritional state. Dysphagia persisted in 29 patients, exerting a major negative effect on socioprofessional activities in 1 patient, and a minor impact on 15 patients. The esophageal eosinophilic infiltration persisted in all symptomatic patients, but cell numbers spontaneously decreased significantly (78.7 vs. 40.3 cells/hpf). The inflammatory process evoked fibrosis of the esophageal lamina propria, but did not spread to the stomach or duodenum. During the study period, no case evolved to hypereosinophilic syndrome or developed an esophageal, lympho- or myeloproliferative malignancy.

In healthy individuals, a significant proportion of intestinal, but not blood, eosinophils expressed CD25 and IL-13, suggesting a physiologic activation occurring in the digestive tract and involving an eosinophilic subgroup. Eosinophils infiltrating the inflamed esophageal mucosa of EE patients also demonstrated heterogeneity for CD25 and cytokine expression, but the majority expressed CD25, IL-4, and IL-13. Moreover, IL-13 positive intestinal eosinophils were increased in patients compared to the normal intestinal mucosa (Figure 1).

EE is an increasingly recognized, IL-5 driven [5], inflammatory disorder of the esophagus. Since the publication of several comprehensive series in the early nineties [1, 6, 7], EE has been accepted as unique, well-defined clinico-pathological entity. Our data demonstrate that EE is a primary chronic disease and that the inflammatory process is definitely restricted to the esophagus. The eosinophilic inflammation leads to persistent dysphagia with the imminent risk of food impaction, likely caused by structural alterations of the esophagus with fibrosis of the subepithelial layers. Fortunately, EE has no impact on the nutritional state and to date, no malignant potential has been associated with this disease [8].

The digestive tract is the only nonhematopoietic organ of the human body showing a relevant number of residing eosinophils under healthy conditions [9]. Eosinophils are found between the stomach and the rectum, but not in the uninflamed esophagus [5]. A first important result to arise from this study was that, in healthy individuals, blood eosinophils and "assumed" resting mucosa-dwelling eosinophils expressed activation markers in a strikingly different pattern: In blood eosinophils, CD25 and IL-13 were almost absent, whereas a considerable fraction of eosinophils residing in the intestinal lamina propria expressed these markers under homeostatic conditions. Within the context of the physiologically occurring homing process, a considerable fraction of eosinophils is, therefore, upregulated to a functional state. This so-called *Baseline Activation Pattern* indicates that eosinophils actively participate in the intestinal immuno-homeostasis. Eosinophils infiltrating the esophageal tissue of EE patients had a different pattern of cytokine expression. This so-called *Primary Activation Pattern* reflects the eosinophils' pivotal involvement in inflammation. A third, so-called *Remote Activation Pattern,* was observed in the duodenal mucosa of EE patients, distant to the inflamed esophagus. This pattern is consistent with a systemic activation induced by the esophageal inflammatory process. Moreover, we were surprised to find that all determined activation markers were expressed by only a fraction of the mucosa-dwelling eosinophils. This heterogeneity was found under homeostatic as well as under inflammatory conditions. The simultaneous coexistence of different subpopulations of histomorphological identical-appearing cells is a well-known phenomenon of lymphocytes. Our data clearly demonstrate that mucosal-dwelling eosinophils exhibit the same behavior even though cells with a different immunophenotype coexist. It is, therefore, likely that, in analogy to lymphocytes, these subpopulations of eosinophils carry out different functions.

References

1. Attwood SE, Smyrk TC, Demeester TR, Jones JB: Esophageal eosinophilia with dysphagia. A distinct clinicopathologic syndrome. Dig Dis Sci 1993; 38:109–116.
2. Rothenberg ME, Mishra A, Collins MH, Putnam PE: Pathogenesis and clinical features of eosinophilic esophagitis. J Allergy Clin Immunol 2001; 108:891–894.
3. Fox VL, Nurko S, Furuta GT: Eosinophilic esophagitis: it's not just kid's stuff. Gastrointest Endosc 2002; 56:260–270.
4. Arora AS, Yamazaki K: Eosinophilic Esophagitis: asthma of the esophagus? Clin Gastroenterol Hepatol 2004; 2:523–530.
5. Straumann A, Bauer M, Fischer B, Blaser K, Simon HU: Idiopathic eosinophilic esophagitis is associated with a Th2-type allergic inflammatory response. J Allergy Clin Immunol 2001; 108: 954–961.
6. Vitellas KM, Bennett WF, Bova JG, Johnston JC, Caldwell JH, Mayle JE: Idiopathic eosinophilic esophagitis. Radiology 1993; 186:789–793.
7. Straumann A, Spichtin HP, Bernoulli R, Loosli J, Voegtlin J: Idiopathic eosinophilic esophagitis: a frequently overlooked disease with typical clinical aspects and discrete endoscopic findings. Schweiz Med Wochenschr 1994; 124:1419–1429.
8. Straumann A, Spichtin HP, Grize L, Bucher KA, Beglinger C, Simon HU: Natural history of primary eosinophilic esophagitis: A follow-up of 30 adult patients for up to 11.5 years. Gastroenterology 2003; 125:1660–1669.
9. Kato M, Kephart GM, Talley NJ, Wagner JM, Sarr MG, Bonno M, McGovern TW, Gleich GJ: Eosinophil infiltration and degranulation in normal human tissue. Anat Rec 1998; 252:418–425.

Alex Straumann

Department of Gastroenterology, Kantonsspital Olten, Roemerstrasse 7, CH-4600 Olten, Switzerland, Tel. +41 62 212-5577, Fax +41 62 212-5564, E-mail alex.straumann@hin.ch

Histamine Release for Determination of Systemically Absorbed Allergenic Proteins in Humans

C.G. Dirks[1], M.H. Platzer[2], M.H. Pedersen[1], L.B. Jensen[2], C. Bindslev-Jensen[3], L.K. Poulsen[1], and P.S. Skov[2]

[1]Laboratory of Medical Allergology, Allergy Clinic, National University Hospital, Copenhagen, Denmark, [2]RefLab, Copenhagen, Denmark, [3]Allergy Center, Department of Dermatology, Odense University Hospital, Denmark

Summary: *Background:* The amount and quality of absorbed dietary proteins may be important in the development of food allergy. In order to determine absorbed dietary proteins in human serum we developed a biological method. Histamine release (HR) from sensitized human basophils is an established biological method to detect protein allergenicity. The method using passive sensitization of basophils with allergic sera can be modified eliminating the need for fresh blood. *Aim:* To develop a method to detect allergens in human blood after oral intake of highly allergenic proteins such as peanut. *Methods:* Buffy coats from blood donors were used and mononuclear cells containing 1–2% basophils were isolated using a Lymphoprep gradient. IgE was removed from basophils by stripping and these were subsequently passively sensitized by incubation (37 °C/60 min) with serum from a verified peanut-allergic individual. Passively sensitized basophils were challenged with peanut allergens dissolved in buffer or serum from nonatopic individuals. HR was determined by the glass fiber method and expressed in percentage of total histamine content in the cells. A HR10% was considered positive. *Results:* Passive sensitization and direct HR from a peanut-allergic individual were equally sensitive enabling the detection of peanut allergens in concentrations in the low pg/ml-range. Dose response curves of peanut diluted in buffer or in human serum were comparable allowing the detection of peanut allergens in serum. *Conclusions:* Passive sensitization of basophils is a sensitive method for detecting allergens in serum. The method can be used to detect food allergens after oral intake.

Keywords: absorption, peanut, protein, human, HR, basophils, passive sensitization

The amount and quality of absorbed dietary proteins may be important in the development and elicitation of food allergy. Only a few studies have aimed at detection of food allergens in human blood [1, 2]. We used oral administration of defined amounts of peanut to nonallergic adults as a model for studying the uptake of peanut proteins from the human digestive tract. Our first attempt to determine systemically absorbed dietary proteins in human serum was using a newly developed ELISA [3]. In spite of a sensitivity of less than 1 ng/mL, we failed to detect peanut proteins in the serum of some individuals and additionally, an ELISA based on polyclonal rabbit antibodies did not provide information about protein allergenicity.

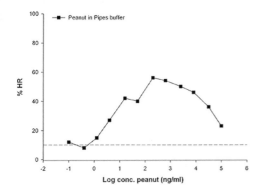

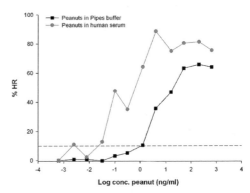

Figure 1. (a) Direct HR. Using fresh blood from a peanut allergic individual, a titration curve showing HR with peanut diluted 3.5-fold in Pipes buffer was performed.

Figure 1. (b) Indirect HR. Titration curves showing HR with peanut diluted as above were performed in buffer and serum by passive sensitization of healthy donor basophils.

Histamine release (HR) from sensitized human basophils is an established biological method to detect protein allergenicity [4–6]. Thus, we aimed at developing a sensitive method for detection of allergens in human blood after oral intake of highly allergenic proteins, such as peanut, by applying the method of passive sensitization of basophils using sera from highly sensitized patients.

Material and Methods

Buffy coat blood from healthy donors was screened and selected for their capability to elicit an anti-IgE response (HR > 30%) and with no HR-reactivity toward peanut allergens. Basophils were obtained by Lymphoprep centrifugation (1.078 g/cm$^{3;}$ 1300 g/15 min/11 °C) and basophil-bound IgE was removed using acid treatment with a phosphate buffer (pH: 3.55). The basophil cells were then passively sensitized with sera from verified peanut allergic patients or sera from nonsensitized controls. Basophils were then incubated with peanut allergens in buffer or in nonallergic human sera. HR was determined by the glass fiber method and expressed in percentage of total histamine content. An HR > 10% was considered positive. For comparison of dose response curves the allergen concentration reducing 50% of the maximal HR ($\frac{1}{2}HR_{max}$) was calculated. Direct HR from fresh blood from a verified peanut-allergic individual was tested with dilutions of a

peanut extract and compared with HR from passively sensitized basophils.

Results

Direct HR

Basophils obtained from fresh blood from a verified peanut-allergic individual were incubated with a peanut extract diluted 3.5-fold in Pipes buffer (Figure 1A). The titration curve shows the detection of allergens demonstrating a typical bell-shaped dose-response curve. The detection limit of peanut allergens in buffer was approximately 1 ng peanut/mL with a cut-off at 10% HR. $\frac{1}{2}HR_{max.}$ was obtained at 4 ng/mL.

Passive Sensitization

The native IgE of healthy donor basophils were stripped and passively sensitized with serum from the peanut allergic individual. For comparison with *direct HR,* a titration curve with peanut diluted as stated and in nonpeanut-sensitized serum was performed. The detection limit in serum was approximately 0.03 ng/mL and $\frac{1}{2}HR_{max.}$ 0.08 ng/mL (Figure 1B). This showed that passive sensitization of healthy donor basophils was superior in sensitivity to direct HR. Control experiments in which basophils were sensitized with a nonatopic serum demonstrated no HR (results not shown).

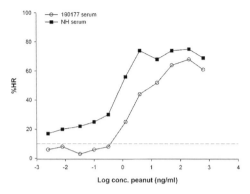

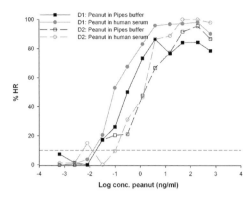

Figure 2. (a) Basophils sensitized with peanut IgE from 2 different patients, "190177" (36 kU$_A$/l) and "NH" (125 kU$_A$/l).

Figure 2. (b) Sensitization of different donor basophils (D1 + D2) with specific peanut IgE from verified peanut allergic individual ("NH"), detecting peanut proteins in pipes buffer and human serum.

To test the influence of the titer of specific IgE, basophils of one donor were sensitized with serum from two different verified peanut-allergic individuals, with specific peanut IgE at 36 kU$_A$/L ("190177") and 125 kU$_A$/L ("NH"). Serum with a high specific IgE had a higher sensitivity (2 pg/mL) compared to serum with lower IgE (1.2 ng/mL). Similarly ½HR$_{max.}$ was reached at 2 ng/mL for "190177"-serum and 0.5 ng/mL for "NH"-serum (Figure 2A).

To test the influence of donor basophils a titration curve in nonsensitized serum and Pipes buffer were made by sensitizing different healthy donor basophils (D1 + D2) with specific peanut IgE from "NH" (Figure 2B). When different donor basophils were used, the sensitivity varied from 0.03 ng/mL (D1) to 0.4 ng/mL (D2) and ½HR$_{max.}$ from 0.085 ng/mL to 1.4 ng/mL in serum.

Discussion

Detection of ingested proteins in serum has been investigated by others using ELISA or enzymatic methods [1]. We used a biological method with passive sensitization of basophils. With a detection of 0.03 ng peanut allergens/mL compared to 1 ng/mL, we confirmed that passive sensitization of stripped basophils is a more sensitive method to detect peanut proteins compared to the direct HR. Although titration curves of peanut allergens in buffer

and serum were comparable, it was also shown that allergen detection was more sensitive in serum. In this study we also clarified the differences in response when two different sera from peanut-allergic patients are used for passive sensitization. Figure 2A shows that the sensitivity is dependent on a high specific IgE level in the serum used for sensitization. Considering the variation in donor responses sensitizing two different basophil donors with the same peanut positive serum (Figure 2B) might have an effect on the results, but in this study the results were comparable. Direct HR is dependent on fresh blood from an allergic individual who also reacts to small amounts of allergens, whereas passive sensitization is a more flexible method as it is possible to select serum from allergic individuals who react to the allergen in question and donors with highly reactive basophils.

In conclusion, passive sensitization of donor basophils is a sensitive biological method to detect food allergens in serum, thereby eliminating the use of fresh blood.

Acknowledgment

This study was supported by the research program EPI-PAT (supported by the Danish Ministry of Food, Agriculture and Fisheries) and the FAREDAT program (EU commission, 5th framework program).

References

1. Castell JV, Friedrich G, Kuhn CS, Poppe GE: Intestinal absorption of undegraded proteins in men: presence of bromelain in plasma after oral intake. Am J Physiol 1997; 273:G139–G146.
2. Husby S: Dietary antigens: uptake and humoral immunity in man. APMIS Suppl 1988; 1:1–40.
3. Poulsen LK, Pedersen MH, Platzer M, Madsen N, Sten E, Bindslev-Jensen C, Dircks CG, Skov PS: Immunochemical and biological quantification of peanut extract. Arb Paul Ehrlich Inst Bundesamt Sera Impfstoffe Frankfurt a. M. 2003; 94:97–105.
4. Luttkopf D, Muller U, Skov PS, Ballmer-Weber BK, Wuthrich B, Skamstrup HK, Poulsen LK, Kastner M, Haustein D, Vieths S: Comparison of four variants of a major allergen in hazelnut (Corylus avellana) Cor a 1.04 with the major hazel pollen allergen Cor a 1.01. Mol Immunol 2002; 38:515–525.
5. Hansen KS, Ballmer-Weber BK, Luttkopf D, Skov PS, Wüthrich B, Bindslev-Jensen C, Vieths S, Poulsen LK: Roasted hazelnuts – allergenic activity evaluated by double-blind, placebo-controlled food challenge. Allergy 2003; 58:132–138.
6. Budde IK, de Heer PG, van der Zee JS, Alberse RC: The stripped basophil histamine release bioassay as a tool for the detection of allergen-specific IgE in serum. Int Arch Allergy Immunol 2001; 126:277–285.

Christina Glattre Dirks

Allergy Clinic, FIN 7551, National University Hospital, Blegdamsvej 9, DK-2100 Copenhagen, Denmark, Tel. +45 35 457555, Fax +45 35 457581, E-mail cglattre@rh.dk

Proton Pump Inhibitors Promote Oral Sensitization to Hazelnut

I. Schöll[1], G. Reese[2], E. Untersmayr[1], N. Bakos[3], F. Roth-Walter[1], A. Gleiss[4], G. Boltz-Nitulescu[1], O. Scheiner[1], and E. Jensen-Jarolim[1]

[1]Center of Physiology and Pathophysiology, Medical University of Vienna, Austria,
[2]Paul-Ehrlich-Institut, Department of Allergology, Langen, Germany,
[3]Department of Dermatology, Hetenyi Geza Hospital, Szolnok, Hungary,
[4]Department of Medical Computer Sciences, Medical University of Vienna, Austria

Summary: *Background:* Two mechanisms are currently proposed for the induction of food allergy. First, allergy can develop directly through oral sensitization with digestion-stable proteins. Second, an initial inhalative sensitization to pollen allergens can lead to cross-reactions elicited by homologous proteins in food. However, we have recently reported a third mechanism by which anti-ulcer drugs can promote oral sensitization to digestion-labile food allergens. *Objectives:* BALB/c mice were fed with hazelnut extract after previous i.m. injection of the proton pump inhibitor omeprazole. In ELISA we found that IgG1 was the predominant subclass of hazelnut-specific antibodies induced by this protocol. Here, we investigated whether these sera also contained hazelnut-specific IgE and tested the respective mouse sera in RBL assays. *Results:* Hazelnut extract elicited β-hexosaminidase release in a dose-dependent manner only when RBL cells were passively sensitized with the serum pool of mice treated with omeprazole, indicating the presence of hazelnut-specific IgE in these sera. *Conclusion:* Our experimental data indicate that medication with anti-ulcer drugs may lead to the induction of IgE-mediated food hypersensitivity towards hazelnut without genuine pollen sensitization.

Keywords: hazelnut, allergy, anti-acids, hypoacidity

In industrialized countries the incidence of allergies, including food allergies, is steadily increasing. To date there are about 2% of the adult population and relatively more children (6–8%) affected by allergic reactions to food [1–3]. For food allergies, two mechanisms have been proposed that seem to be relevant for the sensitization phase. First, some dietary proteins are resistant to peptic or tryptic digestion [4]. These proteins are called "true" food allergens. It is obviously their intact structure which is a precondition for the induction of IgE antibodies and, further, for eliciting allergic symptoms. On the other hand, it has been observed that IgE antibodies of patients who suffer from respiratory allergies also recognize proteins in food which possess homologous structures. Via this mechanism, clinical cross-reactions can be induced, for instance, IgE against Bet v 1 in birch pollen is also cross-linked by the homologous Cor a 1 from hazelnut, Mal d 1 from apple, Dau c 1 from carrot, etc. [5–7]. The reactivity to the crossreactive allergen is often less pronounced than to the genuine allergen, which may be a matter of affinity [8].

Apart from the above described mechanisms, we have shown in recent studies that a third mechanism for food allergy induction exists: medication with anti-acid drugs leads to hypoacidity of the stomach and can thereby hinder the peptic breakdown of food proteins

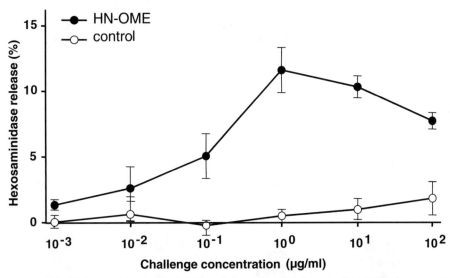

Figure 1. Treatment with Omeprazole promotes induction of allergen-specific IgE in mice. Female BALB/c were pre-treated intramuscularly with the proton pump inhibitor Omeprazole and thereafter fed with hazelnut extract. Their serum pool was capable of inducing β-hexosaminidase release from rat basophil leukemia cells upon stimulation with hazelnut extract (HN-OME). The release (given as percentage of the total β-hexosaminidase content, y-axis) was dependent on the concentration of hazelnut extract (x-axis). In contrast, treatment of cells with preimmune serum of these mice (control) did not elicit mediator release.

[9,10]. As a consequence, the secondary structure of these molecules is presented intact to the immune system and can induce sensitization. This has an important implication for usually harmless digestible proteins, which can thereby be turned into potent allergens, as recently demonstrated for fish allergens [10]. Here, we show that this mechanism is also true for hazelnut proteins when they are prevented from gastric digestion by the proton pump inhibitor Omeprazole.

Four to six-week-old female BALB/c mice ($n = 5$) received Omeprazole i.m. (11.6 μg; Losec, AstraZeneca, Vienna, Austria). After 1 h, these mice were fed hazelnut extract (2 mg in 100 μL PBS). Three of these five mice produced hazelnut-specific IgG1 during anti-acid treatment which were capable of eliciting passive cutaneous anaphylaxis [9]. To examine whether the sera of these mice also contained relevant hazelnut-specific IgE, we subjected them to mediator release experiments on rat basophil leukemia cells expressing FcεRI, but no Fcγ receptors [11–13]. Briefly, RBL-2H3 (DSMZ, Braunschweig, Germany) were plated in flat-bottomed 96-well cell culture plates

(Nunc, Wiesbaden, Germany) at 1.5×10^5 cells per well. The cells were passively sensitized for 1 h with mouse serum pool diluted 1:50. For the mediator release experiments, the sensitized RBL-2H3 cells were challenged with hazelnut extract at concentrations ranging from 10 μg/ml to 1 ng/ml. The antigen-specific release was quantified by measuring β-hexosaminidase activity and expressed as percent of the total β-hexosaminidase content obtained by lysing the cells with Triton-X-100. For measurements of spontaneous release and possible nonspecific effects, naive RBL cells were incubated with Tyrode's buffer, cell culture medium, and control sera, respectively.

In this experiment, a serum pool of the Omeprazole-treated mice actually revealed hexosaminidase releasing capacity, in contrast to their preimmune serum pool, indicating the presence of hazelnut-specific IgE antibodies (Figure 1).

Taken together, our results show that feedings of hazelnut in combination with Omeprazole treatment not only induces IgG1, but also allergen-specific IgE and, therefore, true IgE-mediated type I food allergy. Our data indicate

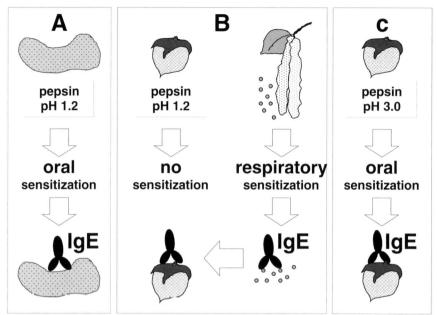

Figure 2. The fate of a protein during gastrointestinal digestion is decisive for its allergenic potential. Panel A: Proteins that resist gastric digestion can sensitize and elicit allergic reactions via the gastrointestinal route, e.g., the peanut allergen Ara h 1. Panel B: Food proteins which are easily degraded by pepsin are likely to be harmless because they are not able to sensitize or elicit allergic reactions via the gastrointestinal route. However, respiratory allergens can induce IgE antibodies crossreacting with homologous proteins in food (e.g., birch pollen allergen Bet v 1 crossreacts with hazelnut allergen Cor a 1), leading to relatively milder clinical reactions at the primary contact sites. Panel C: In settings of elevated gastric pH, pepsins are not activated, normally harmless proteins persist the gastric transit and become sensitizing elicitors of food allergy.

that incomplete protein breakdown, as during treatment with anti-ulcer drugs (proton pump inhibitors, antacids, or H2-receptor blockers) can also promote true food allergy to proteins which are usually digestible, such as those found in hazelnut (Figure 2).

Acknowledgments
This work was supported by the Austrian Science Fund SFB F1808-B04 and the Austrian National Bank grant 10326.

References

1. Sampson HA, Burks AW: Mechanisms of food allergy. Annu Rev Nutr 1996; 16:161–177.
2. Sampson HA: Food allergy. Part 1: immunopathogenesis and clinical disorders. J Allergy Clin Immunol 1999; 103:717–728.
3. Young E, Stoneham MD, Petruckevitch A, Barton J, Rona R: A population study of food intolerance. Lancet 1994; 343:1127–1130.
4. Astwood JD, Leach JN, Fuchs RL: Stability of food allergens to digestion *in vitro*. Nat Biotechnol 1996; 14:1269–1273.
5. Vanek-Krebitz M, Hoffmann-Sommergruber K, Laimer da Camara Machado M, Susani M, Ebner C, Kraft D, Scheiner O, Breiteneder H: Cloning and sequencing of Mal d 1, the major allergen from apple (Malus domestica), and its immunological relationship to Bet v 1, the major birch pollen allergen. Biochem Biophys Res Commun 1995; 214:538–551.
6. Helbling A, Lopez M, Schwartz HJ, Lehrer SB: Reactivity of carrot-specific IgE antibodies with celery, apiaceous spices, and birch pollen. Ann Allergy 1993; 70:495–499.
7. Hirschwehr R, Valenta R, Ebner C, Ferreira F, Sperr WR, Valent P, Rohac M, Rumpold H, Scheiner O, Kraft D: Identification of common allergenic structures in hazel pollen and hazelnuts: a possible explanation for sensitivity to hazelnuts in patients allergic to tree pollen. J Allergy Clin Immunol 1992; 90:927–936.
8. Hantusch B, Schöll I, Harwanegg C, Krieger S, Becker WM, Spitzauer S, Boltz-Nitulescu G, Jensen-Jarolim E: Affinity determinations of purified IgE and IgG antibodies against the major

pollen allergens Phl p 5a and Bet v 1: Discrepancy between IgE and IgG binding strength. Immunol Letters 2004; 97:81–89.

9. Schöll I, Untersmayr E, Bakos N, Walter F, Boltz-Nitulescu G, Scheiner O, Jensen-Jarolim E: Anti-ulcer drugs promote oral sensitization and hypersensitivity to hazelnut allergens in BALB/c mice and humans. Am J Clin Nutr 2005, 81:154–160.

10. Untersmayr E, Scholl I, Swoboda I, Beil WJ, Forster-Waldl E, Walter F, Riemer A, Kraml G, Kinaciyan T, Spitzauer S, Boltz-Nitulescu G, Scheiner O, Jensen-Jarolim E: Antacid medication inhibits digestion of dietary proteins and causes food allergy: a fish allergy model in BALB/c mice. J Allergy Clin Immunol 2003; 112:616–623.

11. Hoffmann A, Jamin A, Foetisch K, May S, Aulepp H, Haustein D, Vieths S: Determination of the allergenic activity of birch pollen and apple prick test solutions by measurement of β-hexosaminidase release from RBL-2H3 cells. Comparison with classical methods in allergen standardization. Allergy 1999; 54:446–454.

12. Hoffmann A, Vieths S, Haustein D: Biologic allergen assay for *in vivo* test allergens with an *in vitro* model of the murine type I reaction. J Allergy Clin Immunol 1997; 99:227–232.

13. Vieths S, Hoffmann A, Holzhauser T, Muller U, Reindl J, Haustein D: Factors influencing the quality of food extracts for *in vitro* and *in vivo* diagnosis. Allergy 1998; 53:65–71.

Erika Jensen-Jarolim

Center of Physiology and Pathophysiology, Medical University of Vienna, Waehringer Guertel 18–20, EBO.3Q, A-1090 Vienna, Austria, Tel. +43 1 40400-5103, Fax +43 1 40400-5130, E-mail erika.jensen-jarolim@meduniwien.ac.at

Oral Threshold Levels and *in vivo* Basophil Activation in Hazelnut Allergic Patients During Oral Provocation Tests

E.-M. Fiedler[1], H. Lee[1], M. Kuhn[2], and M. Worm[1]

[1]*Allergy-Center-Charité, Dpt. of Dermatology and Allergy, Charité – Universitätsmedizin Berlin*
[2]*CONGEN Biotechnologie GmbH, Berlin, both Germany*

Summary: *Background:* Pollen-associated food allergy is common. Symptoms include the oral allergy syndrome (OAS), rhinitis, asthma, urticaria, angioedema, and even anaphylaxis. Such reactions may be induced by small amounts of the allergen and are sometimes life-threatening. The aim of this study was to investigate threshold levels in hazelnut (HN)-allergic patients suffering from OAS. We also tested CD203c expression to evaluate basophil activation before and after the double-blind placebo-controlled food challenge (DBPCFC). *Methods:* The recruited individuals ($n = 30$) had a clinical history of birch pollen and HN allergy. In all patients specific IgE for birch pollen (41.6 ± 6.2 kU/L) and HN (1.6 ± 0.4 kU/L) was detected. After a HN-free diet DBPCFC was performed with increasing amounts of HN (dosage: 0.01 g–10 g). Blood samples were collected before and after the provocation tests for determination of basophil activation using the anti-CD203c-PE by flow cytometric analysis. *Results:* The oral threshold levels eliciting OAS in the study group varied from 0.01–2.0 g (0.4 ± 0.515). The measurement of the basophil activation shows that *in vivo* CD203c expression significantly increased from 38% ($\pm$ 4.9) to 48% (± 4.8). *Conclusions:* Despite the patients developing mild allergic symptoms after exposure to low amounts of HN, a systemic activation of the immune system occurred as indicated by *in vivo* activation of basophils during DBPCFC. Whether CD203c expression may be useful as an *in vitro* test for the prediction of a clinical relevant allergy will need to be determined.

Keywords: oral threshold level, food allergy, hazelnut, double-blind placebo-controlled food challenge, CD203c

Pollen-associated food allergy affects 50–80% of birch pollen-allergic individuals. The patients often suffer from reactions to fruits, but also to tree nuts like HN. Symptoms are the OAS, rhinitis, asthma, urticaria, angioedema, and even anaphylaxis. Such reactions may be induced by small amounts of the allergen and are sometimes life-threatening [1].

The aim of this study was to investigate the oral threshold levels in HN-allergic patients. We

also tested the expression of the basophil activation marker CD203c to evaluate basophil activation *in vivo* before and after the double-blind placebo-controlled food challenge (DBPCFC). CD203c (ecto-nucleotide pyrophosphatase/phosphodiesterase 3), a type II transmembrane protein, has been described as being selectively expressed on basophils, mast cells, and their CD34[+] progenitors. As CD203c is rapidly upregulated after allergen challenge in sensitized

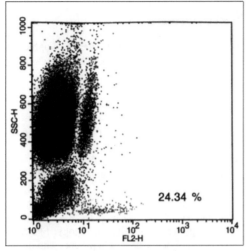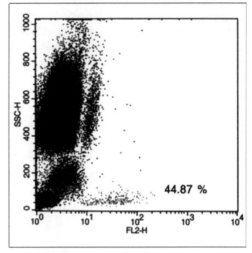

Figure 1. CD203c expression in one patient before and after HN provocation.

patients, it has been proposed as a new tool for allergy diagnosis [2].

Materials and Methods

Subjects

Thirty patients (19 female, 11 male) with a clinical history of birch pollen and HN allergy were included in the study. The mean age was 43 years ranging from 22–65. Twelve healthy, non-birch-pollen-allergic persons, all female, represented the control group; mean age was 33 years ranging from 23–43. Birch pollen and HN sIgE were detected in the sera by using the Pharmacia CAP-System (Freiburg, Germany) in all patients and the control group.

Methods

After a HN-free diet for 1 week SPT was used to confirm the HN sensitization, followed by DBPCFC with increasing amounts of HN (dosage 0.01 g–10.0 g). The DBPCFC was performed according to the EAACI position paper [3]. Heparinized 5 ml blood samples were obtained before and after the provocation test. For the measurement of basophil activation, cells were stained with anti-CD203c-PE and measured by flow cytometric analysis. In the control group SPT and an open food challenge with 10 g of fresh HN was performed.

Results

Oral Threshold Levels in OAS Patients

Of the 30 recruited individuals, 28 suffered from OAS, 26 from seasonal rhinitis, 7 from asthma, and 2 from atopic dermatitis. The mean total IgE levels were 307 ± 85 kU/L and sIgE toward HN were 1.6 ± 0.4 kU/L. SPT was positive in 29 individuals using fresh, native HN. The DBPCFC with different amounts of HN revealed 10 mg as the lowest oral threshold and 2 g as the highest oral threshold (mean 343 ± 100 mg).

Increased CD203c Expression after Oral Provocation Tests

The measurement of the basophil activation after cumulative HN doses in the patient group showed a significant ($p < .05$) increase of *in vivo* CD203c expression from 38% (± 4.9) to 48% (± 4.8). No significant change of the basophil activation was detected in the control group (34% ± 7.7 to 38% ± 7.8).

Discussion

Our results indicate a wide range of threshold levels in HN allergic patients suffering from

OAS. Further investigation is needed to determine the threshold levels in other patients groups, e.g., those suffering from atopic dermatitis. Despite the patients having developed only mild allergic symptoms after exposure to low amounts of HN, a systemic activation of the immune system occurred as indicated by *in vivo* activation of basophils before and after DBPCFC. Whether CD203c expression may be useful as an *in vitro* test for the measurement or the prediction of a clinical relevant allergy will need to be determined by further clinical studies.

Acknowledgment
This study was supported by a grant from the Bundesministerium für Bildung und Forschung (PTJ-BIO/0313013A).

References

1. Ferreira F, Hawranek T, Gruber P, Wopfner N, Mari A: Allergic cross-reactivity: from gene to the clinic. Allergy 2004; 59:243–267.
2. Boumiza R, Monneret G, Forissier MF, Savoye J, Gutowski MC, Powell WS, Bienvenu J: Marked improvement of the basophil activation test by detecting CD203c instead of CD63. Clin Exp Allergy 2003; 33:259–265.
3. Bindslev-Jensen C, Ballmer-Weber BK, Bengtsson U, Blanco C, Ebner C, Hourihane J, Knulst AC, Moneret-Vautrin DA, Nekam K, Niggemann B, Osterballe M, Ortolani C, Ring J, Schnopp C, Werfel T, European Academy of Allergology and Clinical Immunology: Standardization of food challenges in patients with immediate reactions to foods – position paper from the European Academy of Allergology and Clinical Immunology. Allergy 2004; 59:690–697.

Prof. Dr. med. Margitta Worm

Department of Dermatology and Allergy, Charité Campus Mitte, Schumannstr. 20–21, D-10117 Berlin, Germany, Tel. +49 30 450-518105, Fax +49 30 450-518919, E-mail margitta.worm@charite.de

Digestion-Sensitive Wheat Proteins Can Induce Food Allergy

E. Untersmayr[1], N. Bakos[2], I. Schöll[1], M. Kundi[3], F. Roth-Walter[1], K. Szalai[1], A.B. Riemer[1], G. Boltz-Nitulescu, O. Scheiner, and E. Jensen-Jarolim[1]

[1]Center of Physiology and Pathophysiology, Medical University Vienna, Austria,
[2]Department of Dermatology, Hospital of Szolnok, Hungary
[3]Center of Public Health, Medical University of Vienna, Austria

Summary: *Background:* Recently we have demonstrated in an animal model that anti-ulcer drugs promote the development of food allergy. By elevating the gastric pH these drugs hinder peptic digestion and essentially harmless, digestion-labile proteins exhibit sensitizing capacity. The aim of this observational study was to examine whether anti-ulcer drugs support the sensitization toward easily degradable proteins also in humans. *Methods:* We screened 152 adult patients (mean age 65.9 years) without previous history of allergic disorders, who were medicated with H2-receptor blockers or proton pump inhibitors during 3 months due to dyspeptic disorders. Serum samples for determination of specific IgE were taken before, and 3 and 8 months after the beginning of therapy, and SPTs were performed at the 8-month time-point. *Results:* Nine digestion-labile antigens, among them wheat flour, were included in our evaluations. In the 152 acid-suppressed gastroenterological patients, 11% showed *de novo* IgE formation specific for one or more of these digestion-labile dietary compounds without any concomitant inhalative sensitization, and 4.6% formed wheat specific IgE. The patients discontinued anti-acidic treatment after 3 months. Nevertheless, at the 8 months time-point the increase of specific IgE was still significant, e.g., for wheat flour ($p = 0.043$) and sensitization patterns could be confirmed through positive skin prick reactions. *Conclusion:* The presented data demonstrate that anti-ulcer treatment supports sensitization toward digestion-labile dietary compounds such as proteins of wheat. Therefore, we conclude that patients who suffer from dyspeptic complaints and who are continuously acid-suppressed are at risk to develop type I food allergy.

Keywords: food allergy, anti-ulcer drugs, gastric digestion, sensitization, simulated gastric fluid assay

Anti-ulcer drugs are world-wide bestsellers of the pharmaceutical industry. In Taiwan the total consumption of anti-ulcer drugs between 1997 and 2001 was 36.1% [1]. A study performed in Cornwall, United Kingdom, reported that 14% of the total prescription cost and 2% of the health authority budget was spent on prescription of acid-suppression drugs. Furthermore, the authors of this study reported that up to 11% of all patients receive these drugs in a repeated way [2].

This medication reduces the net gastric acid output and is, therefore, applied for antisecretory

therapy of dyspeptic disorders. The highly potent proton pump inhibitors and H2-receptor antagonists are capable of totally abolishing acid secretion [3, 4] and it was demonstrated that a 5-day treatment with the broadly prescribed proton pump inhibitor Omeprazole elevates the gastric pH to an average of 5.0 [5]. Our hypothesis was that conditions with an elevated gastric pH might interfere with the gastric digestion capacity, as the pepsin enzyme activity has a pH optimum between 1.8–3.2 [6].

Digestion stability is a typical feature of "class 1" food allergens, being capable of sensitizing directly via the gastrointestinal tract [7]. In contrast, sensitizing capacity has been doubted for proteins that are susceptible to degradation. They are termed "non-sensitizing elicitors" [8], because food allergic reactions toward these "class 2" food allergens are based on cross-reactivity with pollen allergens as the genuine sensitizers [9]. Therefore, simulated gastric fluid experiments have become standard laboratory protocols employed to characterize known allergens [10] and are part of the decision tree to evaluate the allergenic potential of novel dietary proteins [11]. In these *in vitro* assays, the stability of food proteins is tested with the major gastric protease pepsin at low pH, simulating gastric conditions. However, these tests do not take into consideration conditions with modified gastric acid output, e.g., in atrophic gastritis, partial gastrectomy, or treatment with anti-ulcer drugs, which might affect the gate-keeping function of the stomach.

In previously published studies we demonstrated that the major fish allergen parvalbumin, hazelnut allergens, and also the exclusive food allergen Beluga caviar were degraded within seconds in digestion experiments and thus did not show features of typical class 1 food allergens [12, 13]. Moreover, we revealed that hindering gastric digestion by elevating the gastric pH led to food allergy toward these digestion-sensitive dietary antigens in murine food allergy models. Female BALB/c mice were immunized with the food antigen caviar, with the major fish allergen parvalbumin, or with hazelnut extract, with or without concomitant medication with antacids or antiulcer drugs, such as H2-receptor blockers and proton pump inhibitors. Mice under anti-acidic therapy developed high titers of antigen-specific antibodies of the Th2 type and exhibited positive skin and mucosal challenge results [12, 13]. Furthermore, eosinophilic infiltration of the gastric antrum mucosa was observed exclusively in mice treated with the acid-suppression therapy [14].

To confirm our murine data in human patients, we performed an observational cohort study including 152 adult patients (58 men and 94 women; mean age 65.9 years) from a gastroenterological outpatient clinic [15]. The patients were treated orally for dyspeptic disor-

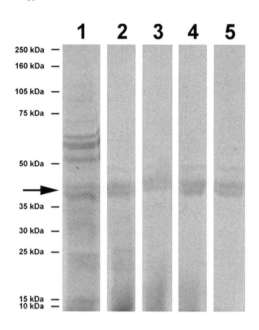

Figure 1. SDS-PAGE analysis of wheat proteins (lane 1) subjected to simulated gastric fluid experiments. Incubation of wheat extract with pepsin at pH. 2.0 results in an immediate fragmentation after 5 sec of digestion (lane 2). After 1 min (lane 3) only small peptide fragments remain to be detected, which are less distinct after 15 min (lane 4) and disappear completely after 2 h (lane 5) of enzymatic digestion. The arrow indicates the pepsin double band at approximately 40 kDa.

ders, such as gastritis, dyspepsia, erosions, gastric ulcers, and reflux for 3 months with the H2-receptor blocker Famotidine (Quamatel® 2 × 40 mg/day; Richter Gedeon RT, Budapest, Hungary) or Ranitidine (Zantac® 2 × 150 mg/day; Pfizer Inc, New York, or Pylorid® 2 × 400 mg/day; GlaxoSmithKline, Brentford, UK) or the proton pump inhibitor Omeprazole (Losec® 1 × 20 mg/day; AstraZeneca, London, UK). Medication compliance was checked in monthly control visits. IgE reactivity toward 19 common dietary antigens (milk, casein, egg white, egg yolk, peanut, walnut, almond, potato, tomato, celery, carrot, apple, orange, wheat flour, rye flour, sesame seed, soy bean, codfish, and crab) was evaluated before (0 months) and after therapy (3 and 8 months) by immunoblotting (AllergyScreen, MEDIWISS analytic, Moers, Germany). Skin tests were performed at the 8-month time-point. To further characterize the food antigens included in our study, digestion experiments with simulated gastric fluid [10] were performed. Nine out of 19 antigens were degraded within 1 min in these experiments. Figure 1 shows the time-dependent digestion of wheat as a paradigm, even though this antigen is one of the most frequent elicitors of allergic reactions [16].

Interestingly, after 3 months of anti-acidic treatment, 11% of all patients showed *de novo* IgE formation toward one or more of these "non-sensitizing elicitors" and 4.6% had formed wheat specific IgE without concomitant inhalative sensitization. For wheat, the increase of IgE was significant both at the 3 months time-point ($p = 0.002$) and still at the 8 months time-point ($p = 0.043$). Moreover, sensitization patterns were confirmed with positive skin reactions for wheat flour 5 months after discontinuation of anti-ulcer therapy.

Taking wheat as an example we conclude from our data that digestion-sensitive food proteins may exhibit sensitizing capacity in situations where gastric digestion is hindered. Thus, long-term acid suppression might be a risk factor for the development of food allergy toward digestion-labile dietary compounds.

Acknowledgments

This work was supported by grants #10326 of the Austrian National Bank "Jubiläumsfond" and SFB F01808–B04 of the Austrian Science Funds.

References

1. Chen TJ, Chou LF, Hwang SJ: Prevalence of anti-ulcer drug use in a Chinese cohort. World J Gastroenterol 2003; 9:1365–1369.
2. Boutet R, Wilcock M, MacKenzie I: Survey on repeat prescribing for acid suppression drugs in primary care in Cornwall and the Isles of Scilly. Aliment Pharmacol Ther 1999; 13:813–817.
3. Sharma BK, Walt RP, Pounder RE, Gomes MD, Wood EC, Logan LH: Optimal dose of oral omeprazole for maximal 24 hour decrease of intra-gastric acidity. Gut 1984; 25:957–964.
4. Chiverton SG, Burget DW, Hunt RH: Do H2 receptor antagonists have to be given at night? A study of the antisecretory profile of SKF 94482, a new H2 receptor antagonist which has a pro-

found effect on daytime acidity. Gut 1989; 30: 594–599.
5. Prichard PJ, Yeomans ND, Mihaly GW, Jones DB, Buckle PJ, Smallwood RA, et al.: Omeprazole: a study of its inhibition of gastric pH and oral pharmacokinetics after morning or evening dosage. Gastroenterology 1985; 88:64–69.
6. Samloff IM: Peptic ulcer: the many proteinases of aggression. Gastroenterology 1989; 96:586–595.
7. Hefle SL: The chemistry and biology of food allergens. Food Tech 1996; 50:86–92.
8. Aalberse RC: Structural biology of allergens. J Allergy Clin Immunol 2000; 106:228–238.
9. Vieths S, Scheurer S, Ballmer-Weber B: Current understanding of cross-reactivity of food allergens and pollen. Ann NY Acad Sci 2002; 964: 47–68.
10. Astwood JD, Leach JN, Fuchs RL: Stability of food allergens to digestion *in vitro*. Nat Biotechnol 1996; 14:1269–1273.
11. Taylor SL, Hefle SL: Will genetically modified foods be allergenic? J Allergy Clin Immunol 2001; 107:765–771.
12. Untersmayr E, Scholl I, Swoboda I, Beil WJ, Forster-Waldl E, Walter F, et al.: Antacid medication inhibits digestion of dietary proteins and causes food allergy: a fish allergy model in BALB/c mice. J Allergy Clin Immunol 2003; 112:616–623.
13. Schoell I, Untersmayr E, Bakos N, Roth-Walter F, Boltz-Nitulecsu G, Scheiner O, Jensen-Jarolim E: Anti-ulcer drugs promote oral sensitization and hypersensitivity to hazelnut allergens in BALB/c mice and humans. Am J Clin Nutr 2005; 81:154–156.
14. Untersmayr E, Ellinger A, Beil WJ, Jensen-Jarolim E: Eosinophils accumulate in the gastric mucosa of food-allergic mice. Int Arch Allergy Immunol 2004; 135:1–2.
15. Untersmayr E, Bakos N, Schoell I, Kundi M, Roth-Walter F, Szalai K, Riemer AB, Ankersmit HJ, Scheiner O, Boltz-Nitulescu G, Jensen-Jarolim E: Anti-ulcer drugs promote IgE formation toward food allergens in adult patients. FASEB J 2005; 19:656–658.
16. Sampson HA: Clinical manifestations of adverse food reactions. Pediatr Allergy Immunol 1995; 6(Suppl. 8):29–37.

Erika Jensen-Jarolim

Center of Physiology and Pathophysiology, Medical University of Vienna, AKH, EBO 3Q, Waehringer Guertel 18–20, A-1090 Vienna, Austria, Tel. +43 1 40400 5103, Fax +43 1 40400 5130, E-mail erika.jensen-jarolim@meduniwien.ac.at

What Can We Learn from the Ratio of IgG1/IgG4 Antibodies to Allergens?

R.C. Aalberse and S.O. Stapel

Sanquin at CLB and Academic Medical Center Amsterdam, The Netherlands

Summary: *Background:* In order to clarify the regulation of B-cell activation in atopy we compared the IgG response to allergens in atopic and nonatopic subjects (both total IgG, as well as IgG4). *Methods:* High-affinity IgG antibodies were measured in serum samples from birth cohorts using purified iodinated allergens from mites, pollen, animal danders, and foods. Subjects were classified according to their IgE antibody status. *Results:* IgG antibodies to allergens from mites or pollen were found almost exclusively in subjects with IgE antibodies to these allergens. In contrast, IgG antibodies to allergens from animal dander or foods were often found in the absence of IgE antibodies. This effect was not restricted to IgG4 antibodies (which represented less than 50% of the IgG antibody response), but was actually more pronounced for the non-IgG4 part of the IgG response (largely IgG1). *Conclusion:* The immune response to classical atopic allergens (from pollen or mites) is distinct from the response to allergens that may induce a *modified Th2* response (i.e., IgG4 without IgE). As a working hypothesis we postulate that an immune response to classical atopic allergens (which is rare in nonatopic subjects) is a low-grade reaction. It largely lacks mature germinal centers and, thus, fails to induce a strong B memory response. In contrast, the modified Th2 response results from a humoral immune response with mature germinal centers (which are unfavorable for the survival of IgE-switched B-cells) and a pronounced B memory response. IgG4-switched B-cells occasionally switch subsequently to IgE.

Keywords: IgG, IgG4, atopy, modified Th2

The focus of this paper will be on antibodies and B-cells (as opposed to T-cells or symptoms). Moreover, we will use IgE antibody primarily for classification of subjects (rather than as an outcome parameter). The outcome parameters are high-affinity IgG and IgG4 antibodies to well-characterized, purified allergens.

Materials and Methods

Purified trace quantity of iodinated fluid-phase allergen in combination with agarose-bound anti-immunoglobulin in suspension.

Results

IgG in Relation to IgE Responses

For some allergens ("classical atopic allergens": pollen, mite) it is rare to find IgG in the absence of IgE. In contrast, for other allergens (nonatopic allergens are modified TH2 inducers: cat, dog) it is common to find IgG in the absence of IgE (but it is still less common and/or the titers are lower in nonatopic than in atopic subjects).

What About IgG4?

It is often assumed that IgG4 dominates the IgG response to atopic allergens. However, this is true only in situations of high (both in terms of dose as well as time) allergen exposure. There is a clear increase in the IgG4/IgG ratio in relation to time of exposure [1]. This increase of the IgG4/IgG ratio with time and exposure is a general phenomenon for Th2-type antigens (i.e., antigens that fail to activate Th1 immune responses; the prototype of a Th1 response is the immune response to bacteria). This increase in IgG4/IgG ratio is a slow process (months to years), which suggests that IgG4-switched B memory cells are reluctant to start terminal differentiation to plasma cells.

Discussion

Atopic vs. Nonatopic, Modified TH2 Humoral Immune Responses

It is becoming increasingly clear that allergens can be subdivided into two categories. On the one hand there are classical atopic allergens such as the major allergens from pollen (grasses, trees, or weeds) and mites. On the other hand there are nonatopic, modified Th2 allergens such as the major allergens from cat or dog. The spectrum of nonatopic allergens gradually merges with antigens that are often not considered to be allergens, such as tetanus toxoid or diphtheria toxoid. The grey area in-between the nonatopic allergens and Th2-inducing antigens contains proteins such as airborne proteins in occupational settings (e.g., in the animal house), proteins in insect venom, and many food proteins. All these antigens induce IgG responses. Initially the IgG4 contribution is only modest, but it may become dominating upon extensive exposure. The distinction is at the IgE/IgG ratio. The classical atopic allergens induce IgG responses almost always in combination with IgE responses ("No IgG without IgE"). In contrast, nonatopic allergens induce IgG responses often in the absence of IgE.

Working Hypothesis

An immune response to classical atopic allergens is a low-grade reaction. It largely lacks mature germinal centers and, thus, fails to induce a strong B memory response. In this environment, direct μ to ε class-switching is not markedly less common than switching to other isotypes. In contrast, the modified Th2 response results from a conventional humoral immune response with mature germinal centers (which are hypothesized to be unfavorable for the survival of IgE-switched B-cells) and a pronounced B memory response. IgG4-switched B-cells occasionally switch subsequently to IgE.

Isotype-switched B-cells have a strikingly different fate, depending on the isotype. IgE-switched B-cells show virtually no clonal expansion or memory, a few switched cells escape negative selection and rapidly differentiate to plasma cell, some of which survive months to years. IgG4-switched B-cells are very different, being predominantly memory B-cells that are hard to activate into fully differentiated plasma cells. IgG1-switched B-cells are intermediate in the sense that these B-cells survive as memory cells, but are more easily activated (and exhausted) than IgG4-switched B-cells.

This hypothesis leads to the following testable predictions: (1) IgE memory B- cells are rare; (2) the ranking of clonal diversity is: IgE > IgG1 > IgG4; (3) direct switching (μ to ε) is more common for classical atopic allergens, whereas indirect switching is more common for nonatopic (modified TH2) allergens.

Acknowledgments
We would like to thank our present and former colleagues at Sanquin/CLB: Henk de Vrieze, Ellen Vermeulen, Astrid van Leeuwen, Peter Calkhoven, Vinay Koshte, and Joost Aalberse. The data on which these concepts are based were largely generated during two cohort studies: The PIAMA project, with thanks to Bert Brunekreef and the other members of the PIAMA study group, and the BOKAAL project, for which we thank Marijke de Jong and

Vera Scharp. International input came from, among others, Stephen Durham, Tom Platts-Mills, and Pat Holt.

References

1. Aalberse RC, Platts-Mills TAE: How do we avoid developing allergy: modifications of the TH2 response from a B-cell perspective. J Allergy Clin Immunol 2004; 113:983–986.

R.C. Aalberse

Department of Immunopathology, Sanquin Research at CLB, Plesmanlaan 125, 1066 CX Amsterdam, The Netherlands, Tel. +31 20 512-3158/3171, Fax +31 20 512-3170, E-mail r.aalberse@sanquin.nl

Immunoglobulin Free Light Chains in Immediate and Delayed Hypersensitivity Reactions

F.A. Redegeld, M.W. van der Heijden, M. Kool, B. Blokhuis,
A.D. Kraneveld, and F.P. Nijkamp

*Department of Pharmacology and Pathophysiology, Utrecht Institute
for Pharmaceutical Sciences, Utrecht University, The Netherlands*

Summary: *Background:* Antibodies play an important role in the humoral response of the adaptive immune system and the isotype determines its effector function. Besides complete Igs, B-cells also produce considerable amounts of Ig free light chains (FLC), which can be found in different body fluids. *Results:* We have shown that FLC can dose-dependently transfer hapten sensitivity upon intravenous/local injection into mice. A second encounter with the cognate antigen induced edema formation (ear swelling). Mast cells were shown to be crucial in this hypersensitivity response. Using *in vitro* cultured primary mast cells provided direct evidence that crosslinking of surface proteins with Ig FLCs stimulated release of granule mediators and production of lipid mediators. Cutaneous sensitization of mice with low molecular weight compounds followed by a second contact with the appropriate antigen on the ear induces contact sensitivity reactions marked by a biphasic ear-swelling response. B-cells were shown to be essential in the development of this typical T-cell-mediated immune response. We have demonstrated that contact sensitization with low molecular weight compounds such as dinitrofluorobenzene, picryl chloride, and oxazolone results in rapid production of antigen-specific FLC. Moreover, we were able to inhibit development of clinical signs of contact sensitivity by treating the sensitized animals with F991, an FLC antagonist. *Conclusions:* In conclusion, we propose that FLC might play a role in both immediate and delayed hypersensitivity responses. These insights in the immunological role of FLC reveal challenging concepts in the treatment of allergic disorders and chronic inflammatory diseases.

Keywords: immunoglobulin free light chains, mast cells, immediate hypersensitivity, delayed hypersensitivity, ear swelling, autoimmune disease

IgE is well known for its central role in allergic responses by activating mast cells and basophils via their FcεRI receptor. Atopy is often referred to as the personal and/or familial predisposition to produce IgE antibodies in response to exposure to allergens and serum levels of total or allergen-specific IgE are commonly determined for the diagnosis of allergy and atopy. However, there seems to be a discordance between the markers of atopy and occurrence of allergic disease. For instance, it has been reported that about 50% of allergic rhinitis patients have serum total IgE in the normal range [1] and also the prevalence of asthma and atopy shows disparities [2]. These discrepancies could be explained by the presence of elevated levels of specific IgE, synthesis of local IgE, induction of strong anti-inflammatory mechanisms, or blockade of IgE receptors by non-antigen-specific IgE. How-

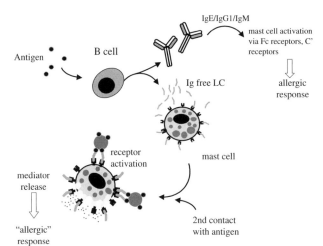

Figure 1. Sequence of events leading to mast cell activation and allergic responses via (a) Fc and C' receptors and (b) Ig FLCs. Antigen contact results in production of complete immunoglobulins and immunoglobulin FLC. FLC sensitize tissue-resident mast cells and second contact with (multivalent) antigen results in crosslinking of surface-bound FLC followed by mast cell activation and the induction of an "allergic" response.

ever, our recent studies suggest that another player might be involved in the induction of hypersensitivity responses, i.e., Ig FLCs [3, 4].

Ig FLCs Elicit Immediate Hypersensitivity-Like Responses

Besides complete immunoglobulins, B-cells also produce considerable amounts of Ig FLCs. Under physiological conditions, free κ and λ light chains can be found in different body fluids [5, 6, 7]. In our recent work, we have shown that Ig FLCs are functionally important and can elicit immediate hypersensitivity reactions [3]. When naïve mice are injected with Ig FLCs, a second encounter with the cognate antigen induced mast cell activation and edema formation (ear swelling) – all features of an immediate hypersensitivity response. Mast cells were shown to be crucial in the response elicited by Ig light chains. We found no response in genetically mast cell-deficient animals and response was restored in mast cell "knock-in" animals. Moreover, mast cells in ear tissue showed morphological signs of anaphylactic degranulation. Using *in vitro* cultured primary mast cells provided direct evidence that crosslinking of surface proteins with Ig FLCs stimulated release of granule mediators and production of lipid mediators. The identity of the receptor for FLCs on mast cells is under investigation. A role for Fc receptors is excluded, because common γ chain-deficient animals (lacking FcεRI and FcγRIII)

exhibit unchanged responses toward Ig FLCs [3].

Ig FLCs Are Crucial in Contact Sensitivity Responses

To investigate the role of FLCs in hypersensitivity disease models, we used a peptide antagonist selectively inhibiting FLC responses. This peptide F991 corresponds with the Ig light chain-binding moiety of Tamm-Horsfall protein [8]. F991 was shown to effectively block the ear-swelling responses induced after topical challenge of FLC-sensitized mice. No effect of F991 was seen on swelling responses elicited in IgM, IgG$_1$, and IgE-immunized animals indicating that it is not interfering with heavy chain-bound light chains in complete immunoglobulins. Cutaneous sensitization of mice with low molecular weight compounds followed by a second contact with the appropriate antigen on the ear induces contact sensitivity reactions marked by a biphasic ear-swelling response. Contact sensitization with low molecular weight compounds such as dinitrofluorobenzene, picryl chloride, and oxazolone results in rapid production of Ig FLCs specific for the hapten used. Indeed, we were able to inhibit development of clinical signs of contact sensitivity by treating the sensitized animals with F991.

In conclusion, we propose that antigen-specific mast cell activation through Ig FLCs may be an alternate pathway to induce hypersensitivity responses. Interference in FLC-induced hypersensitivity responses might, therefore, be an interesting therapeutic target in the treatment "allergic" and chronic inflammatory diseases.

References

1. Sibbald B, Rink E: Epidemiology of seasonal and perennial rhinitis: clinical presentation and medical history. Thorax 1991; 46:895–901.
2. Von Mutius E: Is asthma really linked to atopy? Clin Exp Allergy 2001; 31:1651–1652.
3. Redegeld FA, van der Heijden MW, Kool M, Heijdra BM, Garssen J, Kraneveld AD, Van Loveren H, Roholl P, Saito T, Verbeek JS, Claassens J, Koster AS, Nijkamp FP: Immunoglobulin-free light chains elicit immediate hypersensitivity-like responses. Nat Med 2002; 8:694–701.
4. Redegeld FA, Nijkamp FP: Immunoglobulin free light chains and mast cells: pivotal role in T-cell-mediated immune reactions? Trends in Immunology 2003; 24:181–5.
5. Hannam-Harris AC, Smith JL: Free immunoglobulin light chain synthesis by human foetal liver and cord blood lymphocytes. Immunology 1981; 43:417–423.
6. Bradwell AR, Carr-Smith HD, Mead GP, Tang LX, Showell PJ, Drayson MT, Drew R: Highly sensitive, automated immunoassay for immunoglobulin free light chains in serum and urine. Clin Chem 2001; 47:673–680.
7. Fagnart OC, Sindic CJ, Laterre C: Free κ and λ light chain levels in the cerebrospinal fluid of patients with multiple sclerosis and other neurological diseases. J Neuroimmunol 1988; 19:119–132.
8. Huang ZQ, Sanders PW: Localization of a single binding site for immunoglobulin light chains on human Tamm-Horsfall glycoprotein. J Clin Invest 1997; 99:732–736.

Frank A. Redegeld

Department of Pharmacology and Pathophysiology, Utrecht Institute for Pharmaceutical Sciences, Utrecht University, Sorbonnelaan 16/PO BOX 80082, 3508 TB Utrecht, The Netherlands, Tel. +31 30 253-7355, Fax +31 30 253-7420, E-mail f.a.m.redegeld@pharm.uu.nl

Expression of Plasma Cell Markers CD38, CD138, Intracellular IgE, and XBP-1 in the Plasmacytoid Cell Line U266

L. Hummelshoj[1], L.P. Ryder[2], and L.K. Poulsen[1]

[1]Laboratory of Medical Allergology, Allergy Clinic, National University Hospital, Copenhagen,
[2]Tissue Typing Laboratory, Department of Clinical Immunology, National University Hospital,
Copenhagen, both Denmark

Summary: *Background:* The commitment of a B-cell to ε-isotype class switch and further to an IgE-producing plasma cell is a tightly regulated process, and our understanding of the regulation of IgE-producing cells is essential for the prevention and treatment of atopic disease. However, little is known about the specific differentiation of IgE switched germinal center (GC) B-cells to IgE producing plasma cells or the kinetics of this process. We aimed at designing a method for detection of plasma cells using a plasma cell marker, the transcription factor X-box binding protein I (XBP-1), which is highly expressed during plasmacytic differentiation. *Methods:* The IgE-producing plasma cell line U266 was used to study the expression of intracellular IgE and XBP-1 and the distribution of the plasma cell markers CD38 and CD138. The basophil leukemic cell line KU812 was applied as control. IgE and XBP-1 and surface CD38, CD138, and CD19 were detected by flow cytometry and immunofluorescence microscopy. The expression of XBP-1 was verified by a PCR-based method. *Results:* The methods for detecting intracellular protein and mRNA XBP-1 were optimized and validated. U266 was positive for intracellular IgE, intracellular XBP-1, and CD138. However, only a few cells were positive for CD38, the nonplasma cell marker CD19, and the surface IgE. Furthermore, mRNA XBP-1 was highly expressed in U266 compared to KU812. *Conclusion:* Methods were developed for detecting the plasma cell markers XBP-1, CD38, CD138, and intracellular IgE. XBP-1, IgE, and CD138, but not CD38, were found in the cell line U266, which could be useful as a model for detecting plasma cells.

Keywords: plasma cell, U266, CD138, CD38, XBP-1, IgE, isotype switch

Terminally differentiated antibody-secreting plasma cells are the end-stage effector cells of the humoral immune response but their lifetime is debated [1]. The presence of long-lived IgE producing plasma cells could counteract the effect of immunotherapy treated allergic individuals and could explain the longevity of allergic sensitization in drug-, insect- and food-allergic patients who have not been exposed

for many years. Studies of IgE-producing plasma cells have, however, been hampered by the lack of good markers.

Several molecules have been identified as involved in the regulation of plasma cells including the transcription factor XPB-1, which is essential for their differentiation [2, 3]. Because of the positive effect on differentiation into plasma cells, it would be interesting to

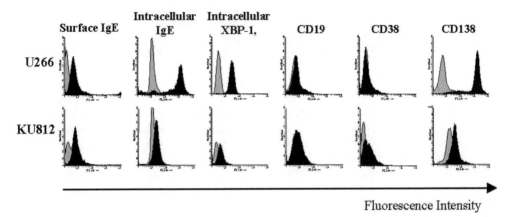

Figure 1. Expression of B-cell markers in U266 and KU812 measured by FACS. Expression of surface IgE, intracellular IgE, XBP-1, CD19, CD38, and CD138 was evaluated by flow cytometry by incubation with specific antibody (black histogram) in comparison with the isotype (grey histogram). The data from one representative experiment of three is shown.

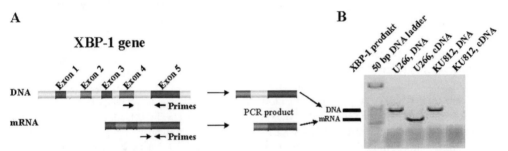

Figure 2. Expression of mRNA XBP-1 in U266 and KU812 measured by PCR. Total RNA and DNA were extracted separately and PCR was conducted using primers spanning two exons in the XBP-1 gene (A) and products run at a 1% agarose gel (B). The data from one representative experiment of three conducted is shown.

examine XBP-1 in more detail. We, therefore, aimed at developing a PCR method for detection of XBP-1 mRNA and a FACS method for measurement of the intracellular protein level of XBP-1 and IgE as well as the plasma cell surface markers CD38 and CD138. As a model system we used the IgE-producing plasma cell line U266, using the basophilic cell line KU812 as a control.

Material and Methods

Total RNA was purified from U266 and KU812 and mRNA were analyzed for XBP-1 by PCR formed with a primer sequence (forward: catggattctggcggtattcact, reverse: acaggttcttccttcactgagacaa) based on a previous study by our group [Hummelshoj L, Ryder LP, Poulsen LK, previously described].

The IgE-producing plasma cell line U266 and the basophilic cell line KU812 were analyzed for intracellular IgE (rabbit antihuman IgE-FITC) and XBP-1 (rabbit antihuman XBP-1, goat antirabbit-FITC) and surface CD38 (mouse antihuman CD38-PE), CD138 (mouse antihuman CD138-CyQ), and CD19 (mouse antihuman CD19-PECy5) by FACS-Scan. Moreover, U266 and KU812 were immunostained with IgE and XBP-1 (same antibodies as above) and visualized in fluorescence microscope.

Results and Discussion

The IgE-producing plasma cell line U266 and the basophilic cell line KU812 were analyzed for intracellular IgE and XBP-1 and surface CD38, CD138, and CD19 by FACS. The methods for detecting intracellular protein and mRNA XBP-1 were optimized and validated. A large fraction of U266 was positive for intracellular IgE (91%), intracellular XBP-1 (82%), and CD138 (89%; Figure 1). However, only 3% of U266 were positive for CD38, which are normally found highly expressed on plasma cells. The B-cell marker CD19 was expressed in less than 3% of the cells.

The basophil cell line, KU812, which served as control, was negative/low for intracellular IgE, intracellular XBP-1, and CD38. KU812 expressed low amounts of CD138 (15%) and no CD19.

U266 and KU812 were immunostained with specific antibodies against intracellular IgE and XBP-1 and visualized in fluorescence microscope (data not shown). As indicated by the FACS results in Figure 1, U266 were positive for intracellular IgE and XBP-1 whereas KU812 were negative for intracellular IgE and slightly positive for XBP-1.

Primers were designed to span over two exons to avoid chromosomal DNA (Figure 2A). DNA and total RNA were purified and PCR used for detection of mRNA XBP-1 (DNA were used as a positive control). mRNA XBP-1 was highly upregulated in U266 and not found expressed in KU812 (Figure 2b). Because of the lack of XBP-1 mRNA expression in KU812, the slightly positive XBP-1 expression observed in FACS and fluorescence microscope could be due an unspecific binding of the antibody. Also, one should keep in mind that XBP-1 is not strictly limited to plasma cells. In adult tissues XBP-1 is expressed ubiquitously, whereas in fetal tissues it is expressed preferentially in exocrine glands, osteoblasts, chondroblasts, and liver [2, 4]. However, the expression of XBP-1 in B-cell lineages is restricted to plasma cells [2].

Conclusion

We have developed a method for detecting the plasma cell markers XBP-1, CD138, and intracellular IgE in the cell line U266 that was not found in KU812. It was not possible to detect CD38 on U266 that are normally found on human plasma cells. The method will be used for detecting plasma cells and for further investigation of the regulation of plasma cells and possible treatment strategies of those cells in allergic disorders.

References

1. Manz RA, Radbruch A: Plasma cells for a lifetime? Eur J Immunol 2002; 32:923–927.
2. Iwakoshi NN, Lee A, Vallabhajosyula P, Otipoby KL, Rajewsky K, Glimcher LH: Plasma cell differentiation and the unfolded protein response intersect at the transcription factor XBP-1. Nature Immunology 2003; 321–329.
3. Reimold AM, Iwakoshi NN, Manis J, Vallabhajosyula P, Szomolanyi-Tsuda E, Gravallese EM, Friend D, Grusby MJ, Alt F, Glimcher LH: Plasma cell differentiation requires the transcription factor XBP-1. Nature 2001; 412:300–307.
4. Clauss IM, Gravallese EM, Darling JM, Shapiro F, Glimcher MJ, Glimcher LH: In situ hybridization studies suggest a role for the basic region-leucine zipper protein hXBP-1 in exocrine gland and skeletal development during mouse embryogenesis. Dev Dyn 1993; 197(2):146–156.

Lone Hummelshoj Jensen

National University Hospital, Laboratory of Medical Allergology, Allergy Clinic 7551, Blegdamsvej 9, 2100 Copenhagen O, Denmark, Tel. +45 35 457593, Fax +45 35 457581, E-mail l.hummelshoj@rh.dk

Improvement of the *in vitro* Diagnostic of Natural Rubber Latex Allergy

Estimation of Cross-Reactivity Through Application of Recombinant and Natural Single Allergens

M. Raulf-Heimsoth[1], H.Y. Yeang[2], M. Lundberg[3], S.A.M. Arif[2], Th. Brüning[1], and H.P. Rihs[1]

[1]*Berufsgenossenschaftliches Forschungsinstitut für Arbeitsmedizin (BGFA), Institut der Ruhr-Universität, Bochum, Germany,* [2]*Rubber Research Institute of Malaysia (RRIM), Kuala Lumpur, Malaysia,* [3]*MIAB, Uppsala, Sweden*

Summary: *Background:* Scientific efforts have resulted in the identification of several latex allergens and their recombinant production. The impact of the single allergens for an advanced *in vitro* natural rubber latex (NRL) diagnostic was studied. *Methods:* Sera of 68 health care workers (HCW) with NRL-related symptoms and a positive NRL skin prick test (SPT) were tested with different latex allergen preparations coupled on ImmunoCAPs (Pharmacia Diagnostics, Uppsala, Sweden). *Results:* 90% of the sera were positive to latex ImmunoCAP spiked with rHev b 5 ("k82 new"). In contrast only 76% of these sera displayed positive specific IgE to latex without additional rHev b 5 (correlation 0.93). Eight out of nine sera with an exclusive IgE-response to the "k82 new" were monosensitized to rHev b 5. A mixture of four recombinant allergens (rHev b 1, 5, 6.01, and 8) coupled to Immuno-CAP advanced the *in vitro* latex-specific IgE-determination compared to the original latex extract preparation, but less efficient than the preparation of latex sap extract including the most important allergens and the addition of rHev b 5. Spiking important but labile recombinant single allergens to native allergen preparations to enhance their amounts has been shown to improve diagnostic sensitivity. *Conclusion:* Based on the analysis of the sensitization profiles Hev b 2, 5, 6.01 and 13 are major allergens for HCW. Together with Hev b 1, the major allergen for spina bifida patients, these allergens should be included in sufficient amounts in a standardized latex diagnostic extract.

Keywords: latex allergy, allergen profile, recombinant allergens

NRL allergy has become a widespread problem with extensive health and economic implications and many efforts have been undertaken to decrease the incidence of latex allergy. The identification of latex allergens, their recombinant production, and the determination of specific sensitization profiles for different patient groups are useful steps toward the understanding of NRL allergy and the improvement of diagnosis and possible treatment [1]. The impact of single allergens for an advanced *in vitro* NRL diagnostic was studied.

For this purpose, sera of 68 latex-allergic HCW who were occupationally exposed to NRL and suffered from NRL-related symptoms (all of them had a positive NRL SPT and

Table 1. Comparison of latex-specific IgE tests

Method	Sensitivity	Specificity	PPV	NPV	Test eff.
"k82 old"	76%	98.3%	98.1%	78.7%	86.7%
k82 + "rHev b 5"	90%	98.3%	98.4%	89.4%	93.8%
rHev b-mix	83.6%	98.3%	98.2%	84.3%	90.6%

PPV = positive predictive value; NPV = negative predictive value; test eff. = test efficiency

a positive challenge test to latex gloves) were collected. These selected HCW belonged to a collective of 128 HCW with suspected latex allergy and established SPT to NRL. *In vitro* testing of the sera had been carried out with latex ImmunoCAP (k82 with and without spiked rHev b 5), with an ImmunoCAP prepared of a mixture of four recombinant latex allergens (rHev b 1, 5, 6.01, and 8; rHev b-mix) and with a panel of single recombinant latex allergens (rHev b 1, 3, 5, 6.01, 7, 8, 9, 10, 11, and 12) using the UniCAP 100 system (Pharmacia Diagnostics, Uppsala, Sweden). All of the recombinant allergens were produced in E.coli in fusion with the maltose-binding protein (MBP) as fusion component. The MBP coupled on ImmunoCAP served as negative control. The native latex allergens nHev b 2 and nHev b 13 were prepared at the Rubber Research Institute in Malaysia, coupled to CNBr-activated paper disks, and their specific IgE-binding was determined in the EAST system.

Positive specific IgE to latex ImmunoCAP k82 (without additional rHev b 5; "k82 old") was found in 52 out of the 68 HCW with a positive SPT indicating a test sensitivity of 76% and a test efficiency of 86.7%. By retesting the 68 sera with the latex ImmunoCAP k82 spiked with rHev b 5 ("k82 new" [2]), 90% of the sera were positive to latex and the test efficiency could be enhanced up to 93.8%. The correlation between the results obtained with "k82 old" and "k82 new" was 0.923; eight out of nine sera with an exclusive IgE-response to the "k82 new" were monosensitized to rHev b 5. Comparison of the results obtained with 59 sera using the latex ImmunoCAP spiked with rHev b 5 and the rHev b-mix CAP demonstrated a good correlation ($r = 0.917$)

between both test systems, but four of the sera showed no IgE binding to the rHev b-mix CAP. These sera were positive to nHev b 2 and/or nHev b 13. The test efficiency using the rHev b-mix ImmunoCAP was enhanced compared to the "k82 old"-ImmunoCAP, but lower than the test efficiency of the latex ImmunoCAP k82 spiked with rHev b 5 (Table 1). To estimate the impact of single profiling for characterization and differentiation of latex risk groups, the specific IgE responses to a panel of single allergens in different latex-allergic patient groups were compared. Using a panel of single latex allergens the following profile was detected in sera of HCW: 17% were positive to rHev b 1, 76% to nHev b 2, 8% to rHev b 3, 67% to rHev b 5, 69% to rHev b 6.01, 14% to rHev b 8, 2% to rHev b 9 and rHev b 10, 22% to rHev b 11 and 83% to nHev b 13.

A subgroup of 14 latex-allergic HCW suffered from additional symptoms when eating various fruits ("latex-fruit syndrome"). Comparing the sensitization profile of this group with latex-allergic HCW without latex-fruit syndrome indicated that sera from latex-allergic HCW without allergic reaction to fruits responded only to nHev b 2, rHev b 5, and rHev b 6.01. No IgE binding was found to the minor allergens rHev b 1, 3, 7, 8, 9, 10, 11 and 12.

The addition of rHev b 5 to the latex ImmunoCAP improved the *in vitro* diagnostic for latex allergy. A mixture of four recombinant allergens advanced the *in vitro* latex-specific IgE determination compared to the original latex extract used for ImmunoCAP (k82) preparation, but was less efficient than the preparation of latex sap extract including the most important allergens and the addition of rHev b 5. Based on the analysis of the sensitization profiles Hev b 2, 5, 6.01 and 13 are major allergens for HCW. Together with Hev b 1, the major allergen for spina bifida patients, this panel should be included in sufficient amounts in a standardized latex diagnostic extract. Further allergens such as Hev b 7, 8, 9, 10, 11, and 12 have to be considered for testing specific cross-reactivities in individual cases.

References

1. Raulf-Heimsoth M, Rihs HP, Brüning T: Latex: a new target for standardization. In J Löwer, W-M Becker, S Vieths (Eds.), Regulatory Control and Standardization of Allergenic Extracts, 10th International Paul-Ehrlich-Seminar. Frankfurt a.M.: Sperlich 2003, pp. 107–115.

2. Lundberg M, Chen Z, Rihs HP, Wrangsjö K: Recombinant spiked allergen extract. Allergy 2001; 56:794–795.

Monika Raulf-Heimsoth

Berufsgenossenschaftliches Forschungsinstitut für Arbeitsmedizin (BGFA), Institut der Ruhr-Universität Bochum, Haus X, Allergologie/Immunologie, Bürkle-de-la-Camp-Platz 1, 44789 Bochum, Germany, Tel. +49 234 302-4582, Fax +49 234 302-4610, E-mail raulf@bgfa.de

Hypersensitivity to NSAID Drugs

A New Integrated Approach to Its Pathophysiological Understanding and Diagnosis

A.L. de Weck[1], M.L. Sanz[2], and P.M. Gamboa[3]

[1]Gerimmun Foundation, Fribourg, Switzerland, [2]Department of Allergology and Clinical Immunology, University of Navarra, Pamplona, Spain, [3]Allergy Division, Hopital Basurto, Bilbao, Spain

Summary: Hypersensitivity to NSAIDs is a well-known syndrome affecting the airways (rhinosinusitis, nasal polyps, asthma) and/or the skin (urticaria, angioedema). Although currently the favorite theory on its pathogenesis is a pharmacogenetic abnormality in the response to cyclooxygenase (COX)-1 inhibitors, much uncertainty remains. Furthermore, it is persistently claimed that only provocation challenge with NSAIDs establishes the diagnosis and that no *in vitro* tests are helpful to ascertain the condition. However, various studies have indicated that blood basophils from patients hypersensitive to NSAIDs may produce, upon stimulation with such drugs *in vitro*, more sulfidoleukotrienes (CAST assay) than patients who tolerate them. This, however, has not been universally confirmed. Our recent study on 60 patients and 30 controls, using a flowcytometric basophil activation test has definitely shown that clinical hypersensitivity to NSAIDs is accompanied by basophil stimulation *in vitro* in about 75% of the cases, with a specificity of 95–100%. A review of known clinical and laboratory findings leads to an integrated view of the syndrome, which requires the joint effects of several factors to be clinically realized. First and foremost, a chronic inflammatory process, which may be of various origins (possibly viral) yields hyperreactive effector cells (mast cells, basophils, eosinophils) either in the skin or in the airways, explaining the final localization of symptoms. On these hyperreactive cells, NSAIDs act on the arachidonic acid metabolism in an altered fashion, most probably based on a pharmacogenetic abnormality leading to increased production of sulfidoleukotrienes. In addition, decreased synthesis of PGE2 removes an essential brake for mediator release by inflammatory cells. The simultaneous intervention of these three factors explains most of the clinical and pathophysiological findings in the NSAID hypersensitivity syndrome and opens logical approaches for diagnosis and treatment.

Keywords: hypersensitivity, NSAIDs, aspirin, sulfidoleukotrienes, CAST, flow cytometry

Hypersensitivity NSAIDs is a well-known syndrome affecting the airways (rhinosinusitis, nasal polyps, asthma) and/or the skin (urticaria, angioedema). It represents about 25% of all adverse reactions to drugs. The favorite theory is that the mechanism of multiple NSAID hypersensitivity is related to the pharmacological activity of the drugs: inhibition of COX-1 causes an imbalance in arachidonic acid metabolism, favoring LTC4 synthesis, probably on a genetic basis [1,2]. Another dogma is that there are no *in vitro* tests for that condition and diagnosis can be established only by provocation challenge [3].

NSAID hypersensitivity has different and, most of the time, exclusive target organs (skin

Allergy Clin Immunol Int: J World Allergy Org, Supplement 2 (2005)

or airways), it usually starts in the 2nd or 3rd decade of life, and is rare in children. Its evolution can vary from very severe to transient; positive provocation may become negative with time [4]. The interval between exposure and symptoms is usually of 30–60 minutes. The clinical features are difficult to reconcile with a strictly pharmacogenetic abnormality. The NSAID hypersensitivity syndrome must be differentiated from anaphylactic reactions to a single NSAID, usually due to specific IgE [6].

The cells involved in NSAID reactions are on the one hand the mast cells, as shown by the presence of tryptase and PGD2 and its metabolites in nasal secretion and/or urine after NSAID challenge [6,7] and the protective effect of disodium cromoglycate. On the other hand, basophils produce increasing amounts of sulfidoleukotrienes (sLT) and 15-HETE [8] upon challenge. Eosinophilia and release of ECP in nasal and bronchial fluid after challenge reveal the participation of eosinophils [1]. Various inflammatory mediators, in particular histamine, tryptase, and sLT, have been detected in nasal fluid, bronchial secretions, or urine after NSAID challenge [9].

There are several hints that some chronic inflammatory process in the airways or in the skin may be a prerequisite for development of the NSAID syndrome. It may follow viral infections [10]; antiviral therapy [11] and steroids have beneficial effects. There is evidence that blood basophils from NSAID hypersensitive patients are hyperreactive to C5a and to other nonspecific stimulants [12–14]. Such patients react to COX-1 inhibitors but usually not to COX-2 inhibitors. The patterns of cross-reactivity are individual and heterogeneous, and are possibly related to the individual effectiveness of COX-1 inhibition. The precise nature of the shift and imbalance in arachidonic acid metabolism of such patients is still not known [1, 2]. Since all patients with chronic airway inflammation and chronic urticaria, possessing hyperreactive basophils, mast cells, and eosinophils, do not become NSAID hypersensitive, it must be postulated that some additional factor explaining the hyperproduction of sLT and other mediators is at play, probably some pharmacogenetic abnormality. A bronchial overexpression of LTC4 synthase [15] and some genetic polymorphism in LTC4 synthase have been described [16] but not confirmed [17]. It is difficult to see how a pharmacogenetic abnormality alone could explain the late onset in life and the organ compartmentalization.

An additional factor is the fact that PGE2, the production of which is markedly impaired by NSAIds, acts as a "brake" on inflammatory cell stimulation [1,18]. A deficiency in PGE2 may, therefore, also contribute to the symptoms.

In vitro Diagnosis by sLT (CAST) and Flowcytometric Basophil Activation

Since 1995, several authors have reported that incubation of blood basophils from NSAID hypersensitive patients with aspirin and other NSAID *in vitro* generated sLTs, which can usually be detected by the commercial CAST test [19,20]. The best documented study in this respect is that of May et al. [21]. However, other authors have obtained entirely negative [22] or less favorable results [23]. We have recently discussed elsewhere [20] the possible reasons for these apparent discrepancies, which seem to rest on technical factors.

Following a number of anecdotal reports [24], we have recently reported a study on 60 confirmed NSAID hypersensitive patients and 30 controls, using flowcytometric basophil activation (FAST alias FLOW CAST) [25] and CAST [20].

The main results, published in detail elsewhere [20,25], are summarized in Table 1.

The main practical conclusion is that the flowcytometric test, using two concentrations of aspirin and diclofenac, yields a sensitivity of 59% and a specificity of 93%. The test is highly correlated to positive provocation tests and may, therefore, confirm diagnosis in a sizeable proportion of cases, although its sensitivity is not ideal. Sensitivity may be increased by adding more NSAiDs but this is at the expense of specificity. The results of CAST, on the other hand, are less impressive

Table 1. Sensitivity and specificity of FAST (FLOW CAST) and CAST in hypersensitivity to NSAIDs.

NSAID	Concentration	Sensitivity (nb positives/nb tested)				Controls	Specificity (Nb positives/nb tested)		
		Patients FAST	CAST	Combi CAST*	Total 2 conc *	FAST	CAST	Combi CAST3	Total 2 conc*
Aspirin	1.25 mg/ml	36.6% (22/60)	20% (12/60)	41.6% (25/60	45% (27/60)	100% (0/30)	85.7% (5/28)	FAST =	100% (0/30)
	0.3 mg/ml	18.3% (11/60)	15% (9/60)	28.3% (17/60)		199% (0/30)	92.8% (2/28)	CAST =	89.5% (2/19)
Paracetamol	1.25 mg/ml	5% (3/60)	8.3% (5/60)	13.3% (8/60)	18.3% 11/60	100% (0/30)	96.4% (1/28)		96.4% (1/28)
	0.3 mg/ml	11.6% (7/60)	6.7% (4)60)	16.7% (10/60)		100% (0/30)	100% (0/28)		
Metamizol	5 mg/ml	8.3% (5/60)	6.3%	(5/60	16.7% (10/60)	25% (15/60)	100% (0/30)		92.8% (2/28)
	0.6 mg/ml	13.3% (8/60)	3.3% (2/60)	16.7% (10/60)		100% (0/30)	96.4% 1/28		92.8% (2/28)
Diclofenac	0.3 mg/ml	36.7% (22/60)	3.3% (2/60)	40% (24/60)	53.3% (32/60)	93.3% (2/30)	85.7% (4/26)		
	0.08 mg/ml	25% (15/60)	13.3% (8/60)	35% (21/60)		96.6% (1/30)	96.4% (1/28)		85.7% (4/28)
Naproxen	1.25 mg/ml	47.6% (20/42)	21.4% 9/42	59.5% (25/42)	76.1% (32/42)	88.8% (3/27)	70.3% (8/27)	59.2% (11/27)	
	0.3 mg/ml	19% (8/42)	28.6% (12/42)	40.5% (17/42)		85.2% (4/27)	88.8% (3/27)	81.5% (5/27)	
4 NSAIDs**	2 conc	66.7% (40/60)	48.3% (28/60)	73.3% (44/60)		93.3% (2/30)	67.8% (9/28)	71.4% (8/28)	
5 NSAIDs***	2 conc	83.3% (35/42)	64.3% (27/42)	95.2% (40/42)		77.2% (6/27)	55.5% (12/24)	44.4% (15/27)	

* FAST and CAST combined, ** Aspirin, paracetamol, metamizol, and diclofenac, *** Naproxen added

but may, in some cases, confirm the FAST tests [20]. Whatever the diagnostic usefulness of these, our studies, as well as others [8,18] confirm that NSAID hypersensitive patients possess in their blood hyperreactive basophils stimulated *in vitro* by NSAIDs.

An Integrated Pathogenetic View of the NSAID Hypersensitivity Syndrome

Most recent authors of reviews or book chapters on aspirin sensitivity bluntly state that "the underlying mechanism of aspirin sensitivity is currently unknown" [26].

This statement may be formally correct, but in view of all facts reviewed above, singularly lacks imagination.

We propose a multifactorial hypothesis, as illustrated in Figure 1. First and foremost, a

chronic inflammatory process, which may be of various origins (possibly viral) yields hyperreactive effector cells (mast cells, basophils, eosinophils) either in the skin or in the airways, explaining the final localization of symptoms. These hyperreactive cells are recognized by their increased reactivity to C5a and other nonspecific stimulants. On these hyperreactive cells, NSAIDs act on the arachidonic acid metabolism in an altered fashion, most probably based on a pharmacogenetic abnormality leading to increased production of sulfidoleukotrienes. In addition, decreased synthesis of PGE2 under the pharmacologic effect of NSAIDs removes an essential brake for mediator release by inflammatory cells. The simultaneous intervention of these three factors explains most of the clinical and pathophysiological findings in the NSAID hypersensitivity syndrome and opens logical approaches for diagnostic and treatment.

It is recognized that this view is still a hypothesis needing confirmation but it has at

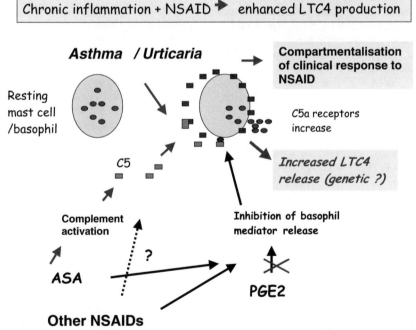

Figure 1. An integrated view of NSAID hypersensitivity. Chronic inflammation in the form of asthma or urticaria induces hyperreactive mast cells/ basophils manifested by an increased sensitivity to C5a and other stimulants. In such hyperreactive cells, NSAID elicit an increased LTC4 production probably on the basis of a pharmacogenetic abnormality. The decrease in PGE2 levels induced by NSAIDs also contributes to enhanced mediator release. The complement activation allegedly induced by aspirin (ASA) may play some additional role.

least the advantage of being logical and suggesting various supporting investigations.

References

1. Szczeklik A, Stevenson D: Aspirin-induced asthma: advances in pathogenesis, diagnosis, and management. J Allergy Clin Immunol 2003; 111: 913–921.
2. Szczeklik A, Gryglewski RJ, Czerniawska-Mysik G: Relationship of inhibition of prostaglandin biosynthesis by analgesics to asthma attacks in aspirin-sensitive patients. Br Med J 1975; 1:67–69.
3. Szczeklik A, Stevenson DD: Aspirin-induced asthma: advances in pathogenesis and management. J Allergy Clin Immunol 1999; 104:5–13.
4. Pleskow WW, Stevenson DD, Mathison DA, Simon RA, Schatz M, Zeiger RS: Aspirin-sensitive rhinosinusitis/asthma: spectrum of adverse reactions to aspirin. J Allergy Clin Immunol 1983; 71:574–579.
5. Blanca M, Perez E, Garcia JJ: Angiedema and IgE antibodies to aspirin: a case report. Ann Allergy 1989; 62:295–298.
6. Fischer AR, Rosenberg MA, Lilly CM, Callery JC, Rubin P, Cohn J, White MV, Igarashi Y, Kaliner MA, Drazen JM, Israel E: Direct evidence for a role of the mast cell in the nasal response to aspirin in aspirin-sensitive asthma. J Allergy Clin Immunol 1994; 94:1046–1056.
7. Mita H, Endoh S, Kudoh M, Kawagishi Y, Kobayashi M, Taniguchi M, Akiyama K: Possible involvement of mast-cell activation in aspirin provocation of aspirin-induced asthma. Allergy 2001; 56:1061–1067.
8. Kowalski ML, Ptasinska A, Bienkiewicz B, Pawliczak R, DuBuske L: Differential effects of aspirin and misoprostol on 15-hydroxyeicosatetraenoic acid generation by leukocytes from aspirin-sensitive asthmatic patients. J Allergy Clin Immunol 2003; 112:505–512.
9. Lee TH, Smith CM, Arm JP, Christie PE: Mediator release in aspirin-induced reactions. J Allergy Clin Immunol 1991; 88:827–829.
10. Szczeklik A: Aspirin-induced asthma as a viral disease. Clin Allergy 1988; 18:15–20.
11. Nakagawa H, Yoshida S, Nakabayashi M, Akahori K, Shoji T, Hasegawa H, Amayasu H: Possible relevance of virus infection for development of analgesic idiosyncrasy. Respiration 2001; 68:422–424.
12. Abrahamsen O, Haas H, Schreiber J, Schlaak M: Differential mediator release from basophils of

allergic and nonallergic asthmatic patients after stimulation with anti-IgE and C5a. Clin Exp Allergy 2001; 31:368–378.
13. Czech W, Schöpf E, Kapp A: Release of sulfidoleukotrienes in vitro: its relevance in the diagnosis of pseudoallergy to acetylsalicylic acid. Inflamm Res 1995; 44:291–295.
14. Wedi B, Kapp A: Aspirin-induced adverse skin reactions: new pathophysiological aspects. Thorax 2000; 55(Suppl 2):S70–S71.
15. Cowburn AS, Sladek K, Soja J, Adamek L, Nizankowska E, Szczeklik A, Lam BK, Penrose JF, Austen KF, Holgate ST, Sampson AP: Overexpression of leukotriene C4 synthase in bronchial biopsies from patients with aspirin-intolerant asthma. J Clin Invest 1998; 101:834–846.
16. Sanak M, Simon H-U, Szczeklik A: Leukotriene C4 synthase promoter polymorphism and risk of aspirin-induced asthma. Lancet 1997; 350: 1599–2000.
17. Van Sambeck R, Stevenson DD, Baldasaro M, Lam BK, Zhao JL, Yoshida S, Yandora C, Dos JM, Penrose JF: 5' Flanking region polymorphism of the gene encoding leukotriene C4 synthase does not correlate with the aspirin-intolerant asthma phenotype in the United States. J Allergy Clin Immunol 2000; 106:72–76.
18. Hecksteden K, Schäfer D, Stuck BA, Klimek L, Hörmann K: Diagnostik der Analgetika-Intoleranz-Syndroms mittels funktioneller Zelltestung (Analgetika-Intoleranz-Test: AIT). Allergologie 2003; 26:263–271.
19. De Weck AL: Zellulärer Allergen De-Stimulierungs-Test (CAST). Eine Übersicht und kritische Auswertung der klinischen Anwendung in der Allergiediagnose. Allergologie 1997; 20:487–502.
20. Sanz ML, Gamboa P, De Weck AL: A new combined test with flowcytometric basophil activation (FAST) and determination of sulfidoleukotrienes (CAST) is useful for in vitro diagnosis of hypersensitivity to aspirin and other nonsteroidal anti-inflammatory drugs (NSAIDs). Int Arch Allergy Immunol 2005; 36:58–72.
21. May A, Weber A, Gall H, Kaufmann R, Zollner TM: Means of increasing sensitivity of an in vitro diagnostic test for aspirin intolerance. Clin Exp Allergy 1999; 29:1402–1414.
22. Pierzchalska M, Mastalerz L, Sanak M, Zalula M, Szczeklik A: A moderate and unspecific release of cysteinyl leukotrienes by aspirin from peripheral blood leukocytes precludes its value for aspirin sensitivity testing in asthma. Clin Exp Allergy 2000; 30:1785–1791.
23. Lebel B, Messaad B, Kvedariene V, Rongier M,

Bousquet J, Demoly P: Cysteinyl-leukotriene release test (CAST) in the diagnosis of immediate drug reactions. Allergy 2001; 56:688–692.

24. Sabbah A, Drouet M, Sainte-Laudy J, Lauret MG, Loiry M: Apport de la cytométrie en flux dans le diagnostic allergologique. Allergie & Immunologie 1997; 29:15–21.

25. Gamboa PM, Sanz ML, Caballero MR, Urrutia I, Antepara I, De Weck AL: The flowcytometric determination of basophil activation induced by aspirin and other non steroidal anti-inflammatory drugs (NSAIDs) is useful for *in vitro* diagnosis of the NSAID hypersensitivity syndrome. Clin Exp Allergy 2004, 34:1448–1457.

26. Bush RK, Asbury DW: Aspirin-sensitive asthma. In WW Busse, ST Holgate (Eds.), Asthma and Rhinitis. Oxford: Blackwell Scientific (2nd ed.), 2000:1315–1325.

A.L. de Weck

Gerimmun Foundation, Beaumont 18, CH-1700 Fribourg, Switzerland, E-mail alain.dew@bluewin.ch

Pollen-Associated Food Allergy

In vitro Diagnosis by Recombinant Allergens and CD63 Expression of Basophils

S.M. Erdmann[1], K. Hoffmann-Sommergruber[2], A. Schmidt[1],
I. Sauer[1], S. Moll-Slodowy[1], O. Scheiner[2], and H.F. Merk[1]

[1]*Department of Dermatology and Allergology, University of Aachen, Germany*
[2]*Department of Pathophysiology, Medical University of Vienna, Austria*

Summary: *Background:* Basophil activation is associated with an increased CD63 expression on basophils. The aim of this study was to investigate whether incubating basophils with the recombinant allergens Bet v 1, Bet v 2, Api g 1, Mal d 1, and Dau c 1 in the basophil activation test based on CD63 expression (BAT) is a useful tool for *in vitro* diagnosis of pollen associated food allergy to celery, apple, and carrot. *Methods:* Thirty patients with an OAS induced by apple, celery, or carrot and 10 controls were selected for this study. Basophils were incubated with Bet v 1, Bet v 2, Api g 1, Mal d 1, and Dau c 1. After double immunostaining with anti-IgE and anti-CD63 monoclonal antibodies CD63 expression was determined by flow cytometry. Results were compared to well established routine diagnostic methods, i.e., SPTs with native foods and measurement of allergen specific serum IgE by the CAP FEIA method. *Results:* Although *in vivo* testing of native foods by SPT showed a sensitivity of 100% with regard to the clinical history of an OAS a combination of both *in vitro* methods – measurement of allergen specific serum IgE and the BAT – showed a sensitivity higher than 90% for all three food allergens investigated. *Conclusion:* The CD63-based BAT is a valuable new *in vitro* method for diagnosis of IgE mediated food allergy and may play a future role particularly if immediate type hypersensitivity cannot be demonstrated by routine methods such as determination of allergen specific serum IgE.

Keywords: food allergy, basophils, basophil activation, recombinant allergens, Bet v 1, CD63, flow cytometry

Recently, it has been reported that the surface marker CD63 is expressed with high density on activated basophils [1]. This new *in vitro* method has been commonly referred to as the CD63-based basophil activation test (BAT) [2]. To date the basophil activation test has not been performed applying purified recombinant allergens in food allergy.

Birch pollen associated allergy to foods such as apple, carrot, and celery is frequently observed in Central and Northern Europe and accounts for a great proportion of all food allergies in adults. In the majority of these cases food hypersensitivity is a result of cross-reactivity to Bet v 1 the major allergen of birch pollen [3]. Homologous proteins to Bet v 1 have been identified in a wide range of flowering plants. Mal d 1, the major allergen from apple, was the first Bet v 1 homologous fruit allergen cloned and produced as recombinant allergen, followed by Api g 1 from celery and Dau c 1 from carrot.

The aim of this study was to investigate whether a two-color flow cytometric method using anti-IgE and anti-CD63 monoclonal antibodies (mAb) could be applied to the diagnosis of birch pollen-associated food allergy to apple, carrot, and celery by use of the recombinant allergens Api g 1, Dau c 1, and Mal d 1, and Bet v 1 and Bet v 2, and to compare sensitivity and specificity with well-established tests such as SPT and measurement of allergen specific serum IgE.

Material and Methods

Thirty patients with a history of an OAS induced by apple, carrot, or celery (20 patients for each food) and 10 controls were selected. All of the patients had a history of seasonal allergic rhinitis or allergic asthma.

Skin Testing and Specific IgE

Patients and controls were skin prick tested with native apple (Golden Delicious), carrot, and celery by using the prick-to-prick technique. In addition all subjects were skin prick tested with birch, grass, and mugwort pollen. Allergen-specific IgE was measured by the CAP FEIA method.

Basophil Activation Test (BAT)

Blood samples from all subjects were drawn into heparinized tubes. 100 µl of whole blood was preincubated with 20 µl of wash buffer containing IL-3 at 37 °C for 10 min. 100 µl of the cell suspension was distributed in microtiter plate wells and mixed in parallel with 100 µl of wash buffer (negative control), 100 µl of fMLP (positive control), and 100 µl of the recombinant allergens Api g 1, Dau c 1, Api g 1, Bet v 1, and Bet v 2 (Biomay, Vienna, Austria). Optimal allergen concentrations for each allergen had been previously established in a pilot study. Plates were incubated for 20 min. at 37 °C. Degranulation was stopped by chilling on ice. Thereafter, phycoerythrin-conjugated anti-IgE (PE-anti-IgE) and FITC-conjugated anti-CD63 mAb were added and incubated for 20 min. on ice. Finally, the heparinized whole-blood samples were lysed, fixed, and washed. Plates were centrifuged and analyzed within 2 h on a FACScan flow cytometer. The basophil population was gated by the expression of PE-anti-IgE. The expression of CD63 was analyzed on this gated cell population. Results were given as percentage of basophils expressing CD63 according to the following formula: number of PE-anti-IgE$^+$ and FITC-anti-CD63$^+$ basophils/number of PE-anti-IgE$^+$ basophils. The cut-off for a positive BAT was 10% CD63$^+$ basophils.

Results

Skin Testing and Specific IgE

SPT with native apple, carrot, and celery showed sensitivities of 100% for all foods. The corresponding specificities were 80%, 90%, and 80%. SPT with birch pollen was positive in all patients, mugwort in 10/30, and grass pollen in 8/30 patients. Measurement of specific IgE against apple, carrot, and celery gave sensitivities of 60%, 70%, and 75% and corresponding specificities of 70%, 100%, and 80%.

Basophil Activation Test (BAT)

In the 30 patients with a history of an OAS the mean percentage of CD63$^+$ basophils (of the total of all IgE$^+$ basophils) after incubating the basophils with wash buffer (negative control) was 2.6% (*SD*: 1.7%) as compared to an average activation of 2.8% of all basophils (*SD*: 1.66%) in the controls.

Incubation of the basophils with fMLP (positive control) resulted in a mean basophil activation of 32.3% (*SD*: 17.08%) in the food allergics.

In the group of food allergics ($n = 20$ for each food) incubating the basophils with the relevant allergen gave the following results with regard to mean basophil activation: Api g 1 49.75% (*SD*: 34.27%), Mal d 1 55.24% (*SD*: 34.54%), and Dau c 1 38.22% (*SD*: 37.02%). In the 10 controls for each food mean basophil activation after incubating with Api g 1, Mal d 1, and Dau c 1 was 13.13% (*SD*: 24.14%), 26.94% (*SD*: 38%), and 2.22% (*SD*: 1.91%), respectively. Comparison of mean percentages of CD63$^+$

basophils showed significant differences between patients and controls in all three allergens. The corresponding p-value of Student's test was < 0.0155 for Mal d 1, < 0.0004 for Api g 1, and < 0.0003 for Dau c 1.

Comparing the rate of concordance between BAT and CAP (both tests negative or positive) in apple allergy in 60% of all subjects, in carrot allergy in 70% of all subjects, and in celery allergy in 75% of all patients both tests gave the same test result. Spearman's correlation coefficients indicated a moderate positive correlation between CAP class and percentage of $CD63^+$ basophils for Dau c 1, Api g 1 and Mal d 1: r(Dau c 1/carrot) = 0.40, r(Api g 1/celery) = 0.58, r(Mal d 1/apple): 0.41. Spearman's correlation coefficients for CAP class and percentage of $CD63^+$ basophils for Bet v 1 and Bet v 2 were 0.53 and 0.38, respectively.

Sensitivity and specificity of Mal d 1 was 75% and 70%, respectively. Sensitivity and specificity of Api g 1 was 75% and 80%, respectively. Sensitivity and specificity of Dau c 1 was 65% and 100%, respectively.

Discussion

In this study flow cytometry was applied to study allergen-induced basophil activation in IgE-mediated food allergy using a double staining method with anti-IgE and anti-CD63 mAb as described in literature [1, 2]. To our knowledge in this study for the first time recombinant allergens were applied in the BAT to study pollen-associated food hypersensitivity. Dose response curves showed that appropriate allergen concentrations varied considerably between the different recombinant allergens applied covering a range between 1 ng/ml (Bet v 1) and

10 µg/ml (Api g 1). Forty-three out of 60 BATs were positive with the relevant food. Interestingly, determination of allergen specific IgE for apple by the well-established CAP-FEIA method was less sensitive than the BAT in detecting sensitization in the group of apple allergics. In our study applying the BAT in conjunction with measurement of allergen-specific IgE, combined sensitivity of *in vitro* diagnosis in apple allergy was 100% (sensitivity of specific IgE: 60%), in carrot allergy 90% (sensitivity of specific IgE: 70%), and in celery allergy 95% (sensitivity of specific IgE: 75%).

Our results suggest that application of recombinant allergens in the BAT is feasible in detecting IgE-mediated food hypersensitivity. When used to evaluate patients with a strong history of pollen-associated food allergy, the BAT reaches the sensitivity of *in vivo* testing of native foods.

References

1. Knol EF, Mul FPJ, Jansen H, Calafat J, Roos D: Monitoring human basophil activation via CD63 monoclonal antibody 435. J Allergy Clin Immunol 1991; 88:328–338.
2. Sanz ML, Maselli JP, Gamboa PM, Oehling A, Dieguez I, de Weck AL: Flow cytometric basophil activation test: a review. J Invest Allergol Immunol 2002; 12:143–154.
3. Breiteneder H, Radauer C: A classification of plant allergens. J Allergy Clin Immunol 2004; 113:821–830.

Stephan Erdmann

Department of Dermatology & Allergology, University Hospital of Aachen, Pauwelsstr. 30, D-52074 Aachen, Germany, E-mail serdmann@ukaachen.de

Immediate Adverse Reactions to Cephalosporins

Study of *in vitro* Crossreactivity by Determining Specific IgE to Different Betalactams

M. Blanca[1], C. Mayorga[2], M.J. Torres[1], J.L. Rodriguez-Bada[2], C. Antúnez[2], J.A. Cornejo-García[2], T. Fernandez[2], R. Rodriguez[2], M.C. Moya[1], and A. Romano[3]

[1]*Allergy Service and* [2]*Research Laboratory for Allergic Diseases, Carlos Haya Hospital, Malaga, Spain,* [3]*Department of Internal Medicine and Geriatrics, UCSC – Allergy Unit, C.I. Columbus, Rome, Italy*

Summary: Second to penicillins, cephalosporins are the betalactams most increasing in consumption and in induction of IgE mediated allergic responses. We examined the importance of different cephalosporin and penicillin determinants in the *in vitro* detection of specific IgE antibodies in the sera of patients with immediate reactions to a cephalosporin derivative. Nineteen patients with a clinical history of immediate allergic reactions to different cephalosporins and with skin test positive to the culprit drug were evaluated. The drugs involved were cefaclor (4), cefonicid (1), cefotaxime (2), ceftazidime (2), ceftriaxone (3) and cefuroxime (7). All patients had specific IgE antibodies, as determined by radioimmunoassay (RAST), to the culprit cephalosporin. Cross-reactivity with penicillins and other cephalosporins was studied by RAST to different betalactams. RAST showed that of the 19 patients, 11 (58%) were only positive to the cephalosporin inducing the allergic reaction and seven (36.8%) had a cross-reaction with a cephalosporin having a similar side chain to that inducing the reaction. No patient was positive to penicillin derivatives. We can conclude that there is high cross-reactivity *in vitro* between cephalosporins, although further studies are needed to determine the clinical value of this *in vitro* crossreactivity. Nevertheless, we detected no crossreactivity between penicillins and cephalosporins in the patients studied, which could imply that this is not as high as generally thought. Thus, to detect specific IgE antibodies in patients with immediate allergic reactions to cephalosporins it is not enough to use just penicillin derivatives; it is also necessary to use at least the culprit cephalosporin.

Keywords: cephalosporins, crossreactivity

Cephalosporins are the second most important betalactams, after penicillins, in terms of increasing consumption and induction of IgE-mediated allergic responses [1]. Study of patients allergic to cephalosporins has shown that three main types of IgE-response exist: patients who have cross-reactivity with BPO, patients who share cross-reactivity between different cephalosporins, and patients who are apparently selective to the target cephalosporin [2]. This last group of patients seems to be increasing, which impedes evaluation if cephalosporin determinants are not included in the study.

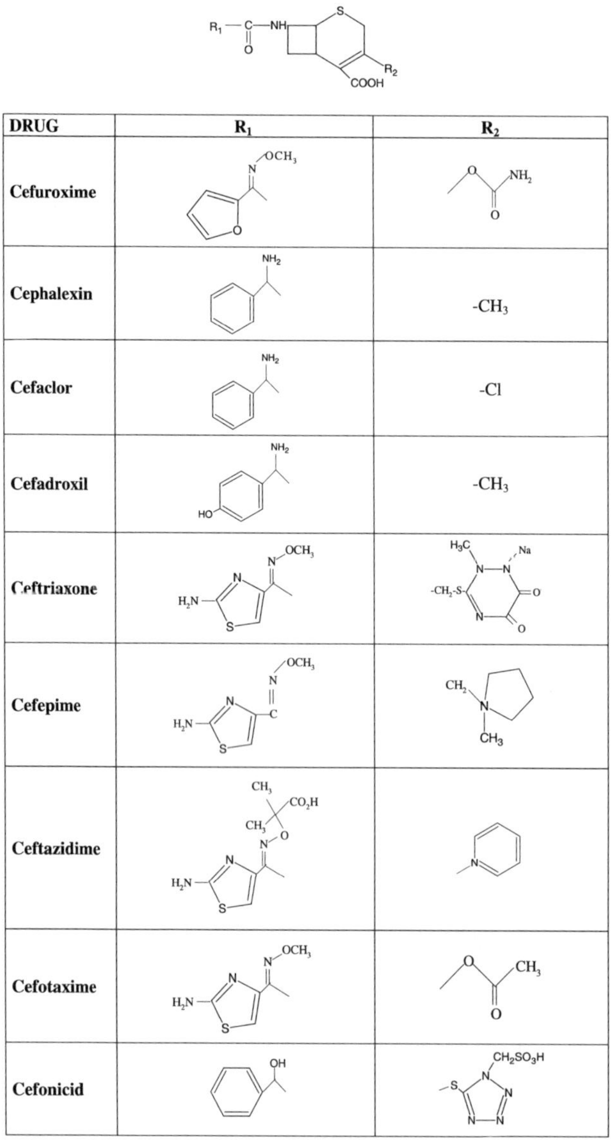

Figure 1. Chemical structure of different betalactams used in the study.

DRUG	R₁	R₂
Cefuroxime		
Cephalexin		-CH₃
Cefaclor		-Cl
Cefadroxil		-CH₃
Ceftriaxone		
Cefepime		
Ceftazidime		
Cefotaxime		
Cefonicid		

We examined the *in vitro* cross-reactivity between different cephalosporin and penicillin determinants in a group of patients with immediate allergic reactions to a cephalosporin derivative with skin test and RAST positive to the target cephalosporin.

Material and Methods

Patients

We studied 19 patients (6 men and 13 women) diagnosed with an immediate allergic reaction to cephalosporins [2] with skin test and RAST positive to the target cephalosporin (Figure 2).

Skin Test

This was carried out as previously reported [2, 3], using benzylpenicilloyl polylysine (BPO-PLL; Allergopharma Merck, Reinbek, Germany; 5×10^{-5}M), minor determinant mixture (MDM; Allergopharma; 2×10^{-2}M), amoxycillin (AX; SB Smithkline Beecham, Madrid, Spain; 20 mg/ml) and ampicillin (AMP; Normon, Madrid; 20 mg/ml), and just the target

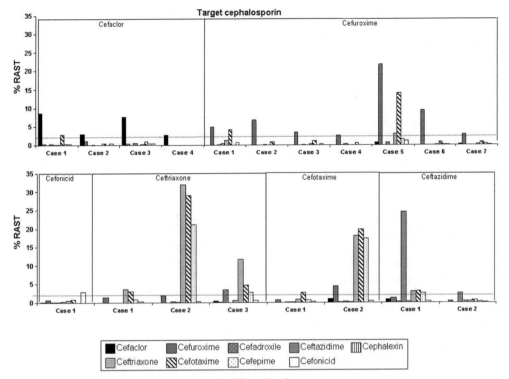

Figure 2. RAST results in the 19 patients evaluated with different betalactams.

cephalosporin (2 mg/ml): cefaclor (Lilly, Madrid), cefonicid (Smithkline), cefotaxime (Roussel Iberica Laboratorios, Madrid), ceftazidime (Glaxo-Wellcome, Madrid), ceftriaxone (Roche, Basel, Switzerland), or cefuroxime (Glaxo).

Radioimmunoassay for IgE Determination

This was made by radioallergosorbent test (RAST) using different penicillins and cephalosporins conjugated to PLL (Sigma, St. Louis, MO) in the solid phase as previously described [2]. Results were calculated as a percentage of the maximum and considered positive if they were higher than 2.5% of label uptake, which was the mean + 2SD of a negative control group.

Results

Of the 19 patients, 6 developed urticaria and 13 anaphylaxis. Skin tests were negative to PPL

and MDM and to the target cephalosporin in all patients; Case 2 was also positive to AMP and Case 11 to AX. RAST results (Figure 2) showed that 11 (58%) were only positive to the target cephalosporin, 7 (36.8%) had a cross-reaction with another cephalosporin having the same or a very similar side chain in R1 to the target cephalosporin, and just one (5.2%) had IgE antibodies to cephalosporin with a different side chain to the target drug (Figure 1). No patient was positive to penicillin derivatives (benzylpenicillin or amoxicillin).

Discussion

Despite structural similarities between penicillins and cephalosporins, the rate of cross-reactivity is not clear. In our study, although two cases were skin test positive to aminopenicillins, no *in vitro* cross-reactivity between penicillins and cephalosporins was detected, probably because of the lower sensitivity of RAST [3]. Nevertheless, the cross-reactivity was lower than expected, indicating the necessity of using the target cephalosporin for diagnosis. This may be explained because both groups of drugs differ in the product obtained from the nucleophillic opening of the betalactam ring. Cephalosporins suffer an extensive fragmentation process in the dihydrothyazine portion, leading to a great number of degradation products and disappearance of the R2 substitution, which makes it unlikely that this structure contributes to the constitution of the antigenic determinant, only the R1 position being relevant [4]. This lack of importance in R2 can be seen from our results, where eight patients had a cross-reaction with a cephalosporin different from the target cephalosporin. In all except one of these patients the cross-reaction was with a cephalosporin that had the same, or a very similar, chemical structure at the R1 position. In the only case in which the cross-reaction was between two cephalosporins with a very different R1 side chain, the R2 side chain was also different, thus, IgE antibodies seem to be directed to the common structure of cephalosporins. However, further studies are needed to determine the clinical value of this *in vitro* cross-reactivity.

Acknowledgments

This study was supported by Fondo Investigacion Sanitaria grant FIS PIO20666.

References

1. McCaig L, Hughes JM: Trends in antimicrobial drug prescribing among office-based physicians in the United States. JAMA 1995; 273:214–219.
2. Romano A, Mayorga C, Torres MJ et al.: Immediate allergic reactions to cephalosporins: cross-reactivity and selective responses. J Allergy Clin Immunol 2000; 106:1177–1183.
3. Torres MJ, Romano A, Mayorga C et al.: Diagnostic evaluation of a large group of patients with immediate allergy to penicillins: the role of skin testing. Allergy 2001; 56:850–856.
4. Sánchez Sancho F, Perez-Inestrosa E, Suau R et al.: Synthesis, characterization, and immunochemical evaluation of cephalosporin antigenic determinants. J Mol Recognition 2003; 16:148–156.

Miguel Blanca

Allergy Service, Hospital Civil, Plaza Hospital Civil s/n, E-29009 Malaga, Spain, Tel. +34 95 1030346, Fax +34 95 1030302, E-mail miguel.blanca.sspa@juntadeandalucia.es

Anti-Interleukin-5 in the Treatment of Hypereosino-philic Skin Diseases

J. Ring[1], S.G. Plötz[1], U. Darsow[1], J. Huss-Marp[1], M. Braun-Falco[1], H.-U. Simon[2], and H. Behrendt[1]

[1]Division Environmental Dermatology and Allergology GSF/TUM, Department of Dermatology and Allergy Biederstein, Technical University of Munich, Germany, [2]Department Pharmacology, University of Bern, Switzerland

Summary: The monoclonal antibody against interleukin-5 (mepolizumab) was used in various hypereosinophilic skin diseases. There was a moderate effect in atopic eczema and a marked improvement in patients with hypereosinophilic syndrome (HES) with skin involvement. On the basis of these results, a multicenter controlled trial with mepolizumab in HES has been started.

Keywords: anti-interleukin-5, mepolizumab, eosinophil, atopic eczema, hypereosinophilic syndrome (HES)

Eosinophil granulocytes represent a major component of the inflammatory infiltrate in various allergic and nonallergic skin diseases. IL-5 has been found to be the relevant cytokine in recruitment and activation of eosinophils [1–4]. We decided, therefore, to study the effect of a monoclonal antibody against IL-5 in diseases with eosinophil participation. Earlier a controlled clinical trial with a human anti-IL-5 monoclonal antibody in allergic bronchial asthma had shown no clinical efficacy in spite of marked reduction of peripheral blood eosinophils [5]. Another study had also found marked reduction of eosinophil counts in the bronchial mucosa after three injections of mepolizumab in an interval of 4 weeks [6]. Here we reflect on the effect of mepolizumab in a variety of skin diseases with eosinophil participation.

Dosage and Application of Anti-IL-5

Patients with either hypereosinophilic syndrome (HES), atopic eczema (AE), or angio-lymphoid hyperplasia with eosinophilia (ALHE) were treated with intravenous injections of 750 mg monoclonal antibody against humanized IL-5 mepolizumab, (GlaxoSmithKline, UK). In some patients, injections were repeated after 4 weeks. Mepolizumab was administered intravenously in a dose of 750 mg diluted in 150 mg physiological saline solution. Each treatment was approved by the local ethics committee after informed consent had been obtained from each patient before treatment. Results and experiences obtained will be discussed briefly regarding the various clinical conditions.

Hypereosinophilic Syndrome (HES)

Results of the first three patients with HES have been published recently [7] and are summarized in Table 1. The intravenous infusions of mepolizumab were followed by a sharp decrease in the number of eosinophils in the peripheral blood as well as in the skin. On the first day blood eosinophils had already dropped dramatically while the total number of leukocytes as well as lymphocytes or lymphocyte subpopulations did not change significantly.

Although lymphocyte stimulation tests revealed unaltered production of Th1 cytokines (IL-2, IFN-γ, TNF-α), there was a decrease in Th2 cytokine secretion (IL-4, IL-5, IL-13). Also, in the serum there was a significant drop in eosinophil cationic protein (ECP), IL-5, and eotaxin as well as thymus-and activation-regulated chemokine (TARC). At the same time, there was a dramatic improvement in itch sensation and amelioration of pruriginous skin lesions.

Over the following weeks, slowly, skin lesions deteriorated in the patients, so that another intravenous infusion was performed. By continuing the treatment in 4-week intervals, long lasting improvement was achieved.

Angiolymphoid Hyperplasia with Eosinophilia (ALHE)

One 67-year-old male patient with a massive soft dermal-subcutaneous tumor behind his left ear was diagnosed as ALHE in histology and immunohistochemistry. Since the patient was not giving consent to an operation and the tumor was growing, treatment with anti-IL-5 was

Table 1. Results of treatment with anti-IL-5 (mepolizumab) in 3 patients with HES.

Decrease in blood eosinophilia	3/3
Marked reduction of itch sensation	3/3
Significant improvement of skin lesions	3/3
Disappearance and reduction of eosinophils and eosinophil products in the skin	2/3
Changes in total leukocytes	0/3
T-lymphocytes	0/3
Cytokine secretion	
Th1 cytokines	0/3
Th2 cytokines	2/3
Systemic side reactions	0/3
Local side reactions	0/3

started for compassionate use. There was a mild reduction in tumor thickness and inflammatory infiltrate, however, no real resolution [8]. The patient did not agree to a second infusion. ALHE is a rare condition of unknown etiopathophysiology. It remains to be seen whether anti-IL-5 applied locally could evolve as a therapeutic modality in this condition.

Atopic Eczema (AE)

A total of 40 patients with moderate to severe atopic eczema were treated in a placebo-controlled randomized clinical trial, receiving two injections (i. v.,) of 750 mg mepolizumab in a 1-week interval, then followed for a period of 30 days with clinical evaluation at Day 16 and Day 30 using the physician's global assessment of improvement scale (PGAI) from 0 = *clear*, 1 = *almost clear*, 2 = *marked improvement*, 3 = *modest improvement*, 4 = *no change*, and 5 = *worse than baseline*. Eosinophils in the blood decreased markedly within 2 days after mepolizumab, while they remained unchanged in the placebo group. Also skin symptoms showed significant improvement more often in the mepolizumab than in the placebo group (72.2% vs. 40% at Day 14). However, there was no significant difference when "marked improvement" or "clearing" were calculated. Improvements in SCORAD were not statistically significant [9].

In the atopy patch test reactivity, there was a trend to a reduction in test reaction intensity toward single allergens in the mepolizumab group compared to placebo [9].

Side Effects

Neither systemic nor local side effects were observed in the patients treated. All patients tolerated the mepolizumab infusion without signs of incompatibility.

Conclusions

Clinical trials with the monoclonal anti-IL-5 antibody mepolizumab in several hypereosinophilic skin diseases yielded differential effects in different skin conditions. While mepolizumab effectively controlled eosinophilic dermatitis in patients with HES and almost completely controlled the severe pruritus leading to considerable clearing of skin lesions, the efficacy of mepolizumab in atopic eczema was less dramatic after two infusions. However, there was significant moderate improvement compared to placebo. The experience with mepolizumab in angiolymphoid hyperplasia with eosinophilia is too limited to allow further conclusions.

Contrary to the results achieved in allergic airway diseases, namely bronchial asthma, anti-IL-5 showed marked or significant moderate clinical efficacy in hypereosinophilic skin diseases. Further studies are necessary to establish the potential role of anti-IL-5 in the treatment of atopic eczema and other hypereosinophilic skin diseases.

In the meantime, a large multicenter controlled trial with mepolizumab in HES has been started at an international level.

Acknowledgments
The authors want to acknowledge the participation of the following centers and coworkers in the atopic eczema trial: M. Oldhoff, E. Knol, M. De Brujin-Weller, C. Brujinzeel-Koomen (Department of Dermatology, University of Utrecht, the Netherlands); K. Breuer, T. Werfel, A. Kapp (Department of Dermatology, University of Hannover, Germany); C. Bucenat, A. Taieb (Department of Dermatology, Bordeaux, France); M. Lahfa, F. Suarez, L. Dubertret (Hôpital St. Louis, Paris, France).

References

1. Brujinzeel-Koomen CA, Van Wichen DF, Spry CJ, Venge P, Bruynzeel PL: Active participation of eosinophils in patch test reactions to inhalant allergens in patients with atopic dermatitis. Br J Dermatol 1988; 118:229–238.
2. Gleich GJ, Leiferman KM, Pardanani A, Tefferi A, Butterfield JH: Treatment of hypereosinophilic syndrome with imatinib mesylate. Lancet 2002; 359:1577–1578.
3. Leiferman KM: A role for eosinophils in atopic dermatitis. J Am Acad Dermatol 2001; 45:S21–S24.
4. Simon HU, Plötz SG, Dummer E, Blaser K: Abnormal clones of T-cells producing IL-5 in idiopathic eosinophilia. New England J Med 1999; 341:1112–1120.
5. Leckie MJ, ten Brinke A, Khan J, Diamant Z, O'Connor BJ, Walls CM, Mathur AK, Cowley HC, Chung KF, Djukanovic R, Hansel TT, Holgate ST, Sterk PJ, Barnes PJ: Effects of an IL-5 blocking monoclonal antibody on eosinophils, airway hyper-responsiveness, and the late asthmatic response. Lancet 2000; 356:2144–2148.
6. Flood-Page PT, Menzies-Gow AN, Kay AB, Robinson DS: Eosinophil's role remains uncertain as anti-IL-5 only partially depletes numbers in asthmatic airway. Am J Respir Crit Care Med 2003; 167:199–204.
7. Plötz SG, Simon HU, Darsow U, Simon D, Vassina E, Yousefi S, Hein R, Smith T, Behrendt H, Ring J: Use of an anti-IL-5 antibody in the hypereosinophilic syndrome with eosinophilic dermatitis. New England J Med 2003; 349: 2334–2339.
8. Braun-Falco M, Fischer S, Plötz SG, Ring J: Angiolymphoid hyperplasia with eosinophilia treated with anti-IL-5 antibody (mepolizumab). Br J Dermatol, in press.
9. Oldhoff JM, Darsow U, Werfel T, Katzer K, Wulf A, Laifaoui J, Hijnen DJ, Plotz S, Knol EF, Kapp A, Bruijnzeel-Koomen CA, Ring J, de Bruijn-Weller MS: Anti-IL-5 recombinant humanized monoclonal antibody (mepolizumab) for the treatment of atopic dermatitis. Allergy 2005; 60:693–696.

Johannes Ring

Department of Dermatology & Allergology, TU Munich, Biedersteiner Str. 29, D-80802 Munich, Germany, Tel. +49 89 4140-3170, Fax +49 89 4140-3171, E-mail Johannes.Ring@lrz.tu-muenchen.de

Lack of Availability of Epinephrine for First-Aid Treatment of Anaphylaxis

F.E.R. Simons

Section of Allergy & Clinical Immunology, Department of Pediatrics & Child Health, University of Manitoba, Winnipeg, Canada

Summary: Epinephrine is life-saving asset in anaphylaxis, which is increasing globally. We ascertained the worldwide availability of epinephrine for first-aid, out-of-hospital use by individuals at risk for anaphylaxis (or, for children, by their caregivers) through a validated e-mail survey of all members of the 2003–2005 World Allergy Organization House of Delegates. The response rate to the survey was 100%. Availability of epinephrine autoinjectors for the first-aid treatment of anaphylaxis varied from country to country. Widespread availability in Europe and some countries such as the United States, Canada, and Australia contrasted with limited availability in Asia, South America, and Africa. The worldwide distribution of epinephrine autoinjectors at reasonable cost should be improved.

Keywords: acute allergic reaction, adrenaline, AnaHelp, Anapen, anaphylaxis, children, epinephrine, EpiPen, EpiPen Jr, food allergy, infant, insect sting allergy

The prevalence of anaphylaxis is increasing globally, in developing nations as well as in developed nations. This medical emergency now occurs more commonly in the community than in a health care setting. Epinephrine (adrenaline), the initial drug of choice in anaphylaxis, can be life-saving if injected promptly by outpatients themselves or, for children, by their caregivers [1]. Epinephrine is listed by the World Health Organization as an essential drug [2], but the extent of its availability for outpatient use is unknown. We hypothesized that availability of epinephrine for use in the first-aid treatment of anaphylaxis might differ from country to country worldwide.

Methods

This hypothesis was tested by designing, validating, and revising a survey instrument that was e-mailed to all members of the 2003–2005 World Allergy Organization House of Delegates, selected as a nonrandomized, fixed-size, convenience sample [3]. The survey included questions about availability of epinephrine in all formulations for out-of-hospital treatment (autoinjectors, ampules, other) and about availability of autoinjectors containing epinephrine doses appropriate for adults, children, and infants. Additional questions included: prescription vs. nonprescription status of autoinjectors, cost of autoinjectors, and whether or not patients got full or partial reimbursement from government or private insurance for the cost. Responses were tabulated by country. For countries with more than one representative in the WAO House of Delegates, the last names of the delegates were arranged in alphabetical order and a single response per country was selected by using a table of random numbers. The accuracy of survey responses was confirmed by contacting epinephrine autoinjector manufacturers and distributors.

Results

Completed self-administered surveys were received from all 75 members of the WAO 2003–2005 House of Delegates, representing 39 countries (100% response rate). At the time of the survey, epinephrine autoinjectors containing a 0.25 or 0.3 mg dose appropriate for use in adults were available in only 56.4% (95% confidence intervals [CI] 40.8–72%) of these countries: Denmark, Finland, France, Germany, Hungary, Italy, The Netherlands, Poland, Portugal, Spain, Sweden, Switzerland, the United Kingdom, the United States, Canada, Australia, Israel, South Africa, and Japan (as of autumn 2003). Epinephrine autoinjectors were said to be available in Brazil, India, and Korea, however, autoinjector manufacturers could not identify any formal distribution channel for them in these countries.

At the time of the survey, epinephrine autoinjectors were not available in Bulgaria, Turkey, Russia, Mexico, Argentina, Chile, Ecuador, Uruguay, Paraguay, Venezuela, Egypt, China, Thailand, Vietnam, the Philippines, Malaysia, or Indonesia.

Epinephrine autoinjectors containing a 0.15 mg dose appropriate for use in some children were available in only 43.6% (CI 28–59.2%) of the 39 countries. Epinephrine autoinjectors containing a dose suitable for use in infants were not available in any country.

In 91% (CI 78.9–100%) of countries where epinephrine autoinjectors were available, a doctor's prescription was required for them. Costs ranged from $30.00 (U.S.) to $110.00 (U.S.). Patients paid the total cost of the epinephrine autoinjector, without financial assistance from government or private insurance, in 27.3% (CI 8.7–45.9%) of the countries. Epinephrine was available *only* in the form of 1 mL ampules for supply to outpatients in 43.6% (CI 28–59.2%) of the countries, and in one of these countries, even the ampules were not reliably available.

Discussion

This survey raises concerns about lack of availability of epinephrine autoinjectors worldwide for outpatients of all ages, especially lack of age- and weight-appropriate epinephrine doses in autoinjectors for children and infants. Lack of availability of epinephrine autoinjectors for first-aid treatment of anaphylaxis is probably under-estimated by the survey, as developing countries where anaphylaxis is an emerging, rather than an established, public health issue are still somewhat under-represented in the WAO House of Delegates. Additional concerns raised by some physicians responding to the survey were: lack of affordability of autoinjectors in many countries where they were available; use of alternatives to autoinjectors, such as having outpatients or their caregivers draw up epinephrine from an ampule, or having physicians pre-fill a needle/syringe unit with epinephrine; and rapid degradation of all epinephrine formulations in tropical climates.

International allergy organizations, manufacturers, government agencies, and humanitarian agencies should work together to improve distribution of epinephrine autoinjectors at reasonable cost worldwide.

References

1. Simons FER: First-aid treatment of anaphylaxis to food: focus on epinephrine. J Allergy Clin Immunol 2004; 113:837–844.
2. Essential medicines. WHO model list (revised April 2003), 13th edition, available from http://www.who.int/medicines/organization/par/edl/eml.shtml (accessed September 13, 2004).
3. Creswall JW: Research design: qualitative, quantitative, and mixed methods approaches (2nd ed). Thousand Oaks, CA: Sage, 2003:153–178.

F. Estelle R. Simons

820 Sherbrook Street, Winnipeg, Manitoba, Canada R3A 1R9, Tel. +1 204 787-2537, Fax +1 204 787-5040, E-mail lmcniven@hsc.mb.ca

A Candidate Vaccine for Specific Immunotherapy in Latex Allergy

Hypoallergenic Variants of Hev b 6.01.

A.C. Drew[1,2,3], N.P. Eusebius[1,2,3], L. Kenins[1,2,3], H.D. de Silva[1,2,3], C. Suphioglu[1,2,3], J.M. Rolland[1,3], and R.E. O'Hehir[1,2,3]

[1]Cooperative Research Centre for Asthma, Sydney, Australia, [2]Department of Allergy, Immunology and Respiratory Medicine, The Alfred Hospital, Melbourne, Australia, [3]Department of Immunology, Monash University Medical School, Melbourne, Australia

Summary: *Background:* Natural rubber latex allergy is a major cause of occupational asthma among latex glove users. Current unfractionated latex extracts are unsuitable for specific immunotherapy because of their high anaphylactic potential. Hypoallergenic mutant recombinant latex allergens with abrogated IgE binding or T-cell epitope-based peptide analogues potentially offer safer alternatives for specific immunotherapy. Hev b 6.01 is one of the two major allergens in latex gloves, with sensitization of 70% of latex glove allergic subjects. The predominant IgE reactivity of Hev b 6.01 is located in the *N*-terminal Hev b 6.02 domain where four disulphide bonds stabilize tertiary conformation. *Methods*: A panel of mutants of recombinant Hev b 6.01 and corresponding synthetic Hev b 6.02 peptides were generated, with successive disruption of the first four disulphide bonds by cysteine to alanine substitutions. The basophil activation test, detecting CD63 surface expression by flow cytometry as a functional marker of basophil activation, was used to assess biological activity. *Results*: The mutants and peptide variants showed markedly decreased basophil activation with the Hev b 6.02 peptide with four cysteine substitutions being unable to activate basophils. Critically, the mutants and peptide variants maintained their T-cell reactivity as shown by induction of T-cell proliferation of oligoclonal CD4[+] latex-specific T-cells from latex-allergic donors. *Conclusions*: The Hev b 6.02 peptide with four cysteine to alanine substitutions, together with the dominant T-cell epitope-based peptides of Hev b 5 that we reported previously, may offer safe and effective specific immunotherapy for latex allergy treatment and/or prevention.

Keywords: latex allergy, molecular biology, basophils, Hev b 6.01

Latex glove allergy is a major cause of occupational asthma among health care workers [1]. Allergen avoidance and symptomatic treatment for adverse reactions form the mainstay of management for latex allergy with no currently available licensed extract for specific immunotherapy [2]. Hev b 6.01 is a 20 kDa protein (prohevein) that is cleaved naturally into a short 43 amino acid protein Hev b 6.02 (hevein) and a larger Hev b 6.03 *C*-terminal fragment. The dominant B-cell epitopes of Hev b 6.01 are contained in the Hev b 6.02 domain with between 75 and 84% of latex-allergic subjects having IgE to the Hev b 6.02 domain and only 30% having IgE to the *C*-terminal fragment [2]. For this reason we targeted the cysteine residues of Hev b 6.02 for site-directed mutagenesis in order to disrupt conformation through progressive interruption of the first four disulphide bridges. Peptide variants of Hev b 6.02 corresponding to two of the mutants were also evaluated. The rHev b 6.01 mutants and Hev b 6.02 peptide variants were demonstrated to be hypoallergenic, with poor activation of basophils, but all retained the desired ability to stimulate T-cells from latex-allergic donors.

Material and Methods

Latex Allergens

Wild-type recombinant Hev b 6.01 (WT rHev b 6.01) [3] was modified by site-directed mutagenesis (QuickChange™XL, Stratagene) with cysteine residues at amino acid residues 3, 12, 17, and 41 sequentially replaced with alanine residues (rHev b 6.01 mutants 1–4 respectively). Hev b 6.02 peptide (43 amino acids) and variants of the peptide with cysteine to alanine substitutions (variant 1, Cys 3 Ala; variant 2, Cys 3, 12, 17, 41 Ala) were synthesized (Mimotopes).

Basophil Activation Test

A whole blood basophil activation test detecting CD63 surface expression by flow cytometry as a functional marker of basophil activation was used to assess biological activity. This assay was modified from Paris-Kohler et al.

[4]. Recombinant antigens were used to stimulate basophils at 10 µg/ml and peptides at 2 µg/ml.

Generation of Latex-Specific T-Cell Lines and T-Cell Proliferation Assays

Hev b 6.01-specific T-cell lines were generated from PBMC and proliferation assays performed using our established methods [3,5]. rHev b 6.01 proteins were sulphonated to improve their solubility [3]. T-cell cultures were stimulated with sulphonated WT rHev b 6.01, sulphonated rHev b 6.01 mutants, and Hev b 6.02 peptides (10 and 30 µg/ml) and proliferation measured by thymidine incorporation. A stimulation index of ≥ 2.5 was defined as positive (stimulation index: counts per minute of antigen-stimulated cultures divided by counts per minute of unstimulated cultures).

Results

Substitution of Cysteine Residues of Hev b 6.01 Reduces Basophil Activation

The basophils of six latex-allergic subjects were stimulated with the rHev b 6.01 proteins and Hev b 6.02 peptides (Table 1). The median

Table 1. Immunological characteristics of rHev b 6.01 mutant proteins and Hev b 6.02 peptide variants.

Antigen		No. of cysteines substituted	[1]Basophil activation	[2]T-cell proliferation
rHev b 6.01 protein	WT	0	++++	+
	Mutant 1	1	++	+
	Mutant 2	2	+	NT
	Mutant 3	3	–	NT
	Mutant 4	4	+	+
Hev b 6.02 peptide	WT	0	+++++	+
	Variant 1	1	+	+
	Variant 2	4	–	+

[1]Median percent activation of basophils from six subjects. –, < 5%; +, 6–19%; ++, 20–39%; +++, 40–59%; ++++, 60–79%; +++++, 80–100%.
[2]Median stimulation index for the proliferative response of Hev b 6.01-specific T-cell lines from five subjects in response to each antigen. +, stimulation index 2.5–10; NT = not tested.

activation of basophils by WT rHev b 6.01 was 73%. Basophil activation was reduced in response to stimulation with mutants of rHev b 6.01 with median activation of 27%, 9%, 2%, and 11% for mutants 1 to 4, respectively.

WT Hev b 6.02 peptide activated basophils from all six subjects with a median value of 81%. Decreased activation was observed after stimulation with Hev b 6.02 peptide variant 1, with a median activation of 18%. Basophil activation was negligible for all six subjects after stimulation with the Hev b 6.02 peptide variant 2, with a median activation of 1%.

T-Cell Proliferation After Stimulation with rHev b 6.01 Mutants and Hev b 6.02 Peptide Variants

Hev b 6.01-specific T-cell lines from five latex-allergic, Hev b 6.01-sensitized subjects were stimulated with WT rHev b 6.01, rHev b 6.01 mutants 1 and 4, WT Hev b 6.02 peptide, and Hev b 6.02 peptide variant 1 and peptide variant 2. Significant proliferation (stimulation index ≥ 2.5) was produced in response to all the rHev b 6.01 mutants and Hev b 6.02 peptide variants (Table 1).

Discussion

The latex allergen Hev b 6.01 is an important cause of latex sensitization in latex-glove users, particularly healthcare workers and laboratory scientists. Current unmodified natural latex extracts are unsuitable for specific immunotherapy because of the high anaphylactic potential.

Highly conformationally dependent molecules such as Hev b 6.01, stabilized by the presence of multiple disulphide bonds, suggest site-directed mutagenesis of cysteine residues to prevent disulphide bridging as a rational strategy for disruption of conformational B-cell epitopes. This approach was utilized to produce hypoallergenic mutants of the major latex allergen Hev b 6.01.

Latex allergy in most individuals results from sensitization to a number of latex allergens [6]. As mono-sensitization to Hev b 6.01 is uncommon [7], any potential immunotherapy preparation would require the use of more than one hypoallergenic recombinant latex allergen or derived synthetic peptide. Hev b 5 and Hev b 6.01, particularly the Hev b 6.02 domain, are the two major allergens for individuals sensitized by latex glove use and these antigens should be targeted in a latex immunotherapy "vaccine" for this patient group [6]. A T-cell stimulatory, hypoallergenic desensitizing "vaccine" targeting both these allergens would be a welcome addition to pharmacotherapy for latex allergy, either as a treatment regimen for patients with confirmed allergy or as a possible preventive option. The combination of the dominant Hev b 5 T-cell epitope peptides reported by us previously [5] and the Hev b 6.02 peptide variant with four cysteine to alanine substitutions described here, would be a strong candidate for inclusion in a therapeutic vaccine.

Acknowledgment

This work was funded by the Cooperative Research Centre for Asthma, Sydney, Australia.

References

1. Kopferschmitt-Kubler MC, Ameille J, Popin E, Calastreng-Crinquand A, Vervloet D, Bayeux-Dunglas MC, Pauli G: Occupational asthma in France: a 1-yr report of the observatoire National de Asthmes Professionnels project. Eur Respir J 2002; 19:84–89.
2. Cullinan P, Brown R, Field A, Hourihane J, Jones M, Kekwick R, Rycroft R, Stenz R, Williams S, Woodhouse C: Latex allergy. A position paper of the British Society of Allergy and Clinical Immunology. Clin Exp Allergy 2003; 33:1484–1499.
3. de Silva HD, Gardner LM, Drew AC, Beezhold DH, Rolland JM, and O'Hehir RE: The hevein domain of the major latex-glove allergen Hev b 6.01 contains dominant T-cell reactive sites. Clin Exp Allergy 2004; 34:611–618.
4. Paris-Kohler A, Demoly P, Persi L, Lebel B, Bousquet J, Arnoux B: *In vitro* diagnosis of cypress pollen allergy by using cytofluorimetric

analysis of basophils (Basotest). J Allergy Clin Immunol 2000; 105:339–345.

5. de Silva HD, Sutherland MF, Suphioglu C, Mc-Lellan SC, Slater JE, Rolland JM, O'Hehir RE: Human T-cell epitopes of the latex allergen Hev b 5 in health care workers. J Allergy Clin Immunol 2000; 105:1017–1024.

6. Sutherland MF, Suphioglu C, Rolland JM, O'Hehir RE: Latex allergy: toward immunotherapy for health care workers. Clin Exp Allergy 2002; 32:667–673.

7. Yip L, Hickey V, Wagner B, Liss G, Slater J, Breiteneder H, Sussman G, Beezhold D: Skin prick test reactivity to recombinant latex allergens. Int Arch Allergy Immunol 2000; 121:292–299.

Robyn E O'Hehir

Director, Department of Allergy, Immunology and Respiratory Medicine, The Alfred Hospital, Commercial Road, Melbourne Vic 3004, Australia, Tel. +61 3 9276 2251, Fax +61 3 9276 2245, E-mail r.ohehir@alfred.org.au

Randomized Controlled Trial of Specific Immunotherapy on Allergic Inflammation

in Atopic Dermatitis Patients with Sensitization to House Dust Mites

T. Werfel[1], K. Breuer[1], F. Ruëff[2], B. Przybilla[2], M. Worm[3], M. Grewe[4], T. Ruzicka[4], R. Brehler[5], H. Wolf[6], J. Schnitker[7], and A. Kapp[1]

[1]*Dermatology and Allergology, Medizinische Hochschule Hannover,* [2]*Dermatology and Allergology, Ludwig-Maximilians-Universität, München,* [3]*Dermatology and Allergology, Humboldt Universität, Berlin,* [4]*Dermatology, Heinrich-Heine-Universität, Düsseldorf,* [5]*Department of Dermatology, Universitätsklinikum Münster,* [6]*Clinical Research, ALK-SCHERAX Arzneimittel GmbH, Hamburg,* [7]*Applied Stastics, Bielefeld, all Germany*

Summary: *Background:* Sensitization to house dust mite allergens (HDM), which is detectable with specific IgE-tests, is very common in patients suffering from atopic dermatitis (AD). Specific immunotherapy is an effective therapy in respiratory IgE-mediated allergic diseases, but has not yet been investigated in double-blind placebo-controlled trials in AD. *Methods:* In a multi-center, double-blind, randomized trial we treated patients who had AD, IgE-mediated sensitization against HDM, and a SCORAD-score greater than 40 points with subcutaneous specific immunotherapy. Patients were randomized into three dose groups with maintenance doses of 20 ("active placebo"), 2000, and 20000 SQ-U ("active treatment") *Dermatophagoides pteronyssinus/farinae* extracts for a 1-year treatment. *Results:* Seventy-nine patients with at least one SCORAD assessment (equivalent to treatment for 2 months up to 1 year) could be evaluated as the *full analysis set* (intention-to-treat). The SCORAD-score declined in all three study groups. The differences in the SCORAD between baseline and the last 3 months of treatment were significantly greater in patients actively treated (2000 and 20000 SQ-U) compared to patients with active placebo (20 SQ-U). The application of topical corticosteroids in the two active treatment groups was significantly reduced compared to active placebo. The final assessment of the physician confirmed better skin condition for patients with active treatment compared with active placebo at the end of the therapy. *Conclusion:* Allergen-specific immunotherapy with HDM is effective in patients with AD who are sensitized to HDM, and may be valuable in the treatment of this chronic skin disease.

Keywords: atopic dermatitis, eczema, house dust mite, specific immunotherapy, hyposensitization, SCORAD

AD is one of the most common skin diseases, which is characterized by a chronic course and intensive itching. Sensitizations to HDM allergens, which are detectable with specific IgE tests, are very common in adolescent and adult patients [1, 2].

A causal therapy for AD is not yet available and the complexity of the disease leads to a polypragmatic therapeutical management [2]. Specific immunotherapy is able to inhibit the progress of IgE-mediated allergic diseases [3, 4]. However, data concerning effects of specific immunotherapy on the course of AD are rare. Published results on this topic are only available within open studies [5–10] or are not based on "classical" protocols of subcutaneous immunotherapy [11, 12].

We investigated the clinical efficacy of a subcutaneously applied immunotherapy in patients with AD using a double-blind placebo-controlled protocol. The study was a multicenter, double-blind trial with patients randomly assigned to treatment with specific immunotherapy with ALK-depot SQ mites and maximum concentrations of 20 SQ-U (active placebo), 2000 SQ-U, and 20000 SQ-U for one year. The double-blind design of the study was realized by a "blind observer" who evaluated the SCORAD.

Prior to the treatment we assessed the patients for inclusion/exclusion criteria. IgE-mediated sensitization against HDMs was verified by CAP RAST FEIA (Pharmacia Freiburg, Germany) (inclusion criterion: class $\geq$ 3). The SCORAD score had to be > 40 points, and age had to be between 18 and 55 years. A chronic course of AD was mandatory. The study was approved by the Ethical Committee of the Hannover Medical University and then subsequently by the Local Ethical Committees of the other study centers.

Patients were randomized into the following three dose groups for treatment with subcutaneous specific immunotherapy with ALK-depot SQ *Dermatophagoides pteronyssinus/farinae* (ALK-SCHERAX, Hamburg, Germany): Group 1 ("active placebo"): constant dose of 20 SQ-U, Group 2: maintenance dose of 2000 SQ-U, and Group 3: maintenance dose 20000 SQ-U. Therapy was started in all groups with 20 SQ-U. All injections were given at weekly intervals. In Groups 2 and 3 the dose was increased in the following way: Injection 2: 40 SQ-U, Injection 3: 80 SQ-U, Injections 4–7: 200 SQ-U, Injection 8: 400 SQ-U, Injection 9: 800 SQ-U, Injections 10–13: 2000 SQ-U. In Group 3 the dose was

further increased from Injections 14 to 17 in 2000 SQ-U steps and from Injection 18 a constant dose of 20000 SQ-U was applied. Identical volumes were applied in all injections by adding the solution of ALK-depot SQ without allergens. Treatment of AD was individually adapted to the clinical severity. Topical corticosteroids of European classes 1 to 3 and nonsedating antihistamines with a short half life (cetiricine, loratadine) were allowed. Moreover, basic treatment of the skin with ointments was allowed.

The full analysis set was defined as the group of patients with at least one control of the SCORAD. The valid case set was defined as the group of patients who finished the study according to protocol after 12 months. The full analysis set consisted of 79 patients. Thirty-one cases dropped out due to reasons other than unsatisfactory efficacy, and six more patients came from four centers, which each contributed only a small number of patients with incompletely frequented dose groups (no active placebo in all four centers). Therefore, the valid case set consisted of 42 patients

There was a decline of the SCORAD score points in all study groups. The differences in the SCORAD between the baseline value and the values in the last 3 months of treatment were, however, significantly greater in Groups 2 ($p = 0.0475$, one-sided t-test) and 3 ($p = 0.0147$, one-sided t-test) compared to Group 1. The response rate as defined above was 66.0% in the pooled Groups 2 and 3 and 46.2% in Group 1 ($p = 0.0454$, one sided χ^2 test).

In the valid case set the differences between the dosage groups were even higher: the decrease from baseline to endpoint of the SCORAD amounted to 8.4 ± 3.6 in Group 1, 15.3 ± 4.3 in Group 2, and 25.9 ± 4.1 in Group 3 ($p = 0.0015$, one-sided Jonckheere-Terpstra test). The response rates were 41.2% in Group 1, 66.7% in Group 2, and 84.6% in Group 3 ($p = 0.0071$, one-sided Cochran-Armitage test).

The decline of SCORAD in the verum groups was significantly higher compared to placebo after only 2 months of treatment ($p < 0.05$). The differences between placebo and verum were maximal after 6 months of treatment ($p < 0.005$). Further differentiation of these data revealed a significantly higher effect in the verum group that had been treated with 20000 SQ-U allergen extract compared to the verum group that had been treated with 2000 SQ-U allergen extract.

There was a significant difference in the application of topical corticosteroids with greater reductions in Groups 2 and 3, but greater increase in Group 1. Similar differences in favor of Groups 2 and 3 were seen in the use of systemic antihistamines, but these were statistically less pronounced.

Markedly more patients assessed their skin to be improved or completely healed in Groups 2 and 3 (61.5% and 70.4%, respectively) compared to Group 1 (38.5%; $p = 0.0097$, Cochran-Armitage test). The final assessment of the "blinded" physician confirmed a better skin condition at the end of therapy for patients from Groups 2 and 3 (53.8% and 70.4%) compared to those from Group 1 (34.6%; $p = 0.0046$, Cochran-Armitage test).

In this study we show for the first time in a double-blind placebo-controlled study that specific immunotherapy is effective in AD. The greater decrease of SCORAD score was reflected by a higher percentage of responders in both groups treated with "active" preparations compared to the "active placebo" group. Indirect evidence of effectiveness of specific immunotherapy in AD comes from differences in the usage of topical corticosteroids and systemic antihistamines in the different groups: patients belonging to the "active placebo" group used significantly more topical corticosteroids and antihistamines compared to patients who were treated with higher concentrations of HDM antigens.

Thus, allergen-specific immunotherapy is effective in patients with AD who are sensitized to HDM allergens and may be valuable in the treatment of this chronic skin disease.

Acknowledgments

ALK-SCHERAX, Hamburg, Germany, provided the immunotherapy preparations.

References

1. Werfel T, Kapp A: Environmental and other major provocation factors in atopic dermatitis. Allergy 1998; 53:731–739.
2. Leung DY, Bieber T: Atopic dermatitis. Lancet 2003; 361:151–160.
3. Malling HJ: Immunotherapy for rhinitis. Curr Allergy Asthma Rep 2003; 3:204–209.
4. Nelson HS: Advances in upper airway diseases and allergen immunotherapy. J Allergy Clin Immunol 2003; 111:793–798.
5. Di Prisco de Fuenmayor MC, Champion RH: Specific hyposensitization in atopic dermatitis. Br J Dermatol 1979; 101:697–700.
6. Ring J: Successful hyposensitization treatment in atopic eczema: results of a trial in monozygotic twins. Br J Dermatol 1982; 107:597–602.
7. Zachariae H, Cramers M, Herlin T, Jensen J, Kragballe K, Ternowitz T, Thestrup-Pedersen K: Nonspecific immunotherapy and specific hyposensitization in severe atopic dermatitis. Acta Derm Venereol Suppl (Stockh) 1985; 114:48–54.
8. Seidenari S, Mosca M, Taglietti M, Manco S, Nume G: Specific hyposensitization in atopic dermatitis. Dermatologica 1986; 172:229.
9. Pacor ML, Biasi D, Malekina T: The efficacy of long-term specific immunotherapy for *Dermatophagoides pteronyssinus* in patients with atopic dermatitis. Recenti Prog Med 1994; 85:273–277.
10. Trofimowicz A, Rzepecka E, Hofman J: Clinical effects of specific immunotherapy in children with atopic dermatitis. Rocz Akad Med Bialymst 1995; 40:414–422.
11. Galli E, Chini L, Nardi S, Benincori N, Panei P, Fraioli G, et al.: Use of a specific oral hyposensitization therapy to *Dermatophagoides pteronyssinus* in children with atopic dermatitis. Allergol Immunopathol 1994; 22:18–22.
12. Leroy BP, Boden G, Lachapelle JM, Jacquemin MG, Saint-Remy JM: A novel therapy for atopic dermatitis with allergen-antibody complexes: a double-blind, placebo-controlled study. J Am Acad Dermatol 1993; 28:232–239.

Thomas Werfel

Department of Dermatology and Allergology, Medizinische Hochschule Hannover, Ricklinger Str. 5, D-30449 Hannover, Germany, Tel. +49 511 924-6276, Fax +49 511 924-6440, E-mail Werfel.Thomas@MH-Hannover.de

Allergy Prophylaxis by DNA Vaccination

Inhibits Specific IgE Response and Lung Pathologic Parameters in a Mouse Model

Y. Darcan[1], U. Seitzer[2], J. Galle[3], W.-M. Becker[1], J. Ahmed[2], and A. Petersen[1]

[1]*Divisions of Biochemical and Molecular Allergology,* [2]*Veterinary Infectiology and Immunology,*
[3]*Clinical and Experimental Pathology, all Research Center Borstel, Germany*

Summary: More than 20% of the Western population suffer from symptoms of type I allergy. Often inhalant allergens induce hypersensitivity, which can lead to the development of asthma. Currently hyposensitization therapy is the only curative treatment, but injection of the allergen bears the risk of anaphylactic side effects and shock. Therefore, improved therapeutic strategies are imperative. DNA vaccination is described to induce a strong Th1-mediated immune response against encoded genes and is, thus, discussed as protection against atopic disorders [1]. We wanted to determine the efficacy of prophylactic DNA vaccination using the major pollen allergen Phl p 5b of timothy grass (*Phleum pratense*) to which more than 90% of grass pollen hypersensitive patients are allergic.

BALB/c mice were preimmunized three times by intradermal injections with 50 or 100 µg of the DNA construct pCI/phl p 5b, or with the pCI vector, before five intraperitoneal injections with 5 µg of Phl p 5b protein. All immunizations were performed without adjuvant to mimic the natural situation. One control group was treated with allergen protein alone. The immune response was monitored by determination of the allergen-specific immunoglobulins. The results obtained showed that the production of allergen-specific IgE and IgG1 is substantially inhibited, while allergen-specific IgG2a is increased. Interestingly, the vector alone at higher doses was also able to partially inhibit the IgE and IgG1 antibody response, suggesting the involvement of innate immunity.

Parallel to this, the DNA vaccination prevented the appearance of pathological reactions in the lung of immunized mice. In contrary, mice that only received the protein showed a high degree of goblet cell hyperplasia, peribronchial inflammation, eosinophilia, and mucus production resembling the histopathology of chronic bronchitis. Mice that were preimmunized with the pCI vector showed a considerable decrease of these investigated parameters, related to the concentration of the vector applied. Taken together these first results demonstrate that pretreatment with pCI/phl p 5b inhibits the production of specific IgE and IgG1 after sensitization with the allergen and completely protected those mice from developing a lung-associated pathology resembling chronic bronchitis after nasal challenge. Vaccination with only the pCI vector resulted in partial protection. This indicates that immunostimulatory DNA sequences, e.g., CpG motifs, in the vector are involved in evoking a predominant Th1-mediated immune response and, thus, in inhibiting a subsequent sensitization with an allergen by weakening a Th2-mediated immune response [2].

Keywords: DNA vaccination, grass pollen allergen, mouse model, Phl p 5b

References

1. Hsu CH, Chua KY, Tao MH, Lai Yl, Wu HD, Huang SK, Hsieh KH: Immunoprophylaxis of allergen-induced IgE synthesis and airway hyperresponsiveness *in vivo* by genetic immunization. Nat Med 1996; 2:540–544.
2. Raz E, Tighe H, Sato Y, Corr M, Dudler JA, Roman M, Swain SL, Spiegelberg HL, Carson DA: Preferential induction of a Th1 immune response and inhibition of specific IgE antibody formation by plasmid DNA immunization. Proc Natl Acad Sci USA 1996; 93:5141–5145.

Arnd Petersen

Biochemical and Molecular Allergology, Research Center Borstel, Parkallee 22, D-23845 Borstel, Germany, Tel. +49 4537 188 497, Fax +49 4537 188 686, E-mail apetersen@fz-borstel.de

Quality of Life and Compliance in Patients Allergic to Grass and Rye Pollen

During a 3-year Treatment with Specific Immunotherapy (The LQC Study)

K.-C. Bergmann[1], H. Wolf[2], J. Schnitker[3], F. Petermann[4], and the LQC Study Group

[1]Allergie-Centrum Charité, Berlin, [2]Klinische Forschung, ALK-SCHERAX Arzneimittel GmbH, Hamburg, [3]Institut für Angewandte Statistik GmbH, Bielefeld, [4]Zentrum für Rehabilitationsforschung der Universität Bremen, all Germany

Summary: *Background:* Quality of life (QoL) and compliance are important parameters for the success of a 3-year specific immunotherapy (SIT). We investigated the disease-specific and general QoL and compliance of patients during routine treatment with SIT. *Methods:* The open, uncontrolled study included 106 allergists and 1257 patients with rhinoconjunctivitis to grass pollen treated with SIT (ALK-depot SQ) for 3 years. Patients retrospectively completed the Rhinitis Quality of Life Questionnaire (RQLQ) and a general questionnaire ("Alltagsleben") for the grass pollen seasons before and during a 3-year SIT. Compliance was assessed according to treatment protocols and discontinuations of treatment. *Results:* The average score over the six RQLQ-domains (scale 0 to 6) improved from 2.91 before SIT to 1.05 after 3 years ($p < 0.0001$). For patients impaired more severely (30.8% with score ≥ 4) the general QoL (scale 1 to 5) improved from 3.60 ± 0.34 before SIT to 4.43 ± 0.45 after 3 years. SIT was discontinued by 3.3% of the patients because of compliance problems and by 18.7% for other reasons; 8.2% did not return. *Conclusion:* A 3-year SIT improves the disease-specific and general QoL in routinely treated patients with rhinoconjunctivitis. Compliance with SIT applied by specialized allergists is very high.

Keywords: specific immunotherapy, quality of life, compliance, grass pollen, rye pollen

SIT or allergy vaccination (SAV) as it is described in the WHO position paper [1] has been shown to be efficacious and safe in several controlled clinical trials with documented improvement in both subjective and objective clinical parameters. In order to assess the patient's perspective on the benefit from SIT validated instruments are available to measure the influence of a therapy on the daily life of patients by exploring both the disease-specific and the general QoL [2].

For SIT, normally applied over at least 3 years, patient compliance is crucial for success of the treatment. In a placebo-controlled double-blind study with Alutard SQ allergens it was shown that patients treated with SIT for 3 years had a significantly higher clinically relevant improvement in their QoL compared with placebo [3]. The aim of the current study was to explore the effect of SIT on disease-specific and general QoL and compliance in a large group of patients treated by allergists.

The open, uncontrolled study was conducted between July 1997 and February 2001. The participating physicians (all allergists) were asked to assess rhinoconjunctivitis symptoms, symptomatic treatment and compliance before the initiation of SIT (1997) and during the first year (1998), second year (1999), and third year of SIT (2000). Patients were asked to assess their disease-specific QoL by means of the RQLQ [4] after the grass pollen season prior to SIT and after each season during the 3-year period of therapy and their general QoL by means of the "Alltagsleben"-questionnaire [5] (42 questions on a 1 to 5 scale). During SIT the actual date of injections, the applied dose, and any allergic reactions to the injections were recorded.

Patients with known contraindications for SIT according to the EAACI position paper [6] were excluded. All reasons for discontinuation of treatment during the 3-year protocol were documented and analyzed with regard to the patient compliance.

SIT was performed with the standardized and characterized extracts ALK-depot SQ Gräser-mischung und Roggen (ALK-SCHERAX, Hamburg, Germany) according to the manufacturer's recommendations.

A total of 106 practicing allergists participated in the first year of the study, 102 in the second, and 95 in the third year. From the original 1257 patients, the RQLQ could be evaluated for 1093 patients (87%). Before SIT, patients felt the most impairments in QoL in the domains Practical problems, Nasal symptoms, and Activities (Figure 1). The average score over all domains improved from 2.91 in 1997 before SIT to 1.05 in 2000 after 3 years of SIT ($p < 0.0001$). The 1.86 change in score is significantly greater than the minimal important difference (MID) of 0.5 defined by the authors of the RQLQ as being clinically relevant [7, 8]. Individually, 88.1% of the patients had an average change in score of ≥ 0.5 over all domains. The largest improvements were observed in the domains Nasal symptoms (2.21), Eye symptoms (1.83), Activities (2.33), and Practical problems (2.14).

The general QoL questionnaire could be evaluated for 1073 (85.4%) of the original 1257 patients. In these patients the mean total score of all six domains before SIT was 4.25

± 0.54 and improved after 3 years of SIT to 4.58 ± 0.38. The total score of a subgroup of 331 patients (30.8%) who had a more severe impairment of the general QoL before SIT (score ≤ 4) improved from 3.60 ± 0.34 before SIT to 4.43 ± 0.45 after 3 years of SIT.

SIT was discontinued solely because of compliance problems in 41 (3.3%) patients. Additionally, 103 patients (8.2%) did not return for further visits. These two reasons were considered related or possibly related to lack of compliance, so that 144 patients (11.5%) discontinued SIT possibly because of non-compliance; 18.7% discontinued SIT for other reasons.

After 3 years the total symptom score was reduced by 68%, the nasal score by 65%, and the eye and bronchial score by 71%.

Use of symptomatic medication decreased from 82.9% before SIT to 43.7% in the last year of SIT (DSCG: 36.4% before SIT vs. 15.3% after 3 years SIT, oral antihistamines: 65.8% vs. 26.8%, topical corticosteroids: 23.5% vs. 7%).

The pollen count during the study changed by –12.8%, + 23.7% and + 7.2% for the three seasons with SIT vs. the season before SIT(1612 pollen/m³). No influence on the mean change of symptoms and QoL assessments by the mean change in pollen count of the seasons with SIT vs. the season before SIT was observed by Spearman-rank correlations.

The present study showed that SIT significantly improves the disease-specific QoL in patients with allergic rhinoconjunctivitis and the general QoL in patients with a more severe impairment treated routinely in the allergist's practice.

The results for the RQLQ are in good agreement with the improvement in clinical symptoms documented by the physician and these data are also consistent with results from a placebo-controlled clinical trial with SIT in patients allergic to grass pollen [9].

Natural variations of the pollen exposure of the patients in the study sites during the treatment period were negligible and had no meaningful influence on the symptoms and QoL data. Patient compliance with SIT performed by allergy specialists over a 3-year period is very high.

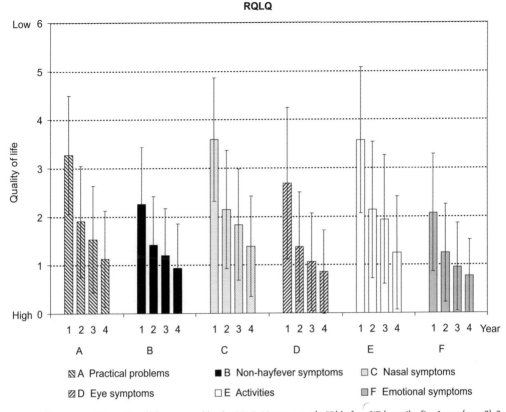

Figure 1. Disease-specific quality of life measured by the RQLQ; Mean scores (± SD) before SIT (year 1), after 1 year (year 2), 2 years (year 3) and 3 years of SIT (year 4).

References

1. Bousquet J, Lockey RF, Malling HJ: WHO position paper Allergen immunotherapy: therapeutic vaccines for allergic diseases. Allergy 1998; 53:1–42.
2. Van Wijk G: Allergy: a global problem. Quality of life. Allergy 2002; 57:1097–1110.
3. Walker SM, Pajno GB, Torres Lima M, Wilson DR, Durham SR: Grass pollen immunotherapy for seasonal rhinitis and asthma: A randomized, controlled trial. J Allergy Clin Immunol 2001; 107:87–93.
4. Juniper EF, Guyatt GH, Dolovich J: Assessment of quality of life in adolescents with allergic rhinoconjunctivitis: development and testing of a questionnaire for clinical trials. J Allergy Clin Immunol 1994; 93:413–423.
5. Bullinger M, Kirchberger I, Steinbüchel N: Der Fragebogen Alltagsleben – ein Verfahren zur Erfassung der gesundheitsbezogenen Lebensqualität. Zeitschrift für Medizinische Psychologie 1993; 2:121–131.
6. Malling HJ, Weeke B: Position paper: Immunotherapy, EAACI Immunotherapy subcommittee. Allergy 1993; 48:7–35.
7. Juniper EF: Quality of life questionnaires: does statistically significant = clinically important? J Allergy Clin Immunol 1998; 102:16–17.
8. Juniper EF, Guyatt GH, Griffith LE, Ferrie PJ: Interpretation of rhinoconjunctivitis quality of life questionnaire data. J Allergy Clin Immunol 1996; 98:843–845.
9. Varney VA, Gaga M, Frew AJ, Aber VR, Kay AB, Durham SR: Usefulness of immunotherapy in patients with severe summer hay fever uncontrolled by antiallergic drugs. Br Med J 1991; 302:265–269.

Karl-Christian Bergmann

Allergie-Centrum Charité, Klinik für Dermatologie und Allergologie, Luisenstr. 2–5, D-10117 Berlin, Germany, E-mail kcbbergmann@hotmail.com

Targeting M-Cells for Induction of a Th1-Immune Response in Allergic Mice

F. Roth-Walter[1], I. Schöll[1], E. Untersmayr[1], G. Boltz-Nitulescu[1], O. Scheiner[1], F. Gabor[2], and E. Jensen-Jarolim[1]

[1]*Center of Physiology and Pathophysiology, Medical University of Vienna, Austria*
[2]*Department of Pharmaceutical Technology and Biopharmaceutics, University of Vienna, Austria*

Summary: *Background:* We aimed here to generate a formulation that serves as a vehicle for orally delivered allergens and allows targeting to M-cells, which are the most effective sites for antigen uptake and transfer into Peyer's patches of the intestine. Several gastrointestinal pathogens, like salmonella, target M-cells and subsequently induce strong Th1-type responses. We investigated whether in a murine model allergen uptake via enterocytes vs. M-cells may be decisive for modulation of an ongoing Th2-response. *Methods:* Microspheres of the PLGA type were loaded with birch pollen proteins, and specifically targeted to enterocytes or to M-cells. BALB/c mice express different carbohydrates on these two cell-types. To target the α-L-fucose on M-cells we functionalized allergen-loaded microspheres with *Aleuria aurantia* lectin (AAL) from an edible mushroom, and with wheat germ agglutinin (WGA) to target the sialylic residues on murine enterocytes. BALB/c mice were first sensitized with BP to induce an allergic phenotype. Subsequently, they were fed with BP-loaded particles functionalized with AAL, WGA, or nonfunctionalized. *Results:* Mice that were fed with AAL-particles developed BP-specific IgG2a-, but no IgG1- or IgE-antibodies. BP-stimulated splenocytes proliferated in a ^{3}H-Thymidin assay specifically. Importantly, AAL-mice produced significantly more INF-γ and IL-10 than the WGA- and control groups. *Conclusion:* Our data indicate that in oral allergen immunotherapy, M-cell targeting is essential to achieve an allergen-specific immune modulation towards the Th1 type.

Keywords: M-cells, *Aleuria Aurantia* lectin, oral immunotherapy, gastrointestinal tract, mucosal targeting, Peyer's patches, birch pollen, microparticle, biodegradable, *Salmonella typhimurium*

Many pathogens like *Salmonella typhimurium*, *Vibrio cholerae*, and reoviruses infect the host via the intestinal route by adhering to M-cells. These cells have a sampling function in the intestine and directly overlie Peyer's patches of the organized mucosal-associated lymphoid tissues (O-MALT). M-cells are a subset within the specialized epithelium covering the organized lymphoid tissues, which is termed follicle-associated epithelium (FAE), and they perform predominantly antigen sampling [1, 2].

In mice, M-cells, but not enterocytes, express α-L-fucose-residues on their apical surface. Our working hypothesis was that, by tar-geting the allergens to M-cells, it should be possible to exploit the oral route for allergen immunotherapy. Here, we chose AAL for M-cell targeting. This lectin derives from the edible orange cup mushroom, it has α-L-fucose specificity [3], and in addition a crystal structure [4, 5] which is very similar to the neuramidase of *Salmonella typhimurium* [3, 6].

To avoid the usage of a potentially harmful carrier for oral allergen immunotherapy, birch pollen allergens were loaded into totally biodegradable poly(D,L-lactic-co-glycolic acid) (PLGA)-microparticles [7]. The microparticles were then functionalized with either AAL

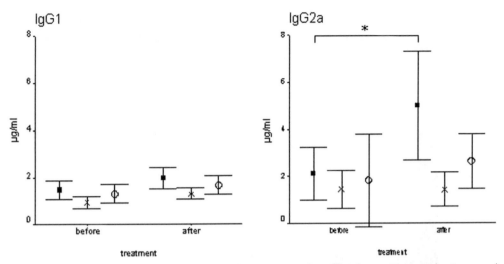

Figure 1. Induction of IgG2a-antibodies by feeding mice with AAL-microparticles. Birch-pollen sensitized mice (*n* = 8 per group) were treated orally with BP-loaded microparticles, functionalized with AAL (■) or WGA (×), or without functionalization (○). Sera before and after treatment were analyzed for BP-specific IgG1- and IgG2a-titers (µg/ml serum) in ELISA. *$p < 0.05$.

or WGA as control lectin, binding to sialylic residues expressed on normal enterocytes [8–11]. In a BALB/c mouse model the humoral and cellular immune responses of birch pollen allergic mice fed with the different allergen-microspheres were investigated.

Methods

Six- to eight-week-old female BALB/c mice were sensitized intraperitoneally (ip) with 10 µg birch pollen proteins in context with Al(OH)$_3$ in saline and subsequently fed with birch pollen-loaded microspheres coated with AAL to target murine M-cells (AAL-MS, *n* = 8), with WGA to target enterocytes (WGA-MS, *n* = 8), and noncoated microparticles (MS, *n* = 8). Birch-pollen loaded microparticles were generated by spray-drying with a size < 10 µm [12]. Blood from the tail vein was taken before and after feedings to investigate serum antibodies of IgE, IgA, IgG1, and IgG2a classes by means of ELISA [7]. After feedings with the different type of microparticles, spleen cells of mice were investigated for birch-pollen specific proliferation and production of IL-4, IFN-γ, and IL-10 [13].

Statistical analysis was performed using

student *t*-test and *p*-values of < 0.05 were considered statistically significant.

Results

Induction of IgG2a in Mice Fed with Microparticles Targeting M-Cells

Sensitization of mice with birch pollen extract and aluminium hydroxide as adjuvant resulted in formation of IgE and IgG1-antibodies in all mice, indicating successful induction of Th2-type immune response. Subsequently, mice were fed with the different microparticles. After five feedings, birch-pollen specific IgG2a levels were significantly higher (*p* = 0.048) in the group fed with AAL-microparticles compared to the other groups of mice (Figure 1). In contrast, no alteration in the serum IgG1 (Figure 1), IgE, and IgA-levels (data not shown) could be observed.

Production of IFN-γ by Birch-Pollen-Sensitized Mice Fed with AAL-Microparticles

Supernatants of birch-pollen stimulated splenocytes of the different mouse groups were an-

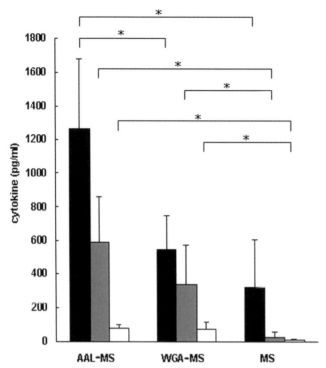

Figure 2. Splenocytes of BP-sensitized mice being treated orally with BP-loaded microparticles ($n = 8$ per group) were analyzed for cytokine production upon stimulation with BP extract. Cells of mice fed with WGA- and AAL-coated microspheres (WGA MS, AAL MS) produced significantly more IL-10 (grey bars) and IL-4 (white bars) than feedings with bare microparticles (MS). Only AAL MS feedings did significantly support IFN-γ production (black bars). * $p < 0.05$.

alyzed for IL-4, IL-10, and INF-γ production. In both targeting strategies, using AAL-MS for M-cells and WGA-MS for enterocytes, IL-10 and IL-4 was significantly elevated. However, as shown in Figure 2, only AAL-feedings markedly induced IFN-γ synthesis.

Discussion

From these data we conclude that induction of Th1 antibody and cytokines in an ongoing Th2 response is possible by targeting M-cells using the oral route. Allergens loaded in AAL-microparticles that bind to α-L-fucose residues expressed on murine M-cells induced INF-γ and in consequence birch-pollen specific IgG2a. This effect could not be seen when enterocytes were targeted with WGA-coated microparticles or without targeting. From lectin-binding studies it is known that in many species and at many O-MALT sites the M-cell surface glycocalyx differ in carbohydrate composition from that of enterocytes, although in humans, no concrete difference could be identified so far

[11, 14–16]. AAL was chosen for targeting M-cells, since (1) it derives from an edible mushroom, (2) it binds to α-L-fucose residues, and (3) its structure is similar to various neuraminidases of pathogens that exploit M-cells for host-invasion like *Vibrio cholerae* [17], *Salmonella typhimurium* [4, 5], paramyxoviruses [18], and influenza viruses, being a well-known virulence factor [19].

Our data demonstrate that antigen delivery to murine M-cells can be mediated by AAL. This lectin is able to target M-cells *in vivo*, and supports IFN-γ and IgG2a production in an ongoing allergic response, at least in an animal model. Therefore, we conclude that AAL-functionalized microspheres may be successfully used for oral allergen immunotherapy. The similarity of AAL with the structure of various neuraminidases of pathogens that invade humans via M-cells suggest that AAL-functionalized microparticles could be useful for mucosal targeting also in human patients.

Acknowledgment

We thank Ing. Magdolna Vermes for excellent technical assistance. This work was supported by BIOMAY manufacturing and trading company and, in part, by the Austrian Science Fund SFB F018 08–B04, Vienna, Austria.

References

1. Clark MA, Hirst BH, Jepson MA: Lectin-mediated mucosal delivery of drugs and microparticles. Adv Drug Deliv Rev 2000; 43:207–223.

2. Jepson MA, Clark MA: Studying M-cells and their role in infection. Trends Microbiol 1998; 6:359–365.

3. Liener IE, Sharon N, Goldstein IJ (Eds.): The lectins: properties, functions, and applications in biology and medicine. Orlando: Academic Press, 1986, pp. 206–207.

4. Wimmerova M, Mitchell E, Sanchez JF, Gautier C, Imberty A: Crystal structure of fungal lectin: six-bladed β-propeller fold and novel fucose recognition mode for *Aleuria aurantia* lectin. J Biol Chem 2003; 278:27059–27067.

5. Fujihashi M, Peapus DH, Kamiya N, Nagata Y, Miki K: Crystal structure of fucose-specific lectin from *Aleuria aurantia* binding ligands at three of its five sugar recognition sites. Biochemistry 2003; 42:11093–11099.

6. Hoyer LL, Roggentin P, Schauer R, Vimr ER: Purification and properties of cloned *Salmonella typhimurium* LT2 sialidase with virus-typical kinetic preference for sialyl α 2–3 linkages. J Biochem (Tokyo) 1991; 110:462–467.

7. Schöll I, Weissenbock A, Förster-Waldl E, Untersmayr E, Walter F, Willheim M, Boltz-Nitulescu G, Scheiner O, Gabor F, Jensen-Jarolim E: Allergen-loaded biodegradable poly(D,L-lactic-co-glycolic) acid nanoparticles downregulate an ongoing Th2 response in the BALB/c mouse model. Clin Exp Allergy 2004; 34:315–321.

8. Gabor F, Stangl M, Wirth M: Lectin-mediated bioadhesion: binding characteristics of plant lectins on the enterocyte-like cell lines Caco-2, HT-29, and HCT-8. J Control Release 1998; 55:131–142.

9. Gabor F, Schwarzbauer A, Wirth M: Lectin-mediated drug delivery: binding and uptake of BSA-WGA conjugates using the Caco-2 model. Int J Pharm 2002; 237:227–239.

10. Gabor F, Wirth M: Lectin-mediated drug delivery: fundamentals and perspectives. STP Pharma Sciences 2003; 13:3–16.

11. Gebhard A, Gebert A: Brush cells of the mouse intestine possess a specialized glycocalyx as revealed by quantitative lectin histochemistry. Further evidence for a sensory function. J Histochem Cytochem 1999; 47:799–808.

12. Walter F, Schöll I, Untersmayr E, Ellinger A, Boltz-Nitulescu G, Scheiner O, Gabor F, Jensen-Jarolim E: Functionalisation of allergen-loaded microspheres with wheat germ agglutinin for targeting enterocytes. Biochem Biophys Res Commun 2004; 315:281–287.

13. Roth-Walter F, Schöll I, Untersmayr E, Fuchs R, Boltz-Nitulescu G, Scheiner O, Weissenböck A, Gabor F, Jensen-Jarolim E: M-cell targeting with *Aleuria aurantia* lectin as a novel approach for oral allergen immunotherapy. J Allergy Clin Immunol 2004; 114:1362–1368.

14. Sharma R, van Damme EJ, Peumans WJ, Sarsfield P, Schumacher U: Lectin binding reveals divergent carbohydrate expression in human and mouse Peyer's patches. Histochem Cell Biol 1996; 105:459–465.

15. Sharma R, Schumacher U, Adam E: Lectin histochemistry reveals the appearance of M-cells in Peyer's patches of SCID mice after syngeneic normal bone marrow transplantation. J Histochem Cytochem 1998; 46:143–148.

16. Gebert A, al-Samir K, Werner K, Fassbender S, Gebhard A: The apical membrane of intestinal brush cells possesses a specialized, but species-specific, composition of glycoconjugates – onsection and *in vivo* lectin labeling in rats, guinea-pigs, and mice. Histochem Cell Biol 2000; 113: 389–399.

17. Crennell S, Garman E, Laver G, Vimr E, Taylor G: Crystal structure of *Vibrio cholerae* neuraminidase reveals dual lectin-like domains in addition to the catalytic domain. Structure 1994; 2:535–544.

18. Crennell S, Takimoto T, Portner A, Taylor G: Crystal structure of the multifunctional paramyxovirus hemagglutinin-neuraminidase. Nat Struct Biol 2000; 7:1068–1074.

19. Smith BJ, McKimm-Breshkin JL, McDonald M, Fernley RT, Varghese JN, Colman PM: Structural studies of the resistance of influenza virus neuraminidase to inhibitors. J Med Chem 2002; 45: 2207–2212.

E. Jensen-Jarolim

Center of Physiology and Pathophysiology, Medical University of Vienna, Währingergürtel 18–20, A-1090-Vienna, Austria, Tel. +43 1 40400-5103, Fax +43 1 40400-5130, E-mail erika.jensen-jarolim@meduniwien.ac.at

Successful Mucosal Immunotherapy in Asthma Induces Tolerance and *M. Vaccae* Potentiates IL-10-Related Tolerance in a Murine Asthma Model

T. Akkoc, N.N. Bahceciler, and I.B. Barlan

Marmara University, Pediatric Allergy & Immunology, Istanbul, Turkey

Summary: *Background:* Allergen specific T-cell responses induced by mucosal immunotherapy can be potentiated by adjuvants. We evaluated the protective effect of intranasal immunotherapy alone or in conjunction with *Mycobacterium (M) vaccae* on airway histopathology and cytokine profile in a murine model of asthma. *Methods:* BALB/c mice were pretreated with either OVA alone or additionally with *M. vaccae* three times, before chronic asthma was established by seven intraperitoneal administrations of OVA, followed by three challenges with intratracheal OVA. Two days later, splenocytes were cultured with PHA, OVA, and *M. vaccae* for cytokine determination and the lungs were histopathologically examined. *Results:* Lung histopathology revealed that all the evaluated parameters were downregulated both in mice pretreated with intranasal immunotherapy alone or in conjunction with *M. vaccae* to the values observed in control mice. The secreted levels of IFN-γ and IL-10 from PHA-stimulated splenocytes were significantly higher in OVA preimmunized mice compared to those with chronic asthma. When compared to controls, OVA preimmunized mice revealed significantly higher spontaneous IL-10 and *M. vaccae* induced-IFN-γ levels. Moreover, mice preimmunized with OVA and pretreated with *M. vaccae* produced higher IL-10 and lower IL-5 and IFN-γ levels. *Conclusions:* We conclude that intranasal immunotherapy is a potential strategy for primary prevention of histopathological changes in asthma. The simultaneous administration of *M. vaccae* upregulates IL-10 production and downregulates both Th1 (IFN-γ and Th2 (IL-5) cytokine secretion by splenocytes. This suggests that *M. vaccae* treatment potentiates the induction of IL-10-secreting regulatory T-cells and development of mucosal tolerance.

Keywords: mycobacterium, immunotherapy, tolerance

M. vaccae has been previously shown to have a potential effect in skewing T-cell responses away from Th2, downregulating IgE response and chronic histopathological changes in airways in murine models of asthma [1–3]. Recently Zuany-Amorim et al. showed the thera-peutic effect of killed *M. vaccae*-suspension, which resulted in induction of allergen-specific CD4+ CD45RB^low regulatory T-cells, with an inhibitory effect on airway inflammation in mice [4].

Mucosal immunotherapy, one of the most

promising therapeutic approaches is suggested to induce allergen-specific T-cell responses which can be potentiated by using adjuvants [5, 6].

In the current study, we aimed to investigate the protective effect of intranasal immunotherapy alone and in conjunction with the adjuvant, *M. vaccae* on parameters of airway histopathology and cytokine responses in the murine model of chronic asthma.

Material and Methods

Animals

Female BALB/c mice (5–6 weeks old) were housed in pathogen-free conditions at the laboratory of Marmara University Research Center in accordance with the guidelines of the animal ethics committee.

Mice were divided into four groups. To establish the chronic asthma model, Groups I, II, and III were immunized with 10 μg of OVA intraperitoneally (i.p.) seven times on each alternate day. Twenty-eight days after the last i.p. injection, they were challenged with 20 μg OVA three times 2 days apart by intratracheal (i.t.) instillation. Mice in group IV served as controls. Mice in Groups I and II were pretreated with either intranasal (in) OVA(100 μg/30 μl) alone on 6 consecutive days (in OVA group) or additionally with 10 μl of 10^7 CFU of *M. vaccae* subcutaneously three times (in the OVA⁺ *M. vaccae* group).

Two days after the last i.t. OVA challenge, lung tissue was sectioned (3–5 μm) and

stained with periodic-acid Schiff. The airways were classified as small (< 500 μm), medium (500–1000 μm) and large (> 1000 μm) according to their circumferences. Measurement of thicknesses of epithelial, basement membrane, smooth muscle, and number of hyperplastic goblet cells of the airways were recorded by using an image analyzer software, adapted to the microscope.

On the same day, splenocytes were cultured with PHA, OVA, and *M. vaccae*. IFN-γ, IL-5, and IL-10 levels were determined in antigen and mitogen stimulated culture supernatants by ELISA.

Results

Histopathology

All of the histopathological parameters in small, medium, and large airways were significantly more in chronic asthma group when compared to healthy mice, indicating that the chronic asthma model was successfully established. All of the histopathological parameters evaluated in small, medium, and large airways showed significant reduction in the OVA-immunized group when compared to those with chronic asthma (Figures 1, 2). Furthermore, no significant difference in any of those parameters was detected when compared with healthy mice, except for epithelial thickness of small and medium airways.

All of the evaluated parameters were significantly less in OVA-immunized, *M. vaccae*

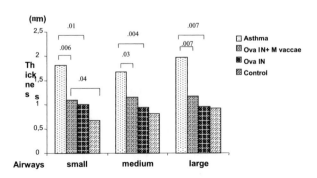

Figure 1. All of the histopathological parameters in small, medium, and large airways were significantly more in chronic asthma group when compared to healthy mice, indicating that the chronic asthma model was successfully established. The thickness of basement membrane evaluated in small, medium, and large airways showed a significant reduction both in OVA-immunized and additionally *M. vaccae*-treated group compared to those with chronic asthma. The OVA-immunized and M. vaccae-treated group was similar to healthy controls except for small-sized airways.

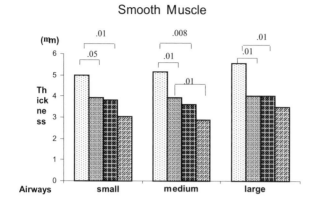

Figure 2. The thickness of smooth muscle was significantly less in OVA-immunized group when compared to asthma group in 3 sized airways, this group was no different than controls. When compared to controls, the *M. vaccae*-treated group had significantly increased thickness only in medium-sized airways. When the same group was compared to asthma group, all sizes of airways had significantly less thickness in smooth muscle.

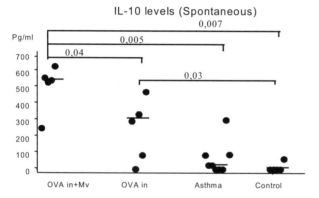

Figure 3. Spontaneous secretion of IL-10 from spleenocytes was higher in OVA-immunized, *M. vaccae*-pretreated mice than in all the other groups, whereas the OVA-immunized group had higher levels compared to controls.

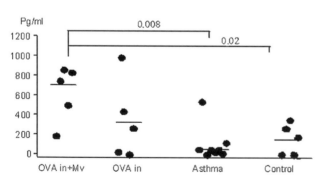

Figure 4. OVA-immunized *M. vaccae*-pretreated mice had significantly higher IL-10 levels from splenocytes upon stimulation with OVA compared to asthma and control groups.

pretreated mice when compared with the of chronic asthma group. Furthermore, OVA-immunized, *M. vaccae* pretreated mice were similar to healthy controls for all the parameters but basal membrane thickness in small airways and smooth muscle thickness in medium airways (Figures 1, 2). Finally, no significant difference was detected in any of the evaluated histopathological parameters in the comparison of OVA-immunized, *M. vaccae* pretreated and nontreated mice.

Cytokine Measurement

Spontaneous IFN-γ ($p = 0.04$) and PHA-stimulated IL-10 ($p = 0.03$) were significantly higher in OVA preimmunized mice when compared to the asthma group. In the comparison of OVA preimmunized mice with healthy controls significantly higher *M. vaccae*-induced IFN-γ ($p = 0.03$) and spontaneous IL-10 ($p = 0.03$) levels were detected (Figure 3).

When compared to the asthma group, mice immunized with OVA and pretreated with *M.vaccae* produced significantly higher IL-10 levels with all the stimulants (Figure 4) and significantly lower OVA-induced IL-5 ($p = 0.02$) and *M. Vaccae*-induced IFN-γ levels ($p = 0.05$). When compared to controls, this group had higher IL-10 levels with all the stimulants (Figure 4) and lower OVA ($p = 0.006$), PHA-induced IL-5 ($p = 0.03$), and spontaneous IFN-γ levels ($p = 0.02$).

When OVA preimmunized and *M.Vaccae* treated and nontreated groups were compared, the first group had significantly higher spontaneous ($p = 0.04$; Figure 3) and PHA-induced IL-10 ($p = 0.03$) and significantly lower spontaneous, PHA ($p = 0.03$) and *M. Vaccae*-induced IFN-γ levels ($p = 0.008$).

Discussion

We concluded that intranasal immunotherapy alone or in conjunction with the adjuvant *M. vaccae* appears to be a potential strategy for primary prevention of histopathological changes in asthma with a corresponding increase in IL-10 production in mice. Simultaneous administration of *M.vaccae* upregulates IL-10 even more and downregulates both Th1 (IFN-γ) and Th2 (IL-5) cytokine secretion by splenocytes, which provides further evidence for induction of IL-10 secreting regulatory T-cells and mucosal tolerance.

References

1. Tukenmez F, Bahceciler NN, Barlan IB, Basaran MM: Effect of preimmunization by killed *M. Bovis* and *vaccae* on IgE response in ovalbumin-sensitized newborn mice. Pediatr Allergy Immunol 1999; 10:107–111.

2. Ozdemir C, Akkoc T, Bahceciler NN, Kucukercan D, Barlan IB, Basaran MM: Clin Exp Allergy 2003; 33:266–270.

3. Wang CC, Rook GAW: Inhibition of an established allergic response to ovalbumin in Balb/c mice by killed *M. vaccae*. Immunology 1998; 93:307–313.

4. Zuany-Amorim C, Sawicka E, Manlius C, Moine A, Brunet L, Kmeny DM, Bowen G, Rook G, Walker C: Suppression of airway eosinophilia by killed *Mycobacterium vaccae*-induced allergen specific regulatory T-cells. Nature Med 2002; 8:625–629.

5. Wiedermann U, Jahn-Schmid B, Bohle B, Repa A, Renz H, Kraft D, Ebner C: Suppression of antigen-specific T- and B-cell responses by intranasal or oral administration of recombinant Bet v 1, the major birch pollen allergen, in a murine model of type 1 allergy. J Allergy Clin Immunol 1999; 103:1202–1210.

6. Jutel M, Akdis M, Budak F, Aebischer-Casaulta C, Wrzyszcz M, Blaser K, Akdis CA: IL-10 and TGF-β cooperate in the regulatory T-cell response to mucosal allergens in normal immunity and specific immunotherapy. Eur J Immunol 2003; 33:1205–1214.

Isil B. Barlan

Division of Pediatric Allergy/Immunology, Marmara University Hospital, Kantarcı sk 5/8 Erenkoy, 81070 Istanbul, Turkey, Tel./Fax +90 216 326-8030, E-mail isilbarlan@marmara.edu.tr

Molecular Basis of the Anti-IgE Therapy

D. Inführ[1], R. Crameri[2], and G. Achatz[1]

[1]*Department of Molecular Biology, University of Salzburg, Austria,* [2] *SIAF, Davos, Switzerland*

Summary: *Background:* Since IgE antibodies play a key role in allergic disorders, a number of approaches to inhibit IgE antibody production are currently being explored. In the recent past the use of nonanaphylactic, humanized anti-IgE antibodies became a systemic therapeutic strategy for allergic diseases. The principle of the idea is that these antibodies bind to the same site on the IgE molecule that interacts with the high-affinity IgE receptor, thereby interfering with the binding of IgE to this receptor without cross-linking the IgE on the receptor. *Results:* Treatment with anti-IgE antibodies leads primarily to a decrease in serum IgE levels. As a consequence, the number of high-affinity IgE receptors on mast cells and basophils decreases, leading to a lower excitability of the effector cells. As a consequence, inflammatory mediator such as histamine, prostaglandins, and leukotrienes will not be triggered. Experimental studies in mice partially indicated that injection of some monoclonal anti-IgE antibodies also inhibited *in vivo* IgE production. *Conclusion:* The biological mechanism remains speculative. An explanation may be that these antibodies can also interact with mIgE on B-cells, which could interfere with the IgE production.

Keywords: anti-IgE antibody, mIgE, B-cell receptor, apoptosis

In 1966 Ishizaka et al. [1] opened a new era in the pathophysiology of immunological disorders when they identified and purified IgE from the serum of allergic patients. Later on it became evident that human IgE molecules, unlike other immunoglobulin classes, bind specifically and with a very high affinity ($K_a = 10^{-9}$M) to receptors (FcεRI) on the surface of human basophils and mast cells [2]. IgE cross-linking of FcεRI+ cells by specific antigens results in the release of a variety of preformed (e.g., histamine) and *de novo* synthesized chemical mediators (e.g., prostaglandins) and cytokines that exert their effects by interacting with specific receptors on target organs. Conventional desensitization immunization with total extracts of allergenic sources [3] often are not effective and go in parallel with anaphylactic reactions. Therefore, a systemic treatment that targets the allergic process, prevents it from occurring, and has fewer side effects than current drugs is desirable. Because IgE is the central macromolecular mediator responsible for the progression of allergic reactions, neu-

tralizing it and inhibiting its synthesis would appear to be a rational approach for the treatment of various allergic diseases.

Several strategies were performed to treat IgE-mediated allergic diseases by down-regulating IgE levels [4–7]. The general concept performed was that chimerized or humanized anti-IgE antibodies with a set of unique binding properties could be used for the isotype-specific control of IgE, and, thus, would seem a logical therapeutic approach to IgE-mediated diseases. What are the demands for an anti-IgE antibody: the anti-IgE antibody must have a high affinity for IgE, should not bind IgE already bound by FcεRI on mast cells and basophils, nor to IgE bound by the low-affinity IgE Fc receptors (FcεRII, also known as CD23) on various other cell types and should bind to membrane-bound IgE (mIgE) on mIgE-expressing B-cells. Summarizing, these antibodies are designed to neutralize free IgE and target IgE-expressing B-cells [4, 6, 8]. If these aims are achieved, the levels of IgE in blood and interstitial fluids for binding to

FcεRI will be greatly reduced, and hence the sensitivity of mast cells and basophils to allergens should be gradually alleviated.

Probably the most readily appreciated pharmacological effect of anti-IgE therapy is its indirect effect on the down-regulation of FcεRI on basophils. In earlier studies, the density of FcεRI on basophils was found to correlate strongly with the level of IgE in blood. In one of the clinical studies [9] and in additional *in vitro* studies [10], it was found that anti-IgE can also down-regulate FcεRI in patients. The results show that the density of FcεRI on basophils had decreased by more than 95%, and in some cases to more than 99%, after anti-IgE was administered to patients for periods of 5 weeks to 3 months [9]. The basophils isolated from patients after anti-IgE treatment were much less sensitive to allergen stimulation. In skin prick tests, it was also found that much larger amounts of allergens were required, indicating that mast cell function was also markedly decreased [9].

Experimental evidence from *in vitro* and *in vivo* studies is generally supportive of the effectiveness of anti-IgE in targeting IgE expressing B-cells and in inhibiting the continual production of IgE. The idea that anti-IgE can cause these effects is based on evidence that anti-IgE binds to mIgE on IgE-expressing B-cells, and as mIgE is a part of the B-cell receptor, anti-IgE may inhibit the B-cells or even cause their lysis, like anti-IgM or anti-IgG [11–13]. However, IgE-secreting plasma cells do not express mIgE and presumably are not affected by anti-IgE. These cells reside in the bone marrow and probably have a life span of several weeks to several months. Since new IgE-secreting plasma cells go through mIgE-expressing B-cell stages during differentiation, if their generation is abrogated by anti-IgE treatment, the existing plasma cells will die off in several weeks to several months, and, thus, the production of IgE will also gradually abate in similar periods. Furthermore, memory B-cells may possibly be affected by anti-IgE. If this occurs, anti-IgE may have long-term effects on the fundamental disease process. The molecular mechanisms leading to the depletion of these cells can be explained by apoptosis and reached by the immunological process of tolerance and/or anergy induction.

Two scenarios of the functioning of an anti-IgE antibody would be possible: First, as shown by self-reacting immature B-cells, cross-linkage of the mIgE receptor without further T-cell support should directly induce apoptosis. Second, as normally shown during the induction of peripheral tolerance of mature B-cells in answer to monovalent (self) antigen, receptor blockage of mIgE by a Fab-fragment should result in an anergic state of the mIgE population. In contrast to normal mature B-cells, which have a half life of 4 to 5 weeks, anergic B-cells were found to last for only 3 to 4 days [14]. Nevertheless, the fate of these anergic B-cells is finally cell death [15].

Like other immunoglobulins, IgE consists of two light chains and two ε-heavy chains and can be detected in two forms, a secreted and a membrane-bound form. mIgE is a transmembrane protein that behaves like a classical antigen receptor on B-lymphocytes [16]. Previous experiments in our and other laboratories showed that the expression of a functional membrane form is essential for generating a humoral IgE and IgG1 response in mice and an IgG2a response in man [17–20]. The transmembrane domain and the cytoplasmic tail are encoded by two exons M1 (transmembrane domain) and M2 (cytoplasmic tail). The cytoplasmic domains of mIgs are different in size and range from only three amino acid residues in the case of mIgM and mIgD to 28 residues for the mIg subclasses. The mIg transmembrane segments are about 25 amino acids long, are highly homologous between the Ig-subclasses and have the potential for interaction with other polypeptides [21]. Beside these 25 membrane-spanning amino acids, M1 additionally encodes isotype-specific extracellular spacer segments. The spacers differ in lengths (13 to 21 amino acids) and show high variability between the different Ig isotypes. It is this extracellular spacer that could be used as target sequence for generating anti-mIgE antibodies with the capacity to inhibit IgE synthesis. First results on this approach were published by Chen et al. [22]. In this study, the ability of an anti-spacer-specific antibody on targeting and lysing mIgE expressing B-cells was examined. Thus, the pharmacological targets are memory B-cells involved in secondary immune responses.

Summarizing, if anti-spacer-specific antibodies indeed inhibit or down-regulate IgE synthesis *in vivo*, these antibodies could be used to treat allergic patients with very high IgE levels. The advantage of this kind therapeutic approach would be the next step in the generation of anti-IgE therapy, with the advantage of inhibiting IgE secretion before secreted IgE production starts.

References

1. Ishizaka K, Ishizaka T, Hornbrook MM: Physicochemical properties of reaginic antibody. V. Correlation of reaginic activity with γ-E-globulin antibody. J Immunol 1966; 97:840–853.
2. Scharenberg AM, Kinet JP: Early events in mast cell signal transduction. Chem Immunol 1995; 61:72–87.
3. Durham SR, Walker SM, Varga EM, Jacobson MR, O'Brien F, Noble W, Till SJ, Hamid QA, Nouri-Aria KT: Long-term clinical efficacy of grass-pollen immunotherapy. N Engl J Med 1999; 341:468–475.
4. Chang TW, Davis FM, Sun NC, Sun CR, MacGlashan DW, Jr., Hamilton RG: Monoclonal antibodies specific for human IgE-producing B-cells: a potential therapeutic for IgE-mediated allergic diseases. Biotechnology (N.Y.) 1990; 8:122–126.
5. Davis FM, Gossett LA, Chang TW: An epitope on membrane-bound but not secreted IgE: implications in isotype-specific regulation. Biotechnology (N.Y.) 1991; 9:53–56.
6. Davis FM, Gossett LA, Pinkston KL, Liou RS, Sun LK, Kim YW, Chang NT, Chang TW, Wagner K, Bews J, et al.: Can anti-IgE be used to treat allergy? Springer Semin Immunopathol 1993; 15:51–73.
7. Chang TW: The pharmacological basis of anti-IgE therapy. Nat Biotechnol 2000; 18:157–162.
8. Heusser C, Jardieu P: Therapeutic potential of anti-IgE antibodies. Curr Opin Immunol 1997; 9: 805–813.
9. MacGlashan DW, Jr., Bochner BS, Adelman DC, Jardieu PM, Togias A, McKenzie-White J, Sterbinsky SA, Hamilton RG, Lichtenstein LM: Down-regulation of Fc(ε)RI expression on human basophils during *in vivo* treatment of atopic patients with anti-IgE antibody. J Immunol 1997; 158:1438–1445.
10. MacGlashan DW, Jr., Bochner BS, Adelman DC, Jardieu PM, Togias A, Lichtenstein LM: Serum IgE level drives basophil and mast cell IgE receptor display. Int Arch Allergy Immunol 1997; 113:45–47.
11. Eray M, Tuomikoski T, Wu H, Nordstrom T, Andersson LC, Knuutila S, Kaartinen M: Crosslinking of surface IgG induces apoptosis in a bcl-2 expressing human follicular lymphoma line of mature B-cell phenotype. Int Immunol 1994; 6:1817–1827.
12. Warner GL, Scott DW: A polyclonal model for B-cell tolerance. I. Fc-dependent and Fc-independent induction of nonresponsiveness by pretreatment of normal splenic B-cells with anti-Ig. J Immunol 1991; 146:2185–2191.
13. Warner GL, Gaur A, Scott DW: A polyclonal model for B-cell tolerance. II. Linkage between signaling of B-cell egress from G0, class II upregulation and unresponsiveness. Cell Immunol 1991; 138:404–412.
14. Fulcher DA, Basten A: Reduced life span of anergic self-reactive B-cells in a double-transgenic model. J Exp Med 1994; 179:125–134.
15. Rathmell JC, Cooke MP, Ho WY, Grein J, Townsend SE, Davis MM, Goodnow CC: CD95 (Fas)-dependent elimination of self-reactive B-cells upon interaction with CD4+ T-cells. Nature 1995; 376:181–184.
16. Reth M: Antigen receptors on B lymphocytes. Ann Rev Immunol 1992; 10:97–121.
17. Achatz G, Nitschke L, Lamers MC: Effect of transmembrane and cytoplasmic domains of IgE on the IgE response. Science 1997; 276:409–411.
18. Kaisho T, Takeda K, Tsujimura T, Kawai T, Nomura F, Terada N, Akira S: IκB kinase α is essential for mature B-cell development and function. J Exp Med 2001; 193:417–426.
19. Knight AM, Lucocq JM, Prescott AR, Ponnambalam S, Watts C: Antigen endocytosis and presentation mediated by human membrane IgG1 in the absence of the Ig(α)/Ig(β) dimer. Embo J 1997; 16:3842–3850.
20. Luger E, Lamers M, Achatz-Straussberger G, Geisberger R, Infuhr D, Breitenbach M, Crameri R, Achatz G: Somatic diversity of the immunoglobulin repertoire is controlled in an isotype-specific manner. Eur J Immunol 2001; 31:2319–2330.
21. Venkitaraman AR, Williams GT, Dariavach P,

Neuberger MS: The B-cell antigen receptor of the five immunoglobulin classes. Nature 1991; 352:777–781.

22. Chen HY, Liu FT, Hou CM, Huang JS, Sharma BB, Chang TW: Monoclonal antibodies against the C(ϵ)mX domain of human membrane-bound IgE and their potential use for targeting IgE-expressing B-cells. Int Arch Allergy Immunol 2002; 128:315–324.

Gernot Achatz

Fachbereich für Molekulare Biologie, Abteilung Allergologie und Immunologie, Hellbrunnerstraße 34, A-5020 Salzburg, Austria, Tel. +43 662 8044-5764, Fax +43 662 8044-144, E-mail gernot.achatz@sbg.ac.at

Inhibition of IgE-Facilitated Allergen Presentation

A Longitudinal Study of Grass Pollen Immunotherapy

L.K. Wilcock, P.A. Wachholz, D. Hae-Won Na, R.C. Aalberse, J.N. Larsen, J.N. Francis, and S.R. Durham

Upper Respiratory Medicine, National Heart and Lung Institute, Imperial College, London, UK

Summary: *Background:* Allergen injection immunotherapy is effective in IgE-mediated atopic disease. Successful treatment is accompanied by increases in allergen-specific IgG, which may act to block IgE-mediated allergen presentation at low allergen levels. *Methods:* In a randomized, placebo-controlled trial of grass pollen immunotherapy, serum samples were taken before and after 2 years of treatment. Serum samples were analyzed for allergen-specific IgG4 and used in an assay of IgE-facilitated allergen presentation, a "functional" measure of IgG blocking activity. *Results:* Subjects who received immunotherapy showed significant increases in IgG4 levels compared to placebo-treated patients ($p < 0.001$). Serum inhibitory activity for allergen-IgE binding to B-cells was also significantly increased ($p < 0.001$). This activity co-eluted with the IgG serum fraction. *Discussion:* Grass pollen immunotherapy induces an IgG-dependent serum inhibitory activity for allergen-IgE binding to B-cells. IgG blocking antibodies could play an important role in the regulation of human T lymphocyte-driven allergic responses.

Keywords: antigen presentation, IgG, allergy, immunotherapy

Allergen immunotherapy is an effective treatment for IgE-mediated disease and provides long-term benefit for at least 3 years after discontinuation [1–4]. Immunotherapy has also been shown to prevent new sensitizations and the progression of rhinitis to asthma in children [5,6]. Immunotherapy has profound effects on the local cellular environment by reducing the number of inflammatory cells and their mediators [7,8]. The mechanisms associated with immunotherapy involve both cellular and humoral responses. Cellular changes include a shift in the local cytokine production to a "protective" Th1 cytokine profile [9–11] and the induction of IL-10-producing regulatory T-cells [12,13]. It is well-established that immu-

notherapy induces significant increases in IgG antibodies [14]. However, immunoreactive IgG levels as detected by ELISA may not correlate with the clinical response to treatment [15]. Facilitated allergen presentation is a mechanism by which IgE captures allergen and, via CD23-dependent binding, allows allergen to be processed and presented to T-cells at 10–100 fold lower concentrations than would occur independent of IgE [16,17]. Serum from patients treated with allergen immunotherapy has been shown to inhibit this process, and this inhibitory activity is contained within the IgG4 fraction [18]. In this study we have further validated this inhibition assay and used it to analyze serum obtained from a double-blind placebo-controlled study of grass-pollen immunotherapy.

Materials and Methods

Serum from an atopic grass-pollen-allergic patient (with Phl p-specific IgE > 100 SU/ml) was incubated with RPMI or with an equal volume of test serum for 1 h at 37 °C with a serial dilution of Phl p allergen extract (ALK Abelló, Hørsholm, Denmark). Epstein-Barr virus-transformed B-cells [16] were washed and 2×10^5 cells were added to the serum/allergen preparation and incubated on ice. Cells were subsequently washed and labeled with anti-IgE-FITC (Dako Cytomation Ltd, Ely, UK). The percentage of cells bound by IgE/allergen complex was assessed by flow cytometry. For validation, allergen dose-response and time-course experiments were performed. CD23-dependency was assessed by preincubation of B-cell lines with anti-CD23 antibody (Dako Cytomation) compared with an isotype control.

Phl p specific IgG4 levels were measured in serum samples by an in-house enzyme-linked immunosorbent assay. 5 μg/ml of Phl p (whole allergen extract, ALK Abelló) was used to coat plates, test serum was diluted 1:100 in PBS and 0.5 μg/ml biotinylated anti-human IgG4 (BD Pharmingen, CA, USA) was used. Tetramethylbenzoate was utilized as a substrate. Data is expressed as arbitrary units compared with known standards.

Clinical details of immunotherapy are published elsewhere [19]. Twenty patients received Phl p extract (Alutard SQ, ALK Abelló) and 17 received placebo injections for 2 years. Subjects were monitored before and 2 years after the start of treatment, both within and outside the grass pollen season.

Results

Binding of serum-IgE was dependent on the concentration of allergen used (optimal at 1–3 μg/ml of allergen) and occurred maximally within 30–120 min of incubation (Figure

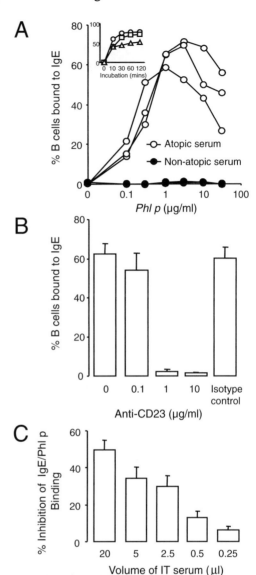

Figure 1. (A) Optimal allergen-IgE binding occurs at 3 μg/ml (n = 3 atopic serum) and within 30 min of incubation (insert). (B) Blocking antibodies to CD23 show that complex binding is CD23-dependent (n = 3; different B-cell lines). (C) Inhibitory activity of immunotherapy serum is concentration-dependent (n = 3; IT serum).

1A). All subsequent experiments used optimal conditions of 3 μg/ml of allergen and 1 h incubation time. Allergen-IgE binding was inhibited in the presence of 1 and 10 μg/ml of blocking CD23 antibody but not with lower concentrations or a control antibody (Figure 1B). Furthermore, allergen-IgE binding correlated

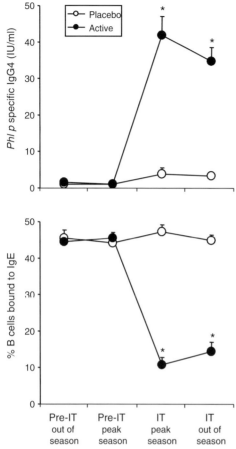

Figure 2. Allergen-specific IgG4 is increased following grass pollen immunotherapy (top panel), and serum inhibitory activity for allergen-IgE binding is increased following treatment (active treatment, *n* = 18; placebo, *n* = 16) (lower panel). Groups were compared using a Mann-Whitney U-test, where * represents *p* < .001.

with the level of CD23 expression on B-cells (data not shown). Addition of serum obtained from subjects receiving grass-pollen immunotherapy inhibited allergen-IgE-binding in a concentration-dependent fashion (Figure 1C).

Fractionation of serum confirmed that this activity was contained largely within the IgG fraction (data not shown). The addition of serum from untreated atopic or nonatopic normal donors demonstrated no inhibitory activity (data not shown).

Grass pollen immunotherapy induced a significant increase in serum allergen-specific IgG4 compared to placebo both within and outside the grass-pollen season ($p < 0.001$,

Figure 2). This increase was accompanied by a significant increase in serum inhibitory activity for the binding of allergen-IgE complexes to B-cells ($p < 0.001$).

Discussion

We have validated an assay that measures allergen-IgE complex binding to the surface of surrogate antigen presenting cells. The assay was shown to be time- and allergen dose-dependent, with binding occurring at very low doses of allergen. Furthermore, the assay was found to be CD23-dependent and inhibited by immunotherapy serum in an IgG-dependent manner.

In a placebo-controlled trial of grass pollen immunotherapy we demonstrated significant increases in serum allergen-specific IgG4 levels that were accompanied by inhibition of allergen-IgE binding to B-cells. Measurement of allergen-specific IgG4 levels after immunotherapy may not be predictive of successful treatment, as no correlation with the clinical response has been shown [15]. Serum inhibitory activity may prove to be a more useful marker of successful treatment compared to IgG4 levels.[18]. Indeed, increased IgG4 levels do not correlate with increased inhibitory activity for allergen-IgE binding (data not shown). Inhibition of allergen-IgE binding can be detected in very dilute serum samples indicating that the overall quantity of allergen-specific IgG4 in immunotherapy serum may be less relevant than its functional qualities. This study demonstrates that allergen-immunotherapy induces "blocking" antibodies that inhibit IgE-facilitated allergen binding to B-cells.

References

1. Varney VA, Gaga M, Frew AJ, Aber VR, Kay AB, Durham SR: Usefulness of immunotherapy in patients with severe summer hay fever uncontrolled by antiallergic drugs. BMJ 1991; 302: 265–269.

2. Bousquet J, Lockey R, Malling HJ, Alvarez-Cuesta E, Canonica GW, Chapman MD, Creticos PJ, Dayer JM, Durham SR, Demoly P, Gold-

stein RJ, Ishikawa T, Ito K, Kraft D, Lambert PH, Lowenstein H, Muller U, Norman PS, Reisman RE, Valenta R, Valovirta E, Yssel H: Allergen immunotherapy: therapeutic vaccines for allergic diseases. World Health Organization. American academy of Allergy, Asthma and Immunology. Ann Allergy Asthma Immunol 1998; 81: 401–405.

3. Durham SR, Walker SM, Varga EM, Jacobson MR, O'brien F, Noble W, Till SJ, Hamid QA, Nouri-Aria KT: Long-term clinical efficacy of grass-pollen immunotherapy. N Engl J Med 1999; 341:468–475.

4. Golden DB, Kwiterovich KA, Kagey-Sobotka A, Valentine MD, Lichtenstein LM: Discontinuing venom immunotherapy: outcome after 5 years. J Allergy Clin Immunol 1996; 97:579–587.

5. Pajno GB, Barberio G, De Luca F, Morabito L, Parmiani S: Prevention of new sensitizations in asthmatic children monosensitized to house dust mite by specific immunotherapy. A 6-year follow-up study. Clin Exp Allergy 2001; 31:1392–1397.

6. Moller C, Dreborg S, Ferdousi HA, Halken S, Host A, Jacobsen L, Koivikko A, Koller DY, Niggemann B, Norberg LA, Urbanek R, Valovirta E, Wahn U: Pollen immunotherapy reduces the development of asthma in children with seasonal rhinoconjunctivitis (the PAT-study). J Allergy Clin Immunol 2002; 109:251–256.

7. Wilson DR, Irani AM, Walker SM, Jacobson MR, Mackay IS, Schwartz LB, Durham SR: Grass pollen immunotherapy inhibits seasonal increases in basophils and eosinophils in the nasal epithelium. Clin Exp Allergy 2001; 31:1705–1713.

8. Durham SR, Varney VA, Gaga M, Jacobson MR, Varga EM, Frew AJ, Kay AB: Grass pollen immunotherapy decreases the number of mast cells in the skin. Clin Exp Allergy 1999; 29:1490–1496.

9. Wachholz PA, Nouri-Aria KT, Wilson DR, Walker SM, Verhoef A, Till SJ, Durham SR: Grass pollen immunotherapy for hayfever is associated with increases in local nasal but not peripheral Th1:Th2 cytokine ratios. Immunology 2002; 105:56–62.

10. Varney VA, Hamid QA, Gaga M, Ying S, Jacobson M, Frew AJ, Kay AB, Durham SR: Influence of grass pollen immunotherapy on cellular infiltration and cytokine mRNA expression during allergen-induced late-phase cutaneous responses. J Clin Invest 1993; 92:644–651.

11. McHugh SM, Deighton J, Stewart AG, Lach-

mann PJ, Ewan PW: Bee venom immunotherapy induces a shift in cytokine responses from a TH-2 to a TH-1 dominant pattern: comparison of rush and conventional immunotherapy. Clin Exp Allergy 1995; 25:828–838.

12. Francis JN, Till SJ, Durham SR: Induction of IL-10⁺ CD4⁺ CD25⁺ T-cells by grass pollen immunotherapy. J Allergy Clin Immunol 2003; 111: 1255–1261.

13. Jutel M, Akdis M, Budak F, Aebischer-Casaulta C, Wrzyszcz M, Blaser K, Akdis CA: IL-10 and TGF-β cooperate in the regulatory T-cell response to mucosal allergens in normal immunity and specific immunotherapy. Eur J Immunol 2003; 33:1205–1214.

14. Aalberse RC, van der Gaarg R, van Leeuwen J: Serologic aspects of IgG4 antibodies. I. Prolonged immunization results in an IgG4-restricted response. J Immunol 1983; 130:722–726.

15. Ewan PW, Deighton J, Wilson AB, Lachmann PJ: Venom-specific IgG antibodies in bee and wasp allergy: lack of correlation with protection from stings. Clin Exp Allergy 1993; 23:647–660.

16. Wachholz PA, Soni NK, Till SJ, Durham SR: Inhibition of allergen-IgE binding to B-cells by IgG antibodies after grass pollen immunotherapy. J Allergy Clin Immunol 2003; 112:915–922.

17. Van Neerven RJ, Wikborg T, Lund G, Jacobsen B, Brinch-Nielsen A, Arnved J, Ipsen H: Blocking antibodies induced by specific allergy vaccination prevent the activation of CD4⁺ T-cells by inhibiting serum-IgE-facilitated allergen presentation. J Immunol 1999; 163:2944–2952.

18. Nouri-Aria KT, Wachholz PA, Francis JN, Jacobson MR, Walker SM, Wilcock LK, Staple SQ, Aalberse RC, Till SJ, Durham SR: Grass pollen immunotherapy induces mucosal and peripheral IL-10 responses and blocking IgG activity. J Immunol 2004; 172:3252–3259.

19. Walker SM, Pajno GB, Lima MT, Wilson DR, Durham SR: Grass pollen immunotherapy for seasonal rhinitis and asthma: a randomized, controlled trial. J Allergy Clin Immunol 2001; 107: 87–93.

Stephen R. Durham

Upper Respiratory Medicine, Allergy and Clinical Immunology, National Heart and Lung Institute, Imperial College London, Dovehouse Street, London, SW3 6LY, UK, Tel. +44 207 352-8121, Fax +44 207 352-8331, E-mail s.durham@imperial. ac.uk

Author Index

Keyword Index